ADOLESCENTS AND ADULTS
WITH LEARNING DISABILITIES
AND ADHD

Adolescents
and Adults
with Learning
Disabilities
and ADHD

Assessment and Accommodation

NOËL GREGG

Foreword by Donald D. Deshler

THE GUILFORD PRESS
New York   London

© 2009 The Guilford Press
A Division of Guilford Publications, Inc.
72 Spring Street, New York, NY 10012
www.guilford.com

Printed in the United States of America

This book is printed on acid-free paper.

Last digit is print number: 9   8   7   6   5   4   3   2   1

Library of Congress Cataloging-in-Publication Data

Gregg, Noël.
    Adolescents and adults with learning disabilities and ADHD : assessment
and accommodation / by Noël Gregg.
        p. cm.
    Includes bibliographical references and index.
    ISBN 978-1-60623-034-3 (hardcover)
    1. Learning disabled—Education.   2. Learning disabled—Services
for.   3. Attention-deficit disorder in adolescence.   4. Attention-deficit
disorder in adults.   I. Title.
    LC4704.5.G74 2009
    371.94—dc22
                                                          2008027887

For Demmie

Every day, every season—a source of inspiration

About the Author

Noël Gregg, PhD, is Distinguished Research Professor in the Departments of Psychology and Communication Sciences and Special Education at the University of Georgia (UGA). She founded the UGA Learning Disabilities Center in 1982 and served as its Director until 1997. From 1993 to 1997, Dr. Gregg served as Director of the Learning Disabilities Research and Training Center. During that period, she produced over 21 videos and teleconferences focusing on the adolescent and adult population with learning disabilities and attention-deficit/hyperactivity disorder (ADHD). Dr. Gregg is also Director of the UGA Regents' Center for Learning Disorders. Her areas of specialization include adolescents and adults with learning disabilities and ADHD, accommodations, alternative media, assessment, written language disorders, and measurement validity. She has been a national expert witness for several key legal cases pertaining to accommodating adults with learning disabilities and ADHD on high-stakes tests. Dr. Gregg has authored *Written Expression Disorders* (1995); coauthored *Adults with Learning Disabilities: Theoretical and Practical Perspectives* (with Cheri Hoy and Alice F. Gay, 1996), *Assessment: The Special Educator's Role* (with Cheri Hoy, 1994), and *Beyond the "SP" Label: Improving the Spelling of Learning Disabled and Basic Writers* (with Patricia J. McAlexander and Ann B. Dobie, 1992); as well as written more than 100 scientific articles and book chapters. She is also a frequent conference presenter and speaker.

Foreword

Historically, the field of disabilities has given less attention to adolescents and adults than to younger children. Most funding initiatives, for example, have been directed at younger students with the assumption (or hope) that if treatment is provided at a young age, many manifestations of learning disabilities (LD) or attention-deficit/hyperactivity disorder (ADHD) may be minimized or eliminated altogether in later years. However, research has shown that adolescents and adults with LD and ADHD have enduring and unique characteristics that are manifested in differing ways as development and setting demands change.

Although the goals of early identification and intervention are important and laudable, there is a potential danger in overemphasizing early treatment at the expense of interventions at later ages. That is, the calls for these early intervention efforts may be misinterpreted as implying that intervening early will ameliorate most of the problems presented by students with LD and ADHD. While this is certainly a desired outcome, Noël Gregg makes a compelling case in this book that the problems identified early in a child's life have a high likelihood of persisting and being manifested at older ages as well. Thus there are at least two reasons for not putting all of our field's "eggs" in the "basket" of early identification and intervention.

First, even though impressive numbers of interventions have been developed for younger students in recent years, it is unlikely that these methods will be successfully implemented on a national scale, given U.S. schools' poor track record of broadly implementing educational innovations. In spite of the effectiveness of the existing interventions, the chances of bringing any innovation to broad-scale implementation with fidelity are slim. Because of the enormous challenges of effecting large-scale implementations, there will be many students who will not receive the intervention and will move on to later grades with significant unaddressed deficits. Second, even if children with LD or ADHD do receive high-quality interventions during their early years, in all likelihood, their disability will endure into adolescence and adulthood. The need for equally effective intervention strategies for these older individuals is as great as (if not greater than) the need for interventions for younger children, because of all the emotional overlays that generally accrue as individuals mature and continue to encounter significant failure. Hence, it is critical that the research and intervention agendas for the LD and ADHD fields be designed to address multiple aspects of these conditions across multiple age ranges. As compelling as the case for early intervention can be, if this case is made at the expense of addressing the equally important set of problems presented by older individuals, the long-term effects of such a policy will be devastating for thousands of older-aged individuals with LD and ADHD.

This book is in a class of its own. Not only does Noël Gregg make a compelling case for the unique and very significant needs of adolescents and adults with LD and ADHD, but she does so in a way that authors of other books do not. The vast majority of books on older individuals with LD and ADHD are somewhat restricted in their focus. That is, they primarily address either the social or the academic or the vocational needs of these individuals, but they do not address all these important areas of inquiry in a comprehensive, integrated manner. Not only does Gregg address each of these areas, but she has accomplished four things that authors of other books on older individuals with LD and ADHD have not done.

First, this book provides an in-depth discussion and analysis of all relevant federal legislative mandates that influence services for adolescents and adults with disabilities. Hence, programming recommendations are strategically positioned in the context of policy realities. Second, this book elegantly integrates relevant literature from the fields of genetics, neurology, biology, disabilities, rehabilitation, and education, to help the reader appreciate the complexity of the problems and the importance of considering varying perspectives on the complex realities behind diagnostic and intervention decision making. Third, each chapter uses a series of case vignettes to contextualize the key constructs presented. These vignettes ground and enhance the reader's understanding of the information that follows. Finally, the information presented on the important role of clinical judgment during the assessment and decision-making process not only is sophisticated and insightful, but represents a topic that has been ignored in much of the literature on LD and ADHD during the past two decades.

Noël Gregg demonstrates throughout this entire volume her remarkable breadth of knowledge about critical learner characteristics, interventions variables, policy requirements, and the interactions among these factors for adolescents and adults with LD and ADHD. She has done a brilliant job of describing the context within which programming solutions must be generated, as well as the form that these solutions must take in order to be embraced by those charged with implementing interventions to significantly improve outcomes.

In light of the way that this book is structured, I am convinced that practitioners will find it to be one of the most valuable resources available to them, for the following reasons:

- It is grounded in the empirical literature; hence, the instructional suggestions can be used with confidence of achieving favorable outcomes.
- It is principle-based.
- It is comprehensive in scope, including a broad array of related resources for extended study of key topical areas.
- It provides clear, step-by-step instructions for how to implement and interpret various assessment protocols and how to link them to program plans and instructional routines.

The organizational framework used in this book is both logical and linked to the field's empirical database. One of the most distinguishing attributes of this book is its comprehensive nature. This book is an extraordinary resource because of Noël Gregg's extensive experience as a scholar, program developer, researcher, and writer. She has a deep understanding of the complexities of secondary and postsecondary school environments, the needs of adolescents and adults with LD and ADHD, and the dynamics that exist between these environments and individuals. Without a doubt, Gregg is one of the brightest and most insightful educators of our time. There is no one better qualified to undertake a project of this scope and complexity.

I believe that this book will provide practitioners, researchers, and policymakers with the foundation that they will need to create the kinds of environments and cultures of learning that will promote academic, social, and employment success for individuals with LD and ADHD. This very readable book is written with passion, vivid examples, and numerous practical suggestions that can be readily implemented. It will add greatly to my abilities as an educator whose career has focused on adolescents and young adults, and it will be a resource to which I will frequently turn.

DONALD D. DESHLER
Director, Center for Research on Learning
Gene A. Budig Professor of Special Education
University of Kansas

Preface

The adolescent and adult populations with learning disabilities (LD) and attention-deficit/hyperactivity disorder (ADHD) represent the largest categories of individuals with disabilities at secondary and post-secondary institutions (educational or employment). Assessing these populations and making decisions about providing appropriate accommodations for them at school and work have become highly controversial topics in recent years. Decision making based on research and best practice is essential for assessing and equitably accommodating individuals with documented disabilities. The outcome data for the secondary and postsecondary populations with LD and ADHD certainly raise concerns about the equity of opportunities for these individuals, and emphasize the necessity of assessments that will support their access to accommodations (see Chapter 1). A primary purpose of this book is to provide professionals with evidence-based research and best-practice resources pertaining to the assessment and accommodation of adolescents and adults with these disorders.

Individuals making the transition from secondary to postsecondary institutions quickly discover that the legal requirements for obtaining accommodation, as well as the comprehensiveness of documentation required for supporting accommodation requests, change radically (see Chapter 2). The problem faced by many individuals with LD and ADHD making the transition to higher education or employment is that their evaluation documentation does not meet the standards set by these institutions or agencies. In an attempt to offer reliable, valid, and practical guidance for professionals involved in providing adequate evaluation documentation for such individuals, a decision-making model based on empirical research and legal mandates is introduced in Chapter 2.

Because adolescents and adults with LD and ADHD comprise a heterogeneous group, different profiles representing a range of abilities and backgrounds are discussed across the chapters to highlight various aspects of assessment and accommodation selection. These narrative and assessment profiles have been chosen to represent the cognitive, affective, language, and achievement abilities characteristic of these individuals.

The effectiveness of a chosen accommodation in enhancing an individual's performance will depend on a professional's knowledge of specific cognitive (Chapter 3), affective (Chapter 4), and language (Chapter 5) processes that influence different types of learning demands. Sensitivity to the processes and factors that influence learning helps professionals determine the type(s) of accommodation(s) most effective for an individual. Reliable and valid assessment decision making is essential to the accommodation process. Throughout this book, resources are provided to aid professionals in selecting evidence-based accommodations by using informed clinical judgment. Within the chapters pertaining to achievement (i.e., Chapters 5 [reading], 6 [writing], and 7 [mathematics, science, and second languages]), decision-making flowcharts guide professionals during the assessment process and in selecting appropriate accommodations.

In secondary and postsecondary education today, debates are raging about the importance of both broad and specific cognitive processing abilities for the diagnosis of LD or ADHD. Despite the controversy, cognitive measures remain significant elements of most assessment batteries, and therefore of making decisions about who is qualified to receive accommodations at the adolescent and adult levels. Chapter 3 provides an overview of research related to both broad cognitive processing (general intelligence) and specific cognitive processes (e.g., working memory, fluid reasoning), and shows how cognitive assessment can be used to support the choice of specific accommodations for adolescents and adults with LD or ADHD.

Unfortunately, the social–emotional well-being and academic competence of individuals with LD and ADHD have often been studied separately, rather than considered within a broader model that accounts for the direct and indirect relationships of one to the other. Follow-up and follow-along studies of adults with LD and ADHD provide evidence that these disabilities exert a lifelong influence, although factors of resilience have been identified as well. The research also indicates that the diagnosis of either LD or ADHD appears to place an individual at a greater risk for other, coexisting psychiatric and/or developmental disorders. Chapter 4 reviews the current research specific to the social and emotional well-being of the adolescent and adult populations with LD and ADHD, and describes effective diagnostic tools and accommodations.

As a result of emerging technologies, a fundamental shift in how we define literacy is taking place in the world of school and work. For adolescents and adults with LD and ADHD, these new technologies offer opportunities to be better prepared for 21st-century education and employment. Many different technologies are being used to accommodate the learning and work environments for these individuals. Universal design for learning (UDL), for instruction (UDI), and for testing (UDT) has begun to emerge in the educational literature, as well as in the philosophy and products of the corporate world. Many of the universal design solutions proposed as effective for the adolescent and adult populations with LD and ADHD involve access to technological tools. Professionals who provide comprehensive evaluations need to think about the specific cognitive, language, and achievement abilities that influence learner performance across both traditional print and alternative media (e.g., electronic text and text-to-speech software) formats. Chapters 5 (reading), 6 (writing), and 7 (mathematics, science, and second languages) provide specific assessment considerations pertaining to the influence of format (print or alternative media) on learner performance, as well as lists of technology accommodations effective for adolescent and adult populations.

Because of standards-based educational reforms and evolving professional licensing requirements, large-scale assessments have increasingly become the gateways to promotion, graduation, and career attainment. Chapter 8 reviews the evidence-based literature pertaining to the accommodation of adolescents and adults with LD and ADHD in such large-scale assessments. Test accommodations adjust the manner in which testing situations are presented and/or evaluated, so that individuals with disabilities can access and/or demonstrate knowledge in a fair and equitable manner.

In the final analysis, the future success of adolescents and adults with LD and ADHD lies within the creative talents of these individuals. However, securing the rights due to these populations requires the determination of all involved (consumers, professionals, systems, etc.) to work toward inclusiveness and collaboration, rather than to focus on boundaries and separateness. The ultimate purpose of this book is to provide professionals with resources to accomplish these goals.

NOËL GREGG

Acknowledgments

Many individuals aided in the preparation of this book. I would like to first recognize the adolescents and adults with LD and ADHD who over my career have shared their experiences with me, informing my understanding and recognition of their strengths and motivation to learn.

Countless professional relationships and scores of research studies across the disciplines of psychology, education, linguistics, and neurology provide the foundation for the ideas discussed throughout this book. One of the primary purposes of this volume is to encourage ongoing cross-disciplinary dialogue pertaining to the assessment and accommodation of adolescents and adults with LD and ADHD. The willingness of professionals across disciplines to value varying perspectives improves the chances for reform to take focus within a changing lens.

I extend a sincere thank you to my editor at The Guilford Press, Rochelle Serwator, who is one of the most outstanding editors with whom I have been privileged to work. She believed in and supported my passion for the ideas presented throughout this book. In addition, I thank Marie Sprayberry for her professional and expeditious copyediting. Her knowledge of the field contributed to very important changes that help make many ideas clearer to the reader. I also thank Laura Specht Patchkofsky, Senior Production Editor, for her expertise in shepherding the text through the publication process.

Finally, I acknowledge the encouragement of my family, who have been steadfast in their support and tolerance of my preoccupation with this project. In particular, I thank Demmie, Anna, Amy, and Debbie. They have exceeded expectations in the love and joy they bring to my life.

Contents

CHAPTER ONE

Why Are Accommodations Important?

Maxine, a European American senior in high school, has significant problems in the area of reading and writing. Her learning disabilities (LD) in the areas of phonemic and orthographic awareness provide support for her right to specific accommodations in the classroom and in testing situations. Several of her accommodations include extra time on tests that require reading or writing; use of alternative media (e.g., electronic text read-alouds); and use of a word processor for content area coursework (science, math, and history). Her problems with processing sounds and matching these sounds to letters are so severe that she has been allowed to substitute other college preparation courses for foreign language courses.

Hamid, a junior in college who immigrated from Iran when he was 3 years old, has been diagnosed with attention-deficit/hyperactivity disorder (ADHD) and generalized anxiety disorder. His ADHD and anxiety disorder functionally limit his learning abilities and provide support for his right to specific accommodations in the classroom and in testing situations. Among the most significant of Hamid's accommodations documented by a comprehensive evaluation include extra time, use of a private testing room, and frequent breaks during testing situations.

The accommodations made in instructional and testing situations for students like Maxine and Hamid have generated a great deal of debate from methodological, policy, and legal perspectives. The most significant barrier facing individuals qualified to receive specific accommodations

1

is the lack of professional knowledge about issues pertaining to these accommodations. Without an understanding of these complex issues, accommodations may be overused, underused, or misused. Thoughtful decision making based on research and best practice is essential to ensure that individuals with documented disabilities will be accommodated appropriately and equitably. It is critical to begin debates about the fairness of accommodations with an accurate understanding of what "accommodations" are and what they are intended to accomplish, as well as with a reflection on our own perceptions of the meanings of such constructs as "reading," "writing," "merit," "equity," and "fairness."

Accommodations adjust the manner in which instructional or testing situations are presented and/or evaluated, so that individuals with documented disabilities can learn and/or demonstrate their learning in a fair and equitable fashion. For Maxine, her significant deficits in phonemic and orthographic awareness functionally limit her ability to decode and spell words in English and to learn another language. However, she demonstrates above-average verbal reasoning, listening comprehension, and executive processing. It is therefore critical to provide Maxine access to information that other students receive through reading printed text, so that her knowledge base will not be influenced by her poor reading decoding and spelling abilities. Using alternative media (e.g., electronic text and text-to-speech software) to take in new content (e.g., science, history) gives her equal access to information. In a testing situation, if we are evaluating (for example) science competencies, the only equitable solution is to provide Maxine with read-alouds and other assistive technologies that will allow her to demonstrate her proficiencies in science. The information being tested is her science knowledge—not her ability to read or spell.

Outcome Data

Outcome data pertaining to secondary and postsecondary populations with LD and ADHD certainly raises concerns about the equity of educational opportunities for these individuals and supports the necessity of providing access to evidence-based accommodations (National Council on Disability, 2003; Wagner, Newman, Cameto, Garza, & Levine, 2005; Young & Browning, 2005). For instance, individuals with LD drop out of high school at a rate two to three times higher than that of their peers (U.S. General Accounting Office, 2003; Young & Browning, 2005); enroll in college and postsecondary training at one-tenth the rate of the general population (Stodden, Jones, & Chang, 2002; Wagner et al.,

2005; Young & Browning, 2005); constitute 20–60% of persons access-ing welfare programs (Burgstahler, 2003; Young & Browning, 2005); and serve time in correctional institutions at significantly elevated rates (Burrell & Warboys, 2000; Christle, Jolivette, & Nelson, 2000; National Council on Disability, 2003; Stenhjem, 2005).

Adolescents and adults with ADHD demonstrate similar dismal outcomes. In comparison to their peers, this population is at greater risk for grade retention, suspension, expulsion, and dropping out of sec-ondary schools (Barkley, 2006; Pagani, Tremblay, Vitaro, Boulerice, & McDuff, 2001; Wagner et al., 2005); for poor postsecondary educational outcomes (Lambert, 1988; Mannuzza, Gittelman-Klein, Bessler, Malloy, & LaPadula, 1993; Wagner et al., 2005; Weiss & Hechtman, 1993); for substance use and abuse (Barkley, 2006); for teen pregnancy (Barkley, 2006; Weiss & Hechtman, 1993); for driver's license suspensions (Bar-kley, 2004); and for employment difficulties (Barkley, 2006; Weiss & Hechtman, 1993).

Although employment outcome studies suggest that adults with LD or ADHD appear to function as well as their peers in obtaining jobs upon graduation, these statistics are misleading if taken only at face value (Wagner et al., 2005). Since no comprehensive study of employ-ment outcomes for adults with LD and/or ADHD has been conducted, our knowledge about the world of work for these populations is based primarily on their own experience and that of professionals working with them (Young & Browning, 2005). The empirically based employ-ment data available are certainly limited in scope.

The employment research we do have available provides evidence that the majority of jobs taken by adolescents and/or adults with LD and/or ADHD are often semiskilled and usually part-time positions (Barkley, 2006; Wagner et al., 2005). Wagner and colleagues (2005) found that while 86% of young adults with LD and/or ADHD earned more than minimum wage, only about 36% of them worked full time. In addition, they found that there was no real change in earnings for youth with LD and ADHD from the original National Longitudinal Transitional Study (NLTS; the 1987 figures were used) to the second study (NLTS-2; the 2003 data were used), even when wages were adjusted for inflation (Wagner et al., 2005).[1] A more shocking finding is that the majority of these individuals' wages are below the federal poverty threshold (U.S. Bureau of the Census, 2004). The earning power gap between youth with LD and/or ADHD and their nondisabled peers is growing wider,

[1]The original NLTS ran from 1985 to 1993; the NLTS-2 was begun in 2000 and is still continuing.

mainly because of disparity between the two groups' educational attainments (Day & Newburger, 2002; Wagner et al., 2005). Lack of participation by youth with LD and ADHD in rigorous secondary curricula, and their limited access to effective postsecondary accommodations, contribute to poor retention in secondary and postsecondary learning environments (Gregg, 2007). Wagner and colleagues also found that only 4% of young adults with LD and ADHD reported availability of accommodations on the job. This limited access to effective employment accommodations contributes to reports from higher percentages of adults with LD and ADHD that they receive poor job evaluations, remain overlooked for career advancements, and are frequently fired (Barkley, 2006; Frank, Sitlington, & Carson, 1995; Wagner et al., 2005; Weiss & Hechtman, 1993).

Clearly, the limited postsecondary educational attainment for adults with LD and ADHD is directly related to their poor employment outcomes. Despite state and federal efforts to improve the career and transitional competencies of individuals with these and other disabilities, the educational achievement of individuals with LD and ADHD remains substantially below that of the general population (Barkley, 2006; Wagner et al., 2005). Several disturbing outcome figures listed in Table 1.1 illustrate the need for professionals to ensure equal and fair access to learning. Providing evidence-based testing and instructional accommodations for adolescents and adults with LD and ADHD, so that they can improve their ability to learn and to demonstrate their knowledge, is essential to improving their secondary and postsecondary outcomes.

TABLE 1.1. National Longitudinal Transitional Study 2 (NLTS-2) Outcome Benchmarks

Benchmark	Percentage with LD meeting benchmark	Percentage with ADHD meeting benchmark
Completing high school	74	59
Dropping out	26	41
Attending 2-year college	23	30
Attending 4-year college	11	6
Attending vocational, technical, or business college	4	7
Earning more than minimum wage	87	86
Working full time	38	37
Males earning more than minimum wage	87	87
Females earning more than minimum wage	79	79

Note. Adapted from Wagner, Newman, Cameto, Garza, and Levine (2005).

Secondary and Postsecondary Demographics

A full and balanced view of the academic and employment needs of persons with LD and/or ADHD requires, first of all, an understanding of the political, geographic, economic, and cultural milieus in which these individuals are currently living. It is important for educators, policymakers, researchers, and other service providers to be cognizant of societal patterns influencing the adolescent and adult populations with LD and ADHD who are historically served and underserved by current systems.

Historically Served Populations with LD and ADHD

Historically served populations with LD or ADHD at the secondary level are those students who have officially qualified for services as defined by federal and state mandates. However, it is important to anchor our understanding of these populations in the context of the general population of secondary students. The students enrolled in high schools today reflect the gradual increase in diversity being manifested in the general U.S. population (National Association for College Admission Counseling, 2006; National Center for Education Statistics [NCES], 2007). In 2007, 57% of U.S. high school students were white, 19% Hispanic, 17% black, 4.6% Asian/Pacific Islander, and 1% Native American (NCES, 2007). Unfortunately, this increase in diversity has not been matched by an increase in educational attainment. A national awareness of low literacy skills and declining graduation rates for the general population of secondary students has led politicians, policymakers, and educators alike to call for secondary school reform (Biancarosa & Snow, 2004; Bridgeland, Dilulio, & Morison, 2006; Educational Testing Service, 2005; Harvey & Housman, 2004; National High School Alliance, 2005; Tucker, 2004). Ineffective secondary curricula, poverty, and lack of student–adult connections appear to be contributing most significantly to these poor outcomes for transitioning adolescents (Morocco, Aguilar, Clay, Brigham, & Zigmond, 2006).

Results from the NLTS-2 provide demographics for the secondary population with LD and/ or ADHD mirroring those for their general-population peers (Wagner et al., 2005). In regard to literacy abilities for secondary students with LD, Wagner and colleagues (2005) found that over 50% of such students performed below the 16th percentile on reading comprehension measures, placing them in the lowest 25th percent of the general population. Approaching the problem from a more positive perspective, Brigham, Morocco, Clay, and Zigmond (2006) summarize the findings from a study of three high schools identified as secondary programs that do make a difference for students with LD.

Similar to the findings of researchers studying the general population of secondary students, they stress the need for more rigorous and motivating curricula, as well as for meaningful student–adult dialogic experiences.

At the postsecondary level, 14 million undergraduates are enrolled in 2- and 4-year colleges in the United States, and the number is expected to reach 16 million by 2015 (*Chronicle of Higher Education*, 2007). Historically served students at the postsecondary level are defined as students making the transition from secondary to postsecondary schools with little or no break in their education, and meeting the more stringent documentation requirements at this level (see Chapter Two). Of the historically served population of students with documented disabilities, individuals with LD make up the largest group of college freshmen (NCES, 2007). Among the population with LD, approximately 17% will take college entrance exams, and 11% of those who graduate from high school will go on to 4-year institutions (Wagner et al., 2005). These figures are substantially lower than those for college-bound students without disabilities. The greatest growth in postsecondary attendance by students with LD or ADHD was experienced at 2-year colleges (Wagner et al., 2005).

Historically Underserved Adolescents and Adults with LD and/or ADHD

Historically, several factions of adolescents and adults with LD and ADHD have been underserved by policymakers, service providers, researchers, and agencies. These groups include (but are not limited to) adults of nontraditional student age (i.e., over 30), females, dropouts, ethnic/racial minorities, and individuals with fewer economic resources. The absence of attention to the specific needs of these groups has commonly resulted in their lack of preparation for advanced educational attainment and/or satisfying careers. Generalizing from research or best practice with historically served individuals to these underserved groups is questionable and ill advised.

Historically underserved students often delay postsecondary enrollment at least 1 or 2 years past high school graduation, enroll part time, remain fully employed, are single parents, and/or do not have high school diplomas (Compton, Cox, & Laanan, 2006; NCES, 2007). Therefore, as a function of their lifestyle and academic preparation, a greater number of these individuals choose to attend community and technical colleges (Gregg, 2007). Similar to their nondisabled peers, approximately 23% of the population with LD and ADHD who graduate from high school will go on to community colleges—a 20% increase since

1987 (Wagner et al., 2005). However, many community and technical colleges are increasing their academic requirements. Many underserved students cannot meet these higher standards, since many of these students do not complete a college preparatory curriculum with rigorous reading, math, and writing requirements (Green, 2006; Noeth & Wimberly, 2002; Twigg, 2006; Wagner et al., 2005). In addition, many of these students delay college attendance or attend only part-time, contributing further to low completion rates (Chen, 2005).

Students of Lower Socioeconomic Status

The barrier that socioeconomic status (SES) presents to successful postsecondary transition is a critical factor requiring far greater attention than it has received (Gregg, 2007). Even among students in the general population, only 65% of students from lower-SES groups graduate from high school, as compared to 95% from the highest-SES groups (Mortensen, 2001). The fact that SES remains the most significant predictor of occupational aspirations and postsecondary transitional status, but still receives little direct attention from researchers and/or policymakers, is difficult to understand (Rojewski & Kim, 2003). Postsecondary career attainment is highly correlated with "systematic patterns of educational placement and social expectations" that remain indirect functions of SES (Rojewski & Kim, 2003, p. 106).

And the interaction of SES with LD and ADHD is a powerful one. Youth with LD and/or ADHD from low-income households perform less well academically than their peers with or without disabilities, independently of race/ethnicity (Barkley, 2006; Rojewski & Kim, 2003). Wagner and colleagues (2005) report that students with LD from households with low incomes ($25,000 or less per year) scored significantly lower on achievement measures than youth from moderate-income households (those earning $25,000 to $75,000 per year). NLTS-2 data (Wagner et al., 2005) indicated that a "low-income Hispanic youth with disabilities is likely to score 15 points lower on reading comprehension measures than a White peer from a moderate-income household, holding other factors in the analysis constant" (p. 48). Unfortunately, low-SES students in general receive less guidance than those of higher SES on how "to navigate the school-to-work transition" (Herr & Niles, 1997, p. 139), and a similar point can be made about low-SES students with LD and ADHD in need of various forms of assistance. For instance, students with LD and ADHD from the highest-SES groups are often the focus of media attention related to requests for accommodations on high-stakes tests; indeed, these students remain overrepresented in the group that accesses accommodations on college entrance examinations.

Students of Nontraditional Age

Increasing numbers of older adults are pursuing postsecondary education. Causes for this include the return of veterans from war, company outsourcing, and the replacement of jobs by technology (Compton et al., 2006). Older adults attending postsecondary institutions are an extremely heterogeneous group. Adults who already have postsecondary degrees and are simply retraining, as well as individuals who never had the opportunity to graduate from high school (e.g., those with general equivalency diplomas), fall into the category of "students of nontraditional age." Several years ago, the government projected about a 20–30% increase of this group over the next 3 years (U.S. Department of Labor, 2002). Therefore, postsecondary institutions will need to provide curricula and services sensitive to the individualized needs of these different learners. Although demographic data on nontraditional-age students with LD and/or ADHD are scarce, we can make some inferences from college enrollment figures for the general population. In addition, we know that a large percentage of nontraditional-age students with disabilities did not have access to resources during their elementary and secondary education. At the time that many of these adults attended school, federal and state laws for accessing services were not in existence or served only young children. Therefore, this population represents a significant number of unidentified individuals.

Females

Females with LD or ADHD experience greater difficulty then their male counterparts in accessing accommodations. Such women face "multiple oppressions, as women, as individuals with disabilities, and disproportionally as racial or ethnic minorities [if they are members of minority groups]" (Ferri, 1997, p. 39). As the result of misperceptions and of systematic bias, many women who are experiencing difficulty in learning are overlooked and never referred for services.

Since the initial passage of federal laws governing access to services for LD, disproportionately greater numbers of males than of females have been identified as qualifying for these services. Initial prevalence studies reflected the findings that males outnumbered females by just under a 3:1 ratio: Approximately 73% of school-identified students with LD were males (Hallahan, Lloyd, Kauffman, Weiss, & Martinez, 2005). Recent prevalence figures continue to provide evidence that within school-identified populations, males outnumber females identified as having LD by a 2:1 ratio (Wagner et al., 2005). For the population with ADHD, prevalence figures mirror those for individuals with LD. The male-to-female ratio of adults with ADHD, for example, ranges from 1.8:1 to 2.6:1 (Barkley, Murphy, & Kwasnik, 1996; Biederman et al., 1993; Hallahan et al., 2005; Roy-Byrne et al., 1997). However, the gap between male and females identified as having ADHD appears to be declining, suggesting greater acceptance of the existence of ADHD in women (Robison, Skaer, Sclar, & Galin, 2002).

The higher prevalence figures for LD or ADHD among males than among females are often attributed to the biological vulnerability of males (Andersen & Teicher, 2000; Barkley, 2006; Hallahan et al., 2005). However, recent epidemiological studies provide an alternative to the assumption that genetics is the sole factor leading to the disparity between the identification of male and female students. Shaywitz, Shaywitz, Fletcher, and Escobar (1990) compared a sample of individuals meeting federal eligibility criteria for LD to an epidemiological sample. They found that the ratio of males to females was about 4:1 in the school-identified sample, but about 1:1 in the epidemiological sample.

If biological vulnerability is not the sole factor underlying prevalence figure disparities by gender, it appears that the most logical other explanation for it is referral bias. A significant body of research indicates that referrals for special education services appear to be based more on oppositional behavior than on academic need (Abidin & Robinson, 2002; Gregory, 1977; McIntyre, 1988; Naiden, 1976; Shinn, Tindal, & Spira, 1987; Vogel, 1990; Young, Kim, & Gerber, 1999). The identification of behavior as a significant factor contributing to teacher referrals provides strong evidence for systematic bias and discrimination. According to Vogel (1990), when females with LD do receive services in the public schools, they are often significantly lower in intelligence and more academically impaired than their male peers.

Teachers are the primary sources of student identification and referral for special education services in our secondary schools (Anderson, 1997; Flynn & Rahbar, 1994; Young et al., 1999). Therefore, teachers' perceptions and beliefs concerning disability, tolerable behavior, and academic expectations for males and females are extremely important to understand. Maniadaki, Sonuga-Barke, and Kakouros (2006) investigated the self-efficacy and behavior severity perceptions of both educators and mothers in relation to students with ADHD. "Self-efficacy" was defined as the participants' rating of their perceived ability to manage the behavior of males or females with ADHD. They found that mothers were more confident than educators in managing the behaviors of these students, and that both groups believed they were better equipped to manage females than males. However, only the educators rated male behavior as generally more severe than female behavior. Maniadkia and colleagues (2006) conclude that the perceived ability to manage the behavior of an individual with ADHD predicts the perceived severity of the behavior, and that perceived severity predicts referral. Therefore, a student's gender often influenced whether a rater's perceptions of severity led to a referral decision.

Recognition of the disparity across genders in identification practices for LD and/or ADHD is certainly not a new finding (Gregg, 1996; Shaywitz et al., 1990; Vogel, 1990). However, more importantly, Young and colleagues (1999) stress that the long-term practice of this pattern has had extremely negative effects on women. Some researchers suggest that undiagnosed LD or ADHD among females contributes directly and/or indirectly to the high prevalence of teenage motherhood and mothers on welfare (Young et al., 1999). High teenage pregnancy rates are also characteristic of the population of adults with ADHD. Recently, Barkley, Fischer, Smallish, and Fletcher (2006) investigated the sexual activity of adults with ADHD. They found that 68% of the females had been involved in a pregnancy as a biological parent, as compared to 38% of males with ADHD and only 16% of the control group members. The relationship of these findings to the underidentified population of women with LD and ADHD will require more research.

A more positive recent outlook for young women with LD and ADHD is reflected in findings that more females with LD and ADHD in 2003 (a 16-percentage-point increase) were engaging in school, work, or preparation for work after graduating from high school, compared to their cohorts in 1987 (Wagner et al., 2005). The employment gap between males and females identified with LD or ADHD appears from this research to be closing. However, this statistic should be viewed in the context of overall earnings: Wagner and colleagues (2005) also found that a larger proportion of males (87%) than of females (79%) earned above minimum wages.

Minorities

Minority groups are contributing a great deal to the enrollment growth in secondary and postsecondary institutions. It is estimated that by 2015, 80% of the 2.6 million new students in higher education will be ethnic minorities (Bragg, Kim, & Barnett, 2006; Carnevale & Fry, 2000; Laanan, 2006), and similar estimates have been made for secondary enrollment figures (Carnevale & Fry, 2000). The fastest-growing ethnic minority group in secondary and postsecondary education is the Hispanic population: According to Carnevale and Fry (2000), by 2015, one in six undergraduates in higher education will be Hispanic.

Unfortunately, the enrollment and retention rates at both second-ary and postsecondary institutions for minorities still lag behind those of their nonminority peers, and the degree attainment for Hispanics and African Americans of college-going age is less than half than that for European Americans and Asians (Green, 2006). African American and Hispanic students with LD are also less likely to gain access to post-secondary learning environments than their nonminority counterparts (Phelps & Hanley-Maxwell, 1997; Wagner et al., 2005). Outcome data for youth with LD provide evidence that European American students score significantly higher on academic performance measures than their peers with LD who are African American or Hispanic (Wagner et al., 2005). The relationship of race or ethnic differences to academic performance for students with LD and/or ADHD raises particular con-cerns about equity and fairness in accommodating the learning envi-ronment for these individuals (Gregg, 2007; Murray & Naranjo, 2008).

It remains a fact that lack of racial and cultural diversity is charac-teristic of students taking high-stakes college entrance and exit exams, whether or not these students have disabilities. Nevertheless, this soci-etal trend is even more sharply evident among the students who do have disabilities. As an example, Lindstrom (2006) investigated students tak-ing the SAT with and without the accommodation of extended time. Individuals requesting extended time on the SAT in this study were individuals with a diagnosis of either LD or ADHD. The students taking the SAT (with or without accommodations) were not extremely diverse (see Table 1.2). However, the lack of diversity among students with LD or ADHD was even greater than among their nondisabled peers.

TABLE 1.2. Ethnicities in Two Groups of Students (with and without Disabilities) Taking the SAT

Examinees' self-described ethnicity	Students without disabilities ($n = 2,476$)	Students with disabilities ($n = 2,476$)
White	62.2%	73.3%
African American or black	8.2%	4.0%
Asian, Asian American, or Pacific Islander	9.3%	1.7%
Mexican or Mexican American	4.0%	1.1%
Puerto Rican	1.0%	0.8%
Latin American, South American, Central American, Hispanic, or Latino	3.3%	1.7%
Other	2.9%	2.2%

Note. Because some participants did not describe their ethnicity, the entries in each column do not total 100%. From Lindstrom (2006). Used by permission of author.

A special word about the increasing numbers of immigrants in the United States is in order here. Hamid, the student introduced at the opening of this chapter, who immigrated from Iran when he was 3 years old and was later diagnosed with ADHD and generalized anxiety disorder, is representative of this growing population. Unfortunately, many members of these cultures and/or racial groups are reluctant to request evaluations or accommodations for learning, particularly at postsecondary institutions. Therefore, the hidden disabilities of LD and ADHD become even more obscure, concealed as they are by cultural mores. In addition, professional misperceptions and bias pertaining to culturally, ethnically, or racially different individuals can easily influence who is referred for services.

Dropouts

Alarmingly, 7,000 students drop out of high school every day, which has led researchers to term the problem a "silent epidemic" (Alliance for Excellent Education, 2006; Bridgeland et al., 2006). "Each year, almost one third of all public high school students and nearly one half of all blacks, Hispanics, and Native Americans fail to graduate with their class" (Bridgeland et al., 2006, p. 1); although some such students may graduate with a later class, many do not. The most commonly cited causes for this epidemic are the low literacy abilities of many students (Biancarosa & Snow, 2004). Students who enter ninth grade functioning at the lowest 25th percent of their class are 20 times more likely to drop out than their higher-performing peers (Biancarosa & Snow, 2004).

Individuals with LD and ADHD account for a large percentage of this "silent epidemic." As noted earlier, many of these students are functioning at reading levels below the 16th percentile (Wagner et al., 2005). Unfortunately, few of these students receive alternative media (e.g., electronic text) and assistive technologies (e.g., text-to-speech software) as instructional accommodations to aid in their access to or demonstration of knowledge (Wolfe & Lee, 2007). Therefore, the gap between their knowledge and their ability to read and write grows wider as they progress throughout school. Receiving extended time on high-stakes tests will not be enough if access to the knowledge represented on these measures has not been consistently available to learners (Cohen, Gregg, & Deng, 2005).

The high dropout rates for secondary students with LD (26%) and ADHD (41%) should be matters of concern for professionals working with these populations (Wagner et al., 2005), as should the much lower graduation rates for students with LD and ADHD (70%) than for those in the general population (85%) (Kaufman & Alt, 2004). Moreover, these figures do not fully reflect the large number of individuals representing historically underserved groups. For instance, Hispanic students with disabilities show only a 60% high school completion rate.

In particular, the 41% dropout figure for students with ADHD represents a "silent epidemic" hazardous to the welfare of these youth as well as to our society. During the period from 1987 to 2003, students identified with ADHD have shown the greatest growth (630%) across populations of students with disabilities served in our public schools (Carnevale & Fry, 2000; Wagner, Cameto, & Newman, 2003; Wagner et al., 2005). Unfortunately, this group of students has demonstrated no improvement in grades, has experienced the largest increase in the percentage suspended from school, and has participated at very low rates in postsecondary education (Wagner et al., 2003; Wagner, Newman, & Cameto, 2004). Their solution for coping appears to be dropping out of school.

Addressing the significant dropout rates for both students with and without disabilities will require a restructuring of current teaching, curricula, and school climate (Biancarosa & Snow, 2004; Bridgeland et al., 2006; Brigham et al., 2006). For students with LD and ADHD, multiple academic pathways are critical to entering and succeeding in postsecondary academic environments (Gregg, 2007). "Academic pathways" have been defined as "boundary-spanning curricula, instructional and organizational strategies, and meaningful assessments that either link or extend from high school to college, including both two- and four-year institutions" (Bragg et al., 2006, p. 6). The utilization of these pathways will vary across the diverse group of individuals with LD and ADHD. Obviously, our traditional learning environments are ineffective for a significant portion of this population. It is time to create systematic and universal solutions that include multiple options (Gregg, 2007).

Universal Design Solutions

The term "universal design" (UD) was coined more than 30 years ago, when Ronald Mace put forth the revolutionary idea that physical environments should be designed to meet the broadly diverse needs of all individuals who use these spaces (see Wilkoff & Abed, 1994). The UD concept is reflected in the proactive inclusion of accessible design features, which minimize the need for individually retrofitted accommodations, in learning and work environments. Many UD products and environmental features have become increasingly common in our lives: Closed captioning on television sets, which is useful for individuals with hearing impairments, also aids the average person in noisy environments such as airports or restaurants; curb cuts, which are helpful for wheelchair users, also increase accessibility for other individuals, including cyclists and parents with strollers. Through the evolution of UD, additional design concepts—including "UD for learning" (UDL), "UD for instruction" (UDI), and "UD for testing" (UDT)—have begun to emerge in the educational literature, as well as in the philosophy and products of the corporate world. For more comprehensive discussions of UDL or UDI, I suggest that the reader visit the websites of the Center for Applied Special Technology (*www.cast.org*) and the University of Washington's DO-IT Center (*www.washington.edu/doit/Faculty/Strategies/Universal*).

UD Solutions for Accessing Print

For many adolescents and adults with LD or ADHD, difficulties with reading present a substantial barrier to achievement and have a major negative impact on postsecondary work and educational outcomes, as this chapter to this point has made clear (see also Chapter Five). Therefore, UD solutions that provide these individuals with alternative means of accessing print are critically needed in both education and work environments. The term "alternative media" ("alt media") refers to a variety of formats into which printed text can be converted, such as Braille, audiotaped text, and electronic text (e-text). To access e-text, an individual can use several forms of assistive technology (AT) such as text-to-speech (TTS) or speech-to-text (STT) software. The alt media most commonly used by the adolescent and adult populations with LD are e-text and audio files (Wolfe & Lee, 2007). Individuals who choose to access print through e-text have many different types of file formats to choose from, such as Microsoft Word (.doc), rich-text format (.rtf), portable document format (.pdf), hypertext markup language (.html), MPEG-1 audio layer 3 (.MP3), and the Digital Accessible Information System (DAISY), to name a few. Again, these file formats alone do not provide accessibility to print, but when used in conjunction with software like TTS software, they make the world of print information available to those with print-related disabilities (see Wolfe & Lee, 2007, for further discussion). Because technology terminology can be confusing, some of the terms commonly used throughout this book are defined in Table 1.3.

Consumers, researchers, teachers, administrators, federal legislators, task groups, and technical assistance programs have forged strong alliances at both the secondary and postsecondary levels to advocate for the importance of alt media and AT for individuals with reading

TABLE 1.3. Technology Terminology

Term	Meaning
Alternative media (alt media)	The various formats into which printed text can be converted (e.g., audiotape, Braille, electronic text).
ASCII text	Machine-readable text in which only letters and punctuation are stored.
Assistive technology (AT)	According to the Assistive Technology Act of 1998, any "product, device, or equipment, whether acquired commercially, modified or customized, that is used to maintain, increase, or improve the functional capabilities of individuals with disabilities." Also called "adaptive technology."
Blog	Online content that provides commentary or news.
Digital Accessible Information System (DAISY)	A universal format for reading and publishing digital talking books.
Digital audio recorder (DAR)	Hand-held device that converts speech into a digital format and transmits it to a computer or another hand-held device.
Electronic text (e-text)	Printed text made available on machine-readable or computerized formats.
Hypertext markup language (.html)	Tagging system used to turn text into web pages.
Optical character recognition (OCR)	Software that converts scanned images of text into machine-readable formats.
Online chat	Any kind of communication over the Internet, but primarily chat between individuals or groups (e.g., AOL Instant Messenger).
.MP3	A common digital audio encoding and storage format. It is a de facto standard format for the transfer and playback of music on a digital audio player (e.g., an iPod).
Portable Document Format (.pdf)	A file format created by Adobe Systems for document exchange.
Rich Text Format (.rtf)	A free document file format developed by Microsoft for cross-platform document interchange.
Social media	Internet media with interactive properties that enable a user to participate in a wide array of online activities.
Speech-to-text (STT) software	Type of speech synthesis application used to translate speech into e-text.

(continued)

TABLE 1.3. *(continued)*

Term	Meaning
Supported e-text	Integration of e-text with AT software.
Text messaging or texting	Term for sending text messages up to 169 characters from mobile phones.
Text-to-speech (TTS) software	Type of speech synthesis application used to translate e-text into speech.
Wiki	Computer software allowing users to create, edit, and link web pages.

disorders. For example, as a result of the Individuals with Disabilities Education Improvement Act of 2004 (IDEA 2004), state departments of education now have the option to adopt the National Instructional Materials Accessibility Standard (NIMAS) for the purpose of providing instructional materials to blind persons or other persons with print disabilities in the K–12 setting (see *nimas.cast.org*; see also Chapter Two for further discussion).

Unfortunately, there are no federal laws requiring publishers to supply postsecondary educational or employment institutions with electronic copies of publications. However, in 2006, higher education members of the Association of American Publishers announced the launch of their Alternative Formats Solutions Initiative (*www.publisherlookup.org*), a national effort to identify ways to supply print-disabled postsecondary students with alternatively formatted course materials. The initiative garnered the input of college and university faculty and staff, students with and without disabilities, support services professionals, national and state disability advocacy groups, and technology providers in an effort to create a national framework of specific, practical solutions. In addition, several states have adopted alt media laws and/or guidelines to meet the challenges that students face in postsecondary educational settings. Both California (*www.atpc.com*) and Georgia (*www.amac.uga.edu*) have allocated resources to support and implement statewide postsecondary alt media initiatives.

In the corporate environment, businesses like Microsoft, Google, and Apple have integrated UDL accessibility features into their enterprise applications and/or project initiatives. In addition, Microsoft (*www.microsoft.com/enable*) and Apple (*www.apple.com/accessibility*) now include accessibility options in their operating systems. These options provide a wide array of alternatives for accessibility and interaction, as current versions of both Microsoft's and Apple's operating systems can include basic voice recognition programs, word prediction, and abbreviation features. Another excellent UDL resource is the Google Library Project (*books.google.com/googlebooks/library.html*), which has partnered with public libraries to digitize and categorize public domain materials. Although Google's decision to digitally scan library books met with some opposition from the publishing community, the fact that large companies like Google see the importance of providing their customers with access to digital media is a positive sign.

In the corporate environment, the UDL approach has focused on the removal of barriers to technology. Many officers of corporations are acknowledging the value of integrating accessible technology into their organizations. John Cleghorn, former chair and chief executive officer of the RBC Financial Group, stated, "If you want to be a business leader and want access to top talent and enhanced market opportunity, you should absolutely promote accessibility" (quoted in Microsoft, 2002, p. 5). The integration of UDL into workplace environments has three primary elements (Microsoft, 2002):

1. *Accessibility features.* The operating system and software must include features that allow each user to adjust and customize the system and software to meet his or her own accessibility needs.
2. *Individualized AT products.* It must be possible to choose AT products specifically to accommodate an individual's profile.
3. *Compatibility.* The operating system and software must be compatible with specific types of technology products.

With similar UDL philosophies, both the academic and corporate environments are moving toward providing universal access, whether in the classroom or in the office. Indeed, one could argue that over the last several years, a new link has formed between the educational and corporate environments. Businesses are now looking toward education to help understand individual employees' needs, whereas educators are looking toward corporations to feed technology solutions into the classroom curriculum.

Limitations of Traditional Models of Access

Until recently, educators have seen alt media and AT as central to the solutions for helping individuals with LD and ADHD access learning, but there is a growing awareness that simply superimposing these on existing models of access may not be enough in the world of work and education (Banerjee & Brinckerhoff, 2007). The rapid proliferation of technologies has led to a blurring of the line between AT and "mainstream" technologies; the latter are described as traditional information and communication technologies used to manage, instruct, and communicate among participants (Banerjee & Gregg, in press). For instance, the infusion of technology into postsecondary education has fundamentally altered how college instruction occurs (Bruce & Levin, 1997; Chickering & Erhman, 2004) and how students acquire new literacies (Leu, 2006). Increasing numbers of postsecondary instructors use course management systems such as WebCT/Vista and related forms of learning technologies in instruction (Bannan-Ritland, 2002; Vest, 2006). The result is digitalization of printed information. For adolescents and adults with LD and ADHD who have reading difficulties, this new situation can be both a boon and a challenge. Those individuals who are unfamiliar with the skills and strategies needed for reading in open learning environments, like the Internet, may find such environments daunting (Leu, 2006). However, those who are prepared to take advantage of these new developments will find that they provide unprecedented advantages.

Adolescents and adults with LD and ADHD need access that also affords them a competitive edge in learning. Timmer (2007) suggests that when policies and procedures offer traditional accommodations (such as tape-recorded class lectures) that become too onerous to use, students are discouraged from pursuing these options. Adolescents or adults with LD or ADHD also often fail to avail themselves of accessibility options because the protocol for receiving such services is time-consuming. One challenge in particular is the lack of alt media format in real time. Adolescents or adults with print LD or ADHD often have to be satisfied with "parallel reading experiences"—that is, to read only when the material is available in an accessible medium, which may be much later than the rest of the class reads it (Banerjee & Gregg, in press). In other words, even if accessibility exists, it is often not efficient. The distributed model of service delivery, which makes accessibility a schoolwide responsibility (and not the sole charge of the disability service office or special education teacher), is often touted as the "right service model." However, this too can pose unanticipated barriers for some students: When services are distributed across different campus constituencies, such as media services, library, information technology services, student affairs, disability services, and remedial services, students must be adept at negotiating the system (Banerjee & Gregg, in press). Adolescents or adults with LD or ADHD, many of whom lack self-advocacy skills, can find accessing resources from multiple sources particularly challenging.

Accommodation Selection

Understanding the issues surrounding accommodation practices must begin with recognizing the consequences for adolescents and adults with LD and ADHD who are not provided access to, or equal opportunities to demonstrate, their knowledge. As noted throughout this chapter, lack of access to accommodations can have major negative effects on career development and adult income. Future policies and practices pertaining to accommodating learning and work environments for the populations with LD and ADHD should be guided by evidence-based research and by UDL/UDT options.

The effectiveness of an accommodation in enhancing an individual's performance is dependent upon a professional's knowledge of the specific cognitive, affective, and language processes that influence different types of learning demands. Understanding the reason(s) for a person's learning deficits should influence the type(s) of accommodation(s) chosen. Consistent and reliable professional decision making is essential to the accommodation process. Throughout this book, resources are provided to aid professionals in selecting evidence-based accommodations by using informed clinical judgment. Moreover, greater interdisciplinary dialogue and sharing of knowledge are needed among all professionals who work with secondary and postsecondary students. A goal of this volume is to help professionals bridge the "discipline gap," so that adolescents and adults with LD or ADHD will benefit from best practices in determining and supporting accommodation.

CHAPTER TWO

Documentation for Accommodation Access

Dan, a European American junior in high school, has been served by special education since second grade, when he was diagnosed with LD and ADHD. Throughout elementary and secondary school, he was provided such accommodations as extra time, read-alouds, and use of a private room during examinations. He is now beginning to apply to colleges and is concerned about whether he will be able to access the same accommodations he has used in high school.

Vernetta, a 35-year-old African American female, began to experience significant academic problems while enrolled at a technical college. She reported always working twice as hard as her peers in high school in order to maintain passing grades. Vernetta's technical college English teacher suggested that her difficulties in writing appeared to be caused by more than just a lack of instruction. The teacher encouraged Vernetta to go to the college counseling and testing center, to explore the possibility of receiving an evaluation to determine the source of her academic underachievement. Since Vernetta had received no special education services during elementary or high school, she was concerned that the college would not provide her access to accommodations.

Access to accommodations requires that an individual meet specific eligibility criteria as defined by legal mandates. It is very easy to become confused by legal terminology and to misinterpret the meaning of regulations designed to provide equitable learning opportunities for individuals with LD or ADHD. In addition, two entirely different sets of laws

20

and regulations protect individuals with disabilities in high school and in postsecondary settings. Secondary students are protected primarily by the Individuals with Disabilities Education Improvement Act of 2004 (IDEA 2004). Individuals who are attending postsecondary institutions or who are in the workforce are safeguarded by such legislation as the Rehabilitation Act of 1973 and the Americans with Disabilities Act (ADA) of 1990. As a result of all these laws, secondary and postsecondary institutions, as well as employers, are responsible for providing reasonable access to accommodations for qualified individuals.

The legal terminology pertaining to the rights and responsibilities surrounding an individual's ability to access accommodations can be very confusing to anyone outside the legal system. Therefore, a summary of frequently used legal terms is provided in Table 2.1, as a reference for professionals and consumers interested in the statutes, regulations, and litigation that provide the foundation for fair and equitable treatment of individuals with disabilities in school or work settings.

Systematic and attitudinal barriers can be reduced or eliminated when both individuals and institutions obtain an understanding of their legal rights and protections. The profiles of Dan and Vernetta,

TABLE 2.1. Legal Terminology

Term	Description
Law	Four types: constitutional law, state laws, local laws, and case law.
Policy	Rules and regulations developed to implement laws.
U.S. Constitution	The "supreme law of the land."
Case law	Law that emerges from court decisions.
State law	Statutory law enacted at the state level.
Litigation	Court cases (state or federal).
Rational basis test	Test the courts utilize to determine whether a state or state agency has discriminated.
Legislation	Laws enacted by the U.S. Congress and by state and local governments.
Statutes	Laws enacted by the U.S. Congress and by state and local governments.
Regulations	Rules developed to carry out legislation by an executive agency charged to do so.
Judicial interpretations	Commentary following judicial opinions, referred to as "dicta."

introduced at the opening of this chapter, are used later to illustrate the complexities of the laws protecting the rights of individuals with disabilities. However, before I discuss the portions of current federal legislation integral to accessing accommodations for students with LD and ADHD across secondary and postsecondary settings, I provide a discussion of some general factors influencing professional decision making, as a basis for a better understanding of the legal interpretation of disabilities.

LD and ADHD: Myths or Facts?

A great deal of popular mythology about LD and ADHD has resulted in skepticism about the authenticity of these disorders. From social critics (Coles, 1987; Spear-Swerling & Sternberg, 1996) to fringe groups such as the Church of Scientology, uninformed individuals suggest that the labels of LD and ADHD are excuses for simply not trying hard enough, not being smart enough, or not obtaining enough education. Other critics insinuate that a "surge" of students is being overidentified as demonstrating LD or ADHD (Flanagan, Keiser, Bernier, & Ortiz, 2003; Gordon & Keiser, 1998). Until fairly recently, if an institution demonstrated higher-than-expected prevalence figures for LD and ADHD, it was mainly the result of professionals' having made clinical decisions based on inadequate knowledge of the psychological and educational literature. Today, however, a great deal of empirically based literature is available to guide professionals in the selection of tools, processes, and policies so that they can arrive at reliable and valid diagnostic decisions. Therefore, as Barkley (2006) states, "claims that ADHD [and I add LD] is a myth reflect either a stunning level of scientific illiteracy or outright attempts to misrepresent the science of ADHD [and LD] so as to mislead the public with propaganda" (p. 93).

The myth that LD and ADHD are not "*real* disabilities" is best refuted by examining the literature that compares individuals with and without LD or ADHD. If these disabilities were not valid disorders, few differences on cognitive, behavioral, or social measures would be found in such comparisons. However, the literature on LD shows that adolescents and adults with LD typically obtain lower scores than normally achieving peers on measures of phonemic awareness, reading rate, working memory, and processing speed (Gregg et al., 2005; Ofiesh, Mather, & Russell, 2005). Individuals with LD appear to use different, and often less efficient, cognitive and linguistic processes than do their peers without disabilities. In addition, the predictive relationships of cognitive and linguistic measures to reading and written language performance differ significantly between the groups. Adolescents and adults with LD may learn to compensate, but they do not outgrow their problems. Therefore, regarding LD as simply low academic performance or underachievement is a misconception that can limit an individual's chances for equal access (Mather & Gregg, 2006). Although LD results in underachievement, it should not be equated with below-average academic functioning (Kavale & Forness, 2003; Kavale, Fuchs, & Scruggs, 1994; Scruggs & Mastropieri, 2002). An individual can be underachieving academically for a myriad of reasons (e.g., lack of instruction, poor school attendance, affective factors, or health) that have little or nothing to do with LD. The adolescent and adult populations with ADHD also demonstrate significantly different profiles from those of their normally achieving peers. In particular, individuals with ADHD demonstrate significant deficits in behavioral inhibition and in several of the executive functions that are critical for effective self-regulation (Barkley, 2006).

Valid diagnoses of LD and ADHD are dependent upon professionals' recognition of these conditions as developmental disorders. Barkley (2006) provides an excellent discussion of the adolescent and adult population with ADHD that has direct implications for individuals with LD as well. The symptoms demonstrated by an individual with ADHD or LD are, by definition, disordered as compared to age-expected behaviors, and thus cause individuals to be substantially limited in major life activities. Barkley concludes his discussion with two relevant points: (1) The symptoms are not "static pathological states or absolute deficits in formerly typical functioning" (p. 265); and (2) the symptoms must be determined by "age-relative thresholds" (p. 265). The idea that fixed symptom thresholds can be applied across the lifespan often leads to the use of invalid criteria for the adult population (Gregg, Coleman, Lindstrom, & Lee, 2007). The importance of looking at how social/ emotional, cognitive, language, and achievement abilities change and influence each other differently across the lifespan is critical to reliable and valid diagnostic decision making for the adolescent and adult populations.

Prevalence

The prevalence of LD and ADHD among the adolescent and adult populations is more difficult to confirm, as fewer researchers focus on these age groups than on children. We do know that approximately 5.5% of the childhood population demonstrates LD (National Center for Education Statistics [NCES], 2007), and 3–7% ADHD (American Psychiatric Association, 2000; Barkley, 2006). Since LD and ADHD are developmental disorders, the prevalence figures from childhood to adulthood should not significantly change—or, at least, they would not if reliable and valid diagnostic decision making were available to all individuals. As of 2006, Barkley identified only five studies of the prevalence of ADHD in the adult population; however, the findings from this research continue to support a 2–4% prevalence of ADHD among adults.

The prevalence figures for adults with LD vary across agencies serving these individuals. Different eligibility criteria used to identify severity, as well as the different profiles of adults served by an institution, influence these figures. For instance, the U.S. Employment and Training Administration (1991) estimated the incidence of adults with LD among Job Training Partnership Act recipients to be 15–23% (Corley & Taymens, 2002). Participants in many adult basic education are reported to demonstrate LD (Mellard, Patterson, & Prewett, 2007; Snow & Strucker, 2000). According to Corley and Taymens (2002), 10–50% of individuals participating in adult education programs may experience LD. Among the college-bound population, the prevalence of LD is reported to be approximately 3–5% (NCES, 2007).

Determining Severity

Among the most significant factors influencing prevalence figures are the diagnostic criteria professionals set in determining the severity thresholds for symptoms, history, and behaviors (emotional, cognitive, and achievement). In other words, how severe must an individual's deficits in these areas be in order to qualify for a diagnosis of LD or ADHD? The two practices most commonly applied by professionals in identifying severity levels have been (1) examination of discrepancies across performance and (2) cutoff standards. These practices, if used with little other evidence, can lead to professional decisions that either over- or underidentify individuals differing in demographic variables (Barkley, 2006; Brackett & McPherson, 1996; Gregg, Coleman, Lindstrom, & Lee, 2007; Hoy et al., 1996).

Discrepancy Methods

Many types of discrepancies are important in diagnostic decision making. The discrepancy between an individual's ability and achievement scores has traditionally been a critical component of eligibility criteria for the adolescent and adult population—but it should never be the single criterion for an eligibility decision, because although it is sensitive, it is not specific enough for diagnosis. Unfortunately, a discrepancy between full-scale intelligence score and achievement became the hall-mark of LD diagnosis for many years, with little consideration of other diagnostic factors (Mather & Gregg, 2006). I am not going to discuss in depth the problems with ability–achievement discrepancy formulas, since a great deal of literature about their limitations is available (e.g., Berninger, 2001; Fletcher et al., 2001; Fuchs, Mock, Morgan, & Young, 2003; Gregg, Coleman, Lindstrom, & Lee, 2007; Kavale, Kaufman, Naglieri, & Hale, 2005; Mather & Gregg, 2006). What we can conclude from this research is that an LD diagnosis based solely on an ability–achievement discrepancy is not a reliable or valid means of determining severity levels.

Intracognitive, intrabehavior, and intra-achievement discrepancy methods are often used by clinicians. Such within-person discrepancies also have some of the same problems as ability–achievement discrepancies if used as the sole criteria for disability determination (Brackett & McPherson, 1996; Hoy et al., 1996; Mather & Gregg, 2006). Scatter across cognitive, behavior, or achievement measures does not define LD or ADHD any more than a discrepancy between ability and achievement does. In addition, the age of the person (adolescent or adult rather than child), his or her educational attainment, and the task demands are all critical factors in diagnostic decision making. Not all scatter is relevant when age, task, and experience are considered. However, significant scatter across cognitive, behavior, and achievement measures does warrant further investigation.

Cutoff Methods

Cutoff methods have been used alone by some professionals to identify LD or ADHD (Dombrowski, Kamphaus, & Reynolds, 2004; Gordon & Keiser, 1998; Siegel, 1990). That is, arbitrary cutoff levels in isolated academic scores have been used to determine functional limitations in learning (e.g., scores < 16th percentile), and thus to set the standard for severity. However, this approach results in a high false-positive rate for low-achieving adults and a high false-negative rate for high-achieving individuals (Brackett & McPherson, 1996; Hoy et al., 1996). Unfortunately, when LD or ADHD is defined as simply low achievement in the form of test scores below a certain percentile, the condition becomes confounded with a myriad of reasons for low academic performance that are separate from LD or ADHD (e.g., malingering, lack of instruction, poor school attendance, affective factors, or health impairments).

Barkley (2006) suggests that a 1.5 standard deviation (*SD*) cutoff criterion be used to identify the specific ADHD symptoms that are functionally limiting to one or more major life activities. However, he stresses that the criteria from the *Diagnostic and Statistical Manual of Mental Disorders* (currently in the text revision of its fourth edition, DSM-IV-TR; American Psychiatric Association, 2000)—the criteria most often used in the diagnosis of ADHD—become "increasingly insensitive to the disorder with age" (p. 266). This makes it even clearer that multiple sources of information are needed for valid clinical decision making. Identifying functional limitations (severity) in the area of learning requires an examiner to utilize much more information than one behavioral rating scale or achievement measure. As with LD, an individual can receive a diagnosis of ADHD when a 1.5 *SD* cutoff criterion for ADHD symptoms is used, but may not perform below the 16th percentile on achievement tests. In such cases, some professionals consider that the functional limitation in learning is not severe enough for services to be required.

Although some adolescents or adults with LD or ADHD do not score below the 16th percentile on select tests of achievement, this is not evidence that they do not struggle with learning. Through years of special tutoring and persistence, some individuals with LD or ADHD can improve enough academically to "break" the 16th percentile barrier (Mather, Gregg, & Simon, 2005). But this does not mean that a disability is no longer present—only that a person has managed to achieve a certain level of academic success on *some* measure(s). The context, task demands, and format of a test can influence an individual's performance (e.g., use of a multiple-choice format may lead to an overestimate of functional skill). Neither the presence nor absence of underachievement should be the sole discriminator for LD or ADHD.

Integrated Method

Many professionals have proposed that clinicians integrate (1) quantitative data (standardized and/or criterion-referenced test scores), (2) observational data, (3) background information, and (4) research-based evidence into the decision-making process. Researchers supporting such integrated methods emphasize that a single score, formula, or cutoff criterion (e.g., ability–achievement discrepancy) is not a valid means of identifying LD or ADHD (Barkley, 2006; Gregg, Coleman, Lindstrom, & Lee, 2007; Mather & Gregg, 2006); rather, they stress the importance of using multiple data sources in decision making. For instance, in addition to norm-referenced measures, clinicians applying an integrated method should consider an individual's developmental and instructional history, medical and psychological history, family history, and environmental factors. Test results "can be an aid to judgment, but they should not be a substitute" (Mather & Gregg, 2006, p. 100).

Statutes Supporting
the Right to Access Accommodations

The laws protecting the rights of adolescents or adults with LD or ADHD to access accommodations are either "entitlement" or "eligibility" statutes. Under entitlement laws (e.g., IDEA 2004), a student with a disability is eligible for a free, appropriate public education if he or she *needs* special education. However, the fact that a student receives a diagnosis of LD or ADHD does not mean that he or she is automatically eligible for special education and related services under IDEA 2004. Rather, it must be determined that a student *requires* special education and/or related services before he or she can qualify for the free entitlements covered by IDEA 2004 (Wright & Wright, 2007, pp. 49–50). In the situation where a secondary student is determined to have a disability but does not need special education services, protection under Section 504 of the Rehabilitation Act may support access to accommodations. Section 504 is a civil rights statute that protects individuals with disabilities for reasons related to their disabilities (Wright & Wright, 2007). Similar to Section 504 of the Rehabilitation Act, the ADA is an eligibility rather than an entitlement statute. Individuals who are attending postsecondary institutions, or those who are employed, are protected from discrimination by eligibility laws; however, such laws do not entitle the individual to services.

Section 504 of the Rehabilitation Act of 1973

Before the passage of the ADA in 1990, Section 504 of the Rehabilitation Act of 1973 (Public Law No. 93-112) was the most significant piece of legislation protecting the rights of individuals with disabilities—in particular, prohibiting educational and employment discrimination on the basis of disability. Unlike many other pieces of legislation covered in this chapter, Section 504 applies to both children and adults with disabilities. It ensures that a student has equal access to an education through such means as accommodations and/or modifications. In addition, Section 504 covers the federal government, every entity that receives financial assistance from the federal government, and anyone who does business with the federal government. The majority of colleges and universities in this country are recipients of federal financial assistance to some degree, and thus must adhere to this statute. Under Section 506 of the Rehabilitation Act Amendments of 1992, Congress amended Section 504 to achieve greater uniformity with the ADA. Therefore, any institution subject to Section 504 will have its conduct measured by the "standards" of Title I of the ADA.

American with Disabilities Act of 1990

The ADA (Public Law No. 101-336) provides protection for individuals with disabilities across programs and employers not covered by the Rehabilitation Act of 1973. Although the ADA does not replace Section 504, it does build upon this legislation (as well as upon the Civil Rights Restoration Act of 1987). ADA and Section 504 utilize the same language in defining what a disability is and in what manner severity requirements (substantial limitations) must be met under the law.

Individuals with Disabilities Education Improvement Act of 2004

The Education for All Handicapped Children Act of 1975 (Public Law No. 94-142), the predecessor of IDEA 2004, has gone through several reauthorizations since it was first enacted. In 1975, fewer than half of all children with disabilities were receiving an appropriate education. Although great progress has been made since then in improving the rights of children with disabilities, Congress noted the following in the findings for the reauthorization of IDEA 2004: "Implementation of this title has been impeded by low expectations and an insufficient focus on applying replicable research on proven methods of teaching and learning for children with disabilities" (quoted in Wright & Wright, 2007, p. 20).

IDEA 2004 requires that students with disabilities be provided appropriate accommodations across both instructional and testing situations. Students who are found to be eligible for special education services under IDEA 2004 must have their accommodation needs specified in their individualized education programs (IEPs). A student's IEP team (by law) includes at least one general educator, at least one special educator, a representative of the local educational agency, and the parents. The IEP team determines, if appropriate, the need for reasonable accommodations that are consistent with federal and state guidelines. However, a student's right to use an accommodation is not generalizable throughout his or her lifespan, or across different settings or situations. Each combination of the individual, the context, and the accountability system requires ongoing professional decision making and reevaluation. Several significant changes were made to IDEA under the 2004 reauthorization that are directly related to the assessment of, education of, and access to accommodations for students with LD and ADHD. In addition, the term "universal design for learning" (UDL) was included in the IDEA 2004 legislation. States and school districts are required to develop and administer assessments using UDL principles. Therefore, the use of assistive technology (AT) and UDL must be addressed by a student's IEP team.

No Child Left Behind Act of 2001

The No Child Left Behind (NCLB) Act of 2001 (Public Law No. 107-110) is a reauthorization of the Elementary and Secondary Education Act of 1965 (Public Law No. 89-10). However, the law was significantly changed during its reauthorization, to attempt to address the increasing problem of millions of children leaving school without the basic skills required for employment (NCES, 2007). In particular, the significant underperformance of students from low-income families, members of racial minorities, students with disabilities, and English language learners led to a public outcry for equity. Several key components of the NCLB Act are significant for adolescents with LD or ADHD. For instance, the law mandates annual proficiency testing for all individuals, research-based reading programs, and highly qualified teachers for all students. Since all adolescents with LD and ADHD are required to receive annual proficiency testing along with their nondisabled peers, issues surrounding these students' accommodations on such measures have assumed a central role in school programming.

The NCLB Act requires states to measure student proficiency in "mathematical and reading or language arts" to determine whether schools are making "adequate yearly progress" toward academic proficiency for all students, including students with disabilities. However, as a result of the mandatory, standards-driven nature of the NCLB Act, this group of learners has begun "to be acknowledged fully," and "schools and school districts [are being] forced to confront the conceptual and technical issues inherent in implementing reform" (McLaughlin, Embler, & Nagle, 2004, p. 2). Federal legislation does caution, however, that only "appropriate accommodations, where necessary" (IDEA 2004), and "reasonable accommodations necessary to measure academic achievement" (NCLB), should be provided to students. Identifying "reasonable" and "appropriate" accommodations requires professional judgment, as these accommodations must be examined separately for each student. The challenge lies in the provision and implementation of accommodations. Who resolves the question of which accommodations should be provided and under what circumstances? Far too often, a single accommodation is used across a variety of settings (e.g., extra time is granted for instructional and testing situations in reading, mathematics, science, etc.), with little thought given to whether this actually meets a student's needs or whether it compromises the purpose of the learning task.

One positive outcome of the NCLB Act has been an increase in proficiency on statewide assessments for students with disabilities (Thompson, Johnstone, Thurlow, & Altaian, 2005). According to the data that have been collected thus far, the trend has been influenced by the following factors: development of policy for participation in testing; alignment of students' IEPs with curriculum standards; ongoing professional development; development and provision of accommodation policies and procedures; increased access to standards-based instruction; and improved data collection (see Thompson et al., 2005, for an in-depth discussion). According to the Thompson and colleagues (2005) report, states identified the following as emerging needs related to providing accommodations to students with disabilities: technical assistance on appropriate instructional and/or testing accommodations; professional development, particularly for general education; and federal guidance on the degree of specificity required in state guidelines.

Technology-Related Legislation

As discussed throughout this book, technology can be used to accommodate an individual's learning and testing environment. Several legislative mandates provide the resources and protection to ensure that adolescents and adults with LD and ADHD receive appropriate technology accommodations.

Mandates for Instructional Material Accessibility

Several years ago, Congress granted nonprofit and governmental agencies an exemption to copyright laws, in order to convert books to accessible formats (Chafee Amendment to the Copyright Act of 1976 [1996]). However, educational institutions were not specifically authorized as such entities, causing administrators at the postsecondary level a great deal of concern about copyright privileges. Wolfe and Lee (2007) suggest that many postsecondary institutions, following a directive from the Office of Civil Rights, established a student copyright agreement process in order to provide the necessary access to instructional material. However, at the secondary level, as a result of IDEA 2004, the U.S. Department of Education has recently endorsed the adoption of a common file format for conversion of standard print to appropriate alternative formats (NIMAS Development & Technical Assistance Centers, 2006). The National Instructional Materials Accessibility Standard (NIMAS) is a technical standard used by publishers to produce source files, which can then be used to create a number of different types of alternative media, such as Braille, audio files, and talking books (NIMAS, 2006). The NIMAS file sets were established to support K–12 students with print disabilities. The final NIMAS regulations were published on July 19, 2006 (71FR41084), and were incorporated into Appendix C to Part 300 of the National Instructional Materials Accessibility standard published August 14, 2006 (*www.nimas.cast.org/about/regulations*).

Other Mandates

The Technology-Related Assistance for Individuals with Disabilities Act of 1988 (Public Law No. 100-407), better known as the Tech Act of 1988, was designed to meet the AT needs of individuals with disabilities. In 1994, the Tech Act was amended (Public Law No. 103-218) to revise and extend AT programs. Under both versions of the Tech Act, grants were provided to states to support statewide programs of technology-related assistance for individuals with disabilities.

The Carl D. Perkins Vocational and Applied Technology Education Act of 1998 (Public Law No. 105-332) provides resources to individuals with disabilities so that they can purchase technology for the purposes of accessing learning at career and technical institutions (Association for Career and Technical Education, *www.ataporg.org*).

The Assistive Technology Act of 1998 officially ended the Tech Act (P.L. 105-394). Its purpose was to support programs and grants to states to encourage greater participation by individuals with disabilities in accessing technology.

The Assistive Technology Act of 2004 (Public Law No. 108-364) changed the focus of the Tech Act of 1988 from supporting state technology infrastructures to delivering AT to persons with disabilities. States are allowed to use 60% of AT state grants on direct-aid programs, including AT reutilization programs, AT demonstration programs, alternative financing programs, and device loan programs. In addition, states may choose to use 70% of their AT grant funds on direct-aid programs.

Finally, the ADA and Section 508 of the Rehabilitation Act Amendments of 1998 (the latter were incorporated into the Workforce Investment Act of 1998, Public Law No. 105-220) require information technology developed or purchased by federal agencies to be accessible to all individuals with disabilities. Although these laws do not mandate alternative solutions to print material, they do stipulate that federal agencies purchase accessible technology.

Documentation in the Secondary Setting

Greater dialogue and sharing of knowledge are needed between professionals who work with the secondary and postsecondary populations with LD and ADHD. Moreover, there exists a great disconnection between the secondary and postsecondary accommodation practices and what appears in the research literature (Gregg & Lindstrom, 2007; Thurlow, 2006). As noted by the National Joint Committee on Learning Disabilities (NJCLD, 2007), this gap will simply increase as "educational reforms under [the NCLB Act and IDEA 2004] require more instructional and intervention information regarding students' educational outcomes" (p. 2).

As mentioned earlier in this chapter, the rights and responsibilities of students with disabilities in secondary settings are primarily governed by entitlement laws. For those adolescents with LD or ADHD who are found to require special education as provided by IDEA 2004, the focus is on *prescriptive* services. For students in either secondary or postsecondary institutions protected by Section 504, the focus is on *access* to learning. Civil rights statutes do not attach any authorization for funding, whereas entitlement laws (such as IDEA 2004) are supported by federal funds, which are dependent upon state compliance with regulations. The definition of disability, the type of evaluation documentation required, and the eligibility criteria all differ between entitlement and eligibility laws. First, in a secondary setting, it is the responsibility of the school district to identify and evaluate a student, at no expense to the parent or individual. In a postsecondary setting, the individual, not the institution, is responsible for identifying him- or herself and providing documentation of a disability. Moreover, the cost of the evaluation is assumed by the individual, not the institution. Although special education services are not provided under Section 504 or ADA, an institution must provide access to learning by accommodating the learning environment for an otherwise qualified individual.

Definitions of LD and ADHD

The IDEA 2004 regulations (34 Code of Federal Regulations [C.F.R.] § 300) provide specific definitions of the various disabilities covered by this statute. (See Table 2.2 for the IDEA 2004 definition of "specific learning disabilities," as well as the NJCLD definition of LD.) Students with ADHD are usually found eligible for services under the category of "other health impairment," "specific learning disabilities," or "emotional disturbance" (Wright & Wright, 2007), most often the first of these. The three types of ADHD are usually defined according to the diagnostic criteria in the DSM-IV-TR (see Tables 2.3 and 2.4). IDEA 2004 does not provide a definition of ADHD or require that the DSM-IV-TR criteria set be the only guidelines followed by professionals. This practice contributes to inconsistent decision making. In a joint policy memorandum on attention-deficit disorder [ADD] or ADHD in 1991,

TABLE 2.2. Definitions of LD

Individuals with Disabilities Education Improvement Act of 2004
(34 C.F.R. §300.8(c)(10))

Specific learning disability means a disorder in one or more of the basic psychological processes involved in understanding or in using language, spoken or written, that may manifest itself in the imperfect ability to listen, think, speak, read, write, spell, or to do mathematical calculations. [The term includes] conditions such as perceptual disabilities, brain injury, minimal brain dysfunction, dyslexia, and developmental aphasia. [The term] does not include learning problems that are primarily the result of visual, hearing, or motor disabilities, of mental retardation, of emotional disturbance, or of environmental, cultural, or economic disadvantage.

National Joint Committee on Learning Disabilities (1997)

Learning disabilities is a general term that refers to a heterogeneous group of disorders manifested by significant difficulties in the acquisition and use of listening, speaking, reading, writing, reasoning, or mathematical skills.

These disorders are intrinsic to the individual, presumed to be due to central nervous system dysfunction, and may occur across the life span. Problems in self-regulatory behaviors, social perception, and social interaction may exist with learning disabilities but do not, by themselves, constitute a learning disability. Although learning disabilities may occur concomitantly with other disabilities (e.g., sensory impairment, mental retardation, serious emotional disturbance), or with extrinsic influences (such as cultural differences, insufficient or inappropriate instruction), they are not the result of those conditions of influences.

the U.S. Department of Education did clearly state that children with ADD/ADHD may be eligible for services under several existing special education categories (the three listed above). In addition, in a 1992 memorandum, the Office of Civil Rights clearly specified that under Section 504, schools must evaluate children who are suspected of having ADD/ADHD if their parents request it. (See Wright & Wright, 2007, for more details about these memoranda.)

Eligibility Criteria and Evaluation Process

The evaluation guidelines for documenting a disability under IDEA 2004 are provided in 34 C.F. R. §300.301. As a result of debates in the field of LD focusing on the definition and the appropriate evaluation for LD, during the reauthorization of IDEA 2004 changes were made to the guidelines for identifying LD (Holdnack & Weiss, 2006; Schrank, Miller, Caterino, & Desrochers, 2006). Although the definition of LD (see Table 2.2) remained the same in IDEA 2004, specific modifications were made to the law relating to the identification of the disability.

TABLE 2.3. DSM-IV-TR Criteria for ADHD

A. Either (1) or (2):

  (1) Six (or more) of the following symptoms of **inattention** have persisted for at least 6 months to a degree that is maladaptive and inconsistent with developmental level:

  Inattention
  (a) often fails to give close attention to details or makes careless mistakes in schoolwork, work, or other activities
  (b) often has difficulty sustaining attention in tasks or play activities
  (c) often does not seem to listen when spoken to directly
  (d) often does not follow through on instructions and fails to finish schoolwork, chores, or duties in the workplace (not due to oppositional behavior or failure to understand instructions)
  (e) often has difficulty organizing tasks and activities
  (f) often avoids, dislikes, or is reluctant to engage in tasks that require sustained mental effort (such as schoolwork or homework)
  (g) often loses things necessary for tasks or activities (e.g., toys, school assignments, pencils, books, or tools)
  (h) is often easily distracted by extraneous stimuli
  (i) is often forgetful in daily activities

  (2) six (or more) of the following symptoms of **hyperactivity–impulsivity** have persisted for at least 6 months to a degree that is maladaptive and inconsistent with developmental level:

  Hyperactivity
  (a) often fidgets with hands or feet or squirms in seat
  (b) often leaves seat in classroom or in other situations in which remaining seated is expected
  (c) often runs about or climbs excessively in situations in which it is inappropriate (in adolescents or adults, may be limited to subjective feelings of restlessness)
  (d) often has difficulty playing or engaging in leisure activities quietly
  (e) is often "on the go" or often acts as if "driven by a motor"
  (f) often talks excessively

  Impulsivity
  (g) often blurts out answers before questions have been completed
  (h) often has difficulty awaiting turn
  (i) often interrupts or intrudes on others (e.g., butts into conversations or games)

B. Some hyperactive–impulsive or inattentive symptoms that caused impairment were present before age 7 years.

C. Some impairment from the symptoms is present in two or more settings (e.g., at school [or work] and at home).

D. There must be clear evidence of clinically significant impairment in social, academic, or occupational functioning.

E. The symptoms do not occur exclusively during the course of a Pervasive Developmental Disorder, Schizophrenia, or other Psychotic Disorder and are not better accounted for by another mental disorder (e.g., Mood Disorder, Anxiety Disorder, Dissociative Disorder, or a Personality Disorder).

Note. From American Psychiatric Association (2000). Copyright 2000 by the American Psychiatric Association. Reprinted by permission.

TABLE 2.4. Types of ADHD

Code based on type:

314.01 Attention-Deficit/Hyperactivity Disorder, Combined Type: if both Criteria A1 and A2 are met for the past 6 months

314.00 Attention-Deficit/Hyperactivity Disorder, Predominantly Inattentive Type: if Criterion A1 is met but Criterion A2 is not met for the past 6 months

314.01 Attention-Deficit/Hyperactivity Disorder, Predominantly Hyperactive–Impulsive Type: If Criterion A2 is met but Criterion A1 is not met for the past 6 months

Coding note: For individuals (especially adolescents and adults) who currently have symptoms that no longer meet full criteria, "In Partial Remission" should be specified.

Note. From American Psychiatric Association (2000, pp. 92–93). Copyright 2000 by the American Psychiatric Association. Reprinted by permission.

First, the regulations now state that an agency must not necessitate the use of a severe discrepancy between intelligence (IQ) and achievement (§300.307(a)(1)). The problem with IQ–achievement discrepancy models has been discussed previously in this chapter. However, the IDEA 2004 regulations do not suggest that ability–achievement discrepancies or other types of discrepancies (e.g., intracognitive, intra-achievement) are irrelevant to the diagnosis of LD. Rather, the law now reinforces the view that discrepancy alone cannot define LD. Second, for the first time, IDEA 2004 requires states to provide a procedure within the evaluation process that is based on a response to intervention (RTI) (34 C.F.R. §300.307(a)(2)). A great deal of debate about the use of RTI during the evaluation process has been published (see Mather & Kaufman, 2006a, 2006b, for in-depth discussions of the issues). However, it is imperative for professionals to understand that under IDEA 2004, RTI does not replace the need for a comprehensive evaluation (34 C.F.R. §300.307; *Federal Register*, 2006). As stated in the *Federal Register*, a public agency must use a variety of data-gathering tools and strategies even with the RTI process.

A comprehensive evaluation is defined by law as involving more than a single screening instrument or test score (34 C.F.R. §300.304; *Federal Register*, 2006). The regulations also require evaluators to use only technically sound instruments that measure relative contributions of cognitive, language, achievement, and behavioral factors influencing performance. In addition, the assessment process and tools utilized by an examiner must by law not be racially or culturally biased. The importance of cognitive processing to the identification of LD and ADHD is discussed further in Chapter Three. However, IDEA 2004 clearly indicates that cognitive processing is central to the definition of LD and must be measured during a comprehensive assessment. The IDEA 2004 regulations define LD as a "disorder in one or more of the basic psychological processes . . . " (see Table 2.2). Therefore, Section 614(b) (3)(A)(iii) of IDEA 2004 itself states that the assessment of these basic psychological processes must be conducted with "valid and reliable" measures.

Secondary-to-Postsecondary Transition Requirements under IDEA 2004

Under IDEA 2004, the provision of transitional services for students with disabilities is now conceptualized as a "results-oriented process" that "improves the academic and functional achievement" of these students (Wright & Wright, 2007, p. 56). Transition services are defined in the IDEA 2004 regulations as a "coordinated set of activities" to facilitate movement from secondary to postsecondary activities, "including postsecondary education, vocational education, integrated employment (including supported employment), continuing and adult education, adult services, independent living, or community participation" (34 C.F.R. §300.43(a)(1)). The activities as defined in the regulations are to be based on an individual student's needs and to take into account his or her strengths, preferences, and interests. In addition, the law specifies that transitional goals be contained in the IEP by the time an adolescent turns 16.

As students make the transition from secondary to postsecondary education, the comprehensiveness of documentation required to support requests for accommodations radically changes. The supporting evaluation evidence of many secondary students, even though they may have received special education or Section 504 services in high school, may not meet the documentation requirements established by a postsecondary institution (Gregg & Lindstrom, 2008; Madaus & Shaw, 2007). Moreover, secondary school personnel are not required to provide a transition evaluation. What is required under IDEA 2004 is a "summary of performance" (SOP), in which a synopsis of a student's functional performance (achievement, cognitive, behavioral) is described, as well as the recommendations on how to assist the individual in meeting postsecondary goals. However, no specific guidelines are provided by the government in regard to the essential components for an SOP. Although templates are available as resources to professionals in developing SOPs (e.g., National Transition Assessment Summit, 2005), these guidelines are simply recommendations rather than legal standards or regulations (Dukes, Shaw, & Madaus, 2007).

The problem faced by many students with LD and ADHD making the transition from secondary to postsecondary institutions (either higher education or employment) is that their evaluation documentation does not meet the standards set by these institutions or agencies. First, the evaluations completed by secondary schools are usually not sufficiently comprehensive for the criteria set by higher education. In addition, since under IDEA 2004 reevaluations are done only every 3 years, and a transitional evaluation is not required of schools, a secondary school student is at risk of having outdated assessment data. A review of postsecondary documentation criteria follows in the next section.

Documentation in the Postsecondary Setting

The definition of disability in the ADA of 1990 was imported directly from Section 504 of the Rehabilitation Act of 1973. At that time, the legislative focus was primarily on individuals with sensory and physical impairments; adults with "hidden" disabilities such as LD or ADHD were not at the forefront of disability advocates' and policymakers' thinking (Gregg, Coleman, Lindstrom, & Lee, 2007; Mather et al., 2005). Since fewer identified adults with LD or ADHD were attending colleges and universities during that era, there was less concern over accommodating their learning needs. Today, however, individuals with LD or ADHD represent the largest group of students with disabilities attending postsecondary educational institutions (Ward & Berry, 2005). Therefore, these populations also present the greatest number of requests for accommodations on postsecondary entrance and licensure examinations (Brinckerhoff & Banerjee, 2007; Lindstrom & Gregg, 2007). It is understandable why the identification of markers to operationalize certain legal terminology as "substantial limitations" or the "average person" is receiving significant attention (see Gregg, Coleman, Lindstrom, & Lee, 2007).

Legal Issues Influencing Clinical Decision Making

The legal debate in the majority of court cases involving adults with LD or ADHD centers around whether such individuals are entitled to reasonable accommodations under ADA. Entitlement to accommodations requires the individuals to demonstrate proof that they qualify for these—in other words, that they are sufficiently limited to be considered "disabled." Under ADA, a "disability" is defined as "a physical or mental impairment that substantially limits one or more of the major life activities" of an individual (42 U.S.C. §12102(2)(A) [ADA]; 29 U.S.C. §705(9) (B) [Rehab Act]).

The ADA Restoration Act of 2008 will help better clarify the definition of "disability," including what it means to be "substantially limited in a major life activity." In addition, it prohibits the consideration of mitigating measures such as medication or assistive technology in determining whether an individual has a disability. The Restoration Act is supported by a broad coalition of civil rights groups, disability advocates, and employer track organizations. However, neither the text of the ADA, Section 504 nor the Department of Justice's (DOJ) implementing regulations define the term "substantially limits" (see *Bartlett V*, 226 F.3d at 80), but the preamble to the regulations provides: "A person is considered an individual with a disability . . . when the individual's important life activities are restricted as to the conditions, manner, or duration under which they can be performed in comparison to most people" (28 C.F.R. Pt. 35, App. A §35.104. This interpretation of the phrase "substantially limits" is nearly identical to that of the Equal Employment Opportunity Commission (EEOC) in connection with Title I of the ADA (29 C.F.R. §1630.2(j)(1)(ii)) (defining substantially limited as "[s]ignificantly restricted as to the condition, manner, or duration under which an individual can perform a particular major life activity as compared to the condition, manner, or duration that the average person in the general population can perform that same major life activity").

Legal interpretations of what might constitute "substantial limitations" of "major life activities" have differed in recent cases involving the adult population with LD or ADHD. Some courts have adopted an operationalization of "substantial limitations" in learning that is literally based on derived achievement scores that (using the bell curve as the metric) fall below the "average" range of the statistical mean (i.e., below the 16th percentile). Support from the courts for this argument has been documented in several cases: *Gonzales v. National Board of Medical Examiners* (2000), *Love v. Law School Admission Council, Inc.* (2007), *Price et al. v. National Board of Medical Examiners* (1997), and *Wong v. Regents of the University of California* (2004). Other courts have operationalized "substantial limitation" for this group of adults as the documentation of processing deficits that, in the presence of cognitive and linguistic integrities, result in unexpected learning failure (see Kavale et al., 2005; Mather et al., 2005). Proponents of the second argument interpret the ADA as not requiring low performance or a poor outcome as the *sole* determiner of a disability. Rather, they suggest that the ADA requires a comprehensive assessment of the effect of a putative impairment on an adult's life. The focus is on the *condition, manner,* or *duration* of one's performance of a major life activity—not whether one *can* perform it, but *how* one performs it (Mather et al., 2005). Support from the courts for this argument has been documented in several cases (e.g., *Albertsons, Inc., v. Kirkingburg,* 1999; *Bartlett v. New York State Board of Law Examiners,* 1997, 1998, 1999, 2000, 2001).

Postsecondary Documentation Criteria for Accessing Accommodations

A major problem facing adults with LD and ADHD in accessing accommodations involves the eligibility criteria used to operationalize disability definitions. The application of eligibility criteria determines access to modifications and accommodations; therefore, those who apply these criteria are the gatekeepers of services (Gregg, 1994; Gregg, Johnson, & McKinley, 1996; Gregg & Scott, 2000). Eligibility criteria provide the validation for definitions. Many adults with LD and ADHD quickly discover that there is no consistency across institutions, agencies, or professionals in either the type of eligibility criteria or the documentation guidelines they apply (Gregg, Scott, McPeek, & Ferri, 1999; Kochhar-Bryant, 2007). Therefore, an adult may be eligible for services at one agency or institution, but not another. Many agencies and institutions also require documentation to be recent (see Educational Testing Service, 2006a, *www.ets.org/portal/site/ets/menuitem*. Some of the policies governing access to accommodations for individuals with LD or ADHD in vocational rehabilitation (VR) agencies, institutions of higher education, and testing agencies are used below to illustrate some of the documentation dilemmas facing many adolescents and adults.

Before I discuss the documentation guidelines and eligibility criteria used by these agencies and institutions, a clarification of terminology is important. These terms include "disability," "documentation guidelines," and "eligibility criteria." As discussed previously, the definition of "disability" under Section 504 and ADA is broad. No definitions for LD or ADHD are included in the regulations for these statutes, unlike the definition of "specific learning disabilities" in the IDEA 2004 regulations (see Table 2.2). Therefore, postsecondary institutions should provide the specific definitions used to construct their documentation guidelines and eligibility criteria. The definition most commonly used for LD in higher education is that written by the NJCLD (1997) and given in Table 2.2. ADHD is most often defined by the DSM-IV-TR symptoms (see Tables 2.3 and 2.4). Unfortunately, many institutions define disabilities simply according to their own documentation guidelines and procedures.

"Documentation guidelines" provide the information (e.g., background information, cognitive processing measures, rating scales) necessary for a specific agency or institution to make decisions pertaining to the provision of accommodations. However, documentation guidelines do not define a disability or provide the criteria by which professionals determine whether behaviors are functionally limited to learning. The "eligibility criteria" are the methods by which severity is defined. Whether a professional, agency, or institution determines severity by using a discrepancy, cutoff, or integrated model, this must be clearly stated in the documentation guidelines and/or policies. In addition, the means of operationalizing that model must be specified. For example, do evaluators define severity by using a 1.5 *SD* discrepancy criterion or a cutoff score at the 16th percentile? As noted by Flanagan and Mascolo (2005), the development of valid methods for assessment require that evaluators follow criteria based on "operational definitions that are grounded in contemporary theory and research" (p. 522). Professionals should also keep in mind that criteria developed for children are often not as valid for the adult population (Barkley, 2006; Gregg, Coleman, Lindstrom, & Lee, 2007).

Vocational Rehabilitation

VR has a long history of serving the adolescent and adult populations with LD and ADHD (Gregg, Johnson, & McKinley, 1996; Kochhar-Bryant, 2007). VR counselors work closely with secondary and postsecondary professionals in providing services for students with disabilities. However, the funds for special education increased by 333% from 1996 to 2004, while VR funding rose only 22% (Council of State Administrators of Vocational Rehabilitation [CSAVR], 2005). Currently, VR agencies serve approximately 10% of the working-age population with disabilities (CSAVR, 2005; Kochhar-Bryant, 2007; Lamb, 2006). The long-term underfunding of these agencies will have nothing but a negative influence on the populations of adolescents and adults with LD and ADHD. VR agencies operate under a policy referred to as "order of selection," which allows an agency to determine that it cannot serve all eligible individuals because of resource constraints. Obviously, more mildly affected populations are placed at greater risk by this policy.

VR counselors receive diagnostic reports from evaluators (both internal and external to the agencies) representing a variety of training and philosophical assessment backgrounds (e.g., behavioral, neuropsychological, psychodynamic, vocational). The definitions of disability, documentation guidelines, and eligibility criteria can easily be interpreted differently by these different professionals. Therefore, the decisions made by some VR counselors (like those of some other postsecondary service providers) about providing adults access to accommodations may be inconsistent. Vague and broadly defined eligibility criteria allow professional decision making about severity levels to remain idiosyncratic.

Higher Education

Colleges and universities operating under the mandates set forth by Section 504 and ADA will have policies describing their documentation guidelines for students with disabilities requesting access to accommodations. To establish eligibility for accommodations, a student must first provide documentation, at his or her own expense, that supports a stated disability. After the disability is established, the institution must determine whether the student is "otherwise qualified" to carry out the requirements of the program of study, and whether the disability documentation supports the need for the requested accommodations. Case law has supported a postsecondary institution's right to require that documentation be current; state the disability; provide educational, developmental, and medical history; and provide comprehensive psychological data (Rothstein, 2002). Although a student may have been served in high school under IDEA 2004, or may provide the college with a psychological evaluation from a private professional diagnosing a disability, the policy and procedures set forth by a postsecondary institution can lead the institution's service providers to determine that past documentation is not comprehensive enough to support access to accommodations. However, if the institution does not agree with the documentation provided by the student, it has a legal obligation to "work cooperatively with the applicant (and the applicant's clinician) to determine the appropriate accommodation" (Konecky & Wolinsky, 2000, p. 77).

One of the most frustrating aspects for postsecondary service providers, who often are responsible for reviewing the documentation of incoming college students with disabilities, is the inconsistent and inadequate documentation often used to support a diagnosis of LD or ADHD. Therefore, postsecondary institutions have developed documentation guidelines over the years to provide the necessary clinical information for determining whether access to accommodations is appropriate. One of the first systematic sets of documentation guidelines was established by the University System of Georgia Regents' Centers for Learning Disorders (see *www.rcld.uga.edu*). The documentation guidelines established by these centers in 1993 were modeled after the University of Georgia Learning Disabilities Center guidelines written in 1982 (Gregg, Heggoy, Stapleton, Jackson, & Morris, 1996; Gregg, Johnson, & McKinley, 1996).

In 1996, the Association on Higher Education and Disability (AHEAD) published similar documentation guidelines for LD and ADHD (see Brinckerhoff, McGuire, & Shaw, 2002, for an in-depth discussion of these early guidelines). Unfortunately, many of these initial guidelines were misused by some professionals and agencies to deny access to accommodations. Often students with LD and ADHD were held to more stringent eligibility criteria than were individuals with other types of disabilities (e.g., psychiatric disorders, health impairments). The problem with past documentation guidelines is that they have often been used (or abused) as eligibility criteria, rather than simply as the guidelines for comprehensive evaluation documentation. Concerned that documentation guidelines were being used to discriminate against some students, AHEAD (2007) has recently published foundation principles and best practices for the review of documentation (see *www.ahead.org/reasons/bestpractices.htm*). Again, guidelines are simply information required in the assessment documentation used to access accommodations. They do not provide a definition of the disability that can be used to set the criteria necessary for validating the disorder.

Brinckerhoff and colleagues (2002) suggest that the following information be part of any comprehensive evaluation necessary for documenting the need for specific accommodations: (1) recent documentation (no more than 3–5 years old); (2) reason for referral; (3) list of evaluation measures used; (4) developmental, educational, and medical histories; (5) statement of the disability, along with a rule-out statement; (6) use of appropriate measures of performance; (7) test results and clinical summary; and (8) support for accommodation(s). Each postsecondary institution should have policies governing the specific documentation guidelines required for an individual to request accommodations. Adolescents and adults with LD or ADHD should be encouraged to begin developing a documentation portfolio in which to keep information commonly requested by postsecondary agencies. In an attempt to provide some general documentation guidelines to help organize and store information in such a portfolio, two checklists have been developed. Figure 2.1 describes the information usually needed to support LD accommodations, and Figure 2.2 describes the data typically required for supporting ADHD accommodations.

A comprehensive evaluation is critical to determining appropriate accommodations for an individual with LD or ADHD. Unfortunately, the myth that there is testing *for* LD or *for* ADHD has led to much confusion and often misidentification of disabilities. No specific LD or ADHD testing battery exists. A comprehensive evaluation requires that

☑ Compare documentation guidelines to definition of LD provided by institution.

☑ Determine the recency of evaluation requirements (3 years is often the norm).

☑ Identify the eligibility criteria for determining functional limitations used by an institution:

- Discrepancy (type)
- Cutoff (16th percentile or other)
- Integrated

☑ Determine licensure or other credentials required by an institution for professional(s) conducting specific types of evaluations.

☑ Provide information pertaining to history (especially learning) in documentation:

- Medical history
- Psychiatric history
- Educational history (including history of accommodations)
- Other description of learning history

☑ Provide evidence of cognitive and linguistic processing abilities across measures:

- Standardized measures
- Informal information

☑ Provide evidence of academic performance across measures:

- Across reading, written expressions, mathematics
- Across skill, fluency, and application tasks

☑ Provide information to support ruling out other causes of functional limitations.

☑ Provide specific information in documentation to match cognitive, language, and academic performance to support accommodation needs.

FIGURE 2.1. General postsecondary LD documentation checklist. Based on AHEAD (2007); University System of Georgia Regents' Center for Learning Disorders documentation guidelines (*www.rcld.uga.edu*); Educational Testing Service documentation guidelines (*www.ets.org*); College Board documentation guidelines (*www.collegeboard.org*); and Mather and Gregg (2006).

☑ Compare documentation guidelines to definition (symptoms) of ADHD provided by institution.

☑ Determine the recency of evaluation requirements (3 years is often the norm).

☑ Identify the eligibility criteria for determining functional limitations used by an institution:
  • Discrepancy (type)
  • Cutoff (16th percentile or other)
  • Integrated

☑ Determine licensure or other credentials required by an institution for professional(s) conducting specific types of evaluations.

☑ Provide information pertaining to history (especially learning) in documentation:
  • Medical history
  • Psychiatric history
  • Educational history (including history of accommodations)
  • Other description of learning history

☑ Provide self-report of six major behaviors from DSM-IV-TR.

☑ Provide corroboration of behaviors by another adult (parent, spouse, friend with integrity of client).

☑ Provide rating scales documenting ADHD behavior.

☑ Provide evidence of academic performance across measures:
  • Skill
  • Fluency
  • Application

☑ Provide information to support ruling out other causes of functional limitations.

☑ Provide a match of cognitive and behavioral performance to support accommodation determining functional limitations used by an institution.

FIGURE 2.2. General postsecondary ADHD documentation checklist. Based on AHEAD (2007); University System of Georgia Regents' Center for Learning Disorders documentation guidelines (*www.rcld.uga.edu*); Educational Testing Service documentation guidelines (*www.ets.org*); and College Board documentation guidelines (*www.collegeboard.org*).

a professional investigate all aspects of cognitive, language, behavioral, affective, and achievement performance before making any diagnostic decision. Because there is a great deal of comorbidity between LD and ADHD, as well as between each of these disabilities and other disabilities (see Chapter Four), it would be quite unethical for an evaluator not to examine all aspects of abilities. During an initial interview, a professional collects information that will enable him or her to decide which instruments and areas to include in the evaluation. However, the examiner must be careful not to overlook an area simply by allowing only self-reported information to guide the evaluation process. It is well known that adolescents and adults with ADHD often underreport the symptoms of the disorder (Barkley, 2006; Fischer, Barkley, Smallish, & Fletcher, 2002), and adults with LD might be too embarrassed to tell an interviewer about the seriousness of their literacy issues. Unfortunately, far too many evaluators simply include an untimed word-reading or spelling test to investigate literacy. Again, the keys to reliable and valid decision making are a comprehensive evaluation and eligibility criteria that can be operationalized.

Testing Agencies

Standardized testing is the "centerpiece of accountability" for both secondary and postsecondary institutions (Disability Rights Advocates, 2005). When Dan, the young man introduced at the beginning of this chapter, takes his high school graduation examination, he will be provided the accommodations of extra time and text-to-speech technology as specified in his IEP. However, his right to these accommodations when he takes the SAT is not guaranteed, because he will be moving from the protection of IDEA 2004 to that of ADA and Section 504. The College Board has specific documentation guidelines, which he will need to meet in order to access accommodations (*www.collegeboard.com/ssd/student/index.html*).

The most common accommodation provided on college admissions tests is extended time for LD or ADHD (Lindstrom & Gregg, 2007). In fact, the number of SAT examinees requesting extra time grew by about 26% between 1998 and 2003 (Bridgeman, Trapani, & Curley, 2003). Between 1990 and 1995, the percentage of students with LD who took an accommodated SAT Reasoning Test increased by an average of 14% per year, and has since stabilized to approximately 2% of all SAT test takers (Lindstrom & Gregg, 2007). The pattern of an increase in requests by students with LD or ADHD to access accommodations on standardized tests has been noted across undergraduate, graduate, and licensure examinations. For example, according to Brinckerhoff and Banerjee (2007), in 2005 the Educational Testing Service (ETS) received over 10,000 requests for accommodations on its graduate examinations. These authors provide an excellent review of the dilemmas faced by testing agencies overwhelmed with the number of requests for accommodations.

Interestingly, according to Brinckerhoff and Banerjee (2007), "Testing agencies are neutral to the model used to establish learning disabilities" (p. 250). By "model," they are referring to the discrepancy, cutoff, or integrated eligibility model. In fact, they note that the majority of testing agencies support an integrated eligibility model, as indicated by the documentation guidelines provided on the agencies' websites. The ETS and College Board have over the years put a great deal of effort into providing fair documentation guidelines and review processes for students requesting accommodations on the basis of disabilities. However, none of the testing agencies provide guidelines indicating how they operationalize the issue of severity. Although Brinckerhoff and Banerjee state that no one score is used to determine eligibility, they do not state how low level individual or factor scores must be to determine severity. When an individual is turned down for accommodations, it is often unclear what specific definition of severity influenced this decision. Quite often, if academic scores are found to be above the 16th percentile, accommodation requests are not approved. However, until examiners or testing agencies are willing to operationalize their eligibility criteria, individuals with specific disabilities and ability levels are more likely to encounter discriminatory practices (see Gregg, Coleman, Lindstrom, & Lee, 2007).

For example, consider Vernetta, the woman introduced at the beginning of this chapter. She scored at the 90th percentile on the Verbal Intelligence Index of the Reynolds Intellectual Assessment Scales (Reynolds & Kamphaus, 2003). Her reading scores were markedly lower: the 6th percentile on the Word Attack subtest of the Woodcock–Johnson III Tests of Achievement (WJ III ACH; Woodcock, McGrew, & Mather, 2001a); the 10th percentile on the WJ III ACH Letter–Word Identification subtest; the 19th percentile on the Comprehension subtest portion of the Nelson–Denny Reading Test (Brown, Fishco, & Hanna, 1993); and the 25th percentile on the WJ III ACH Reading Fluency subtest. On the basis that her scores on the latter two measures were "average" (>16th percentile), she was denied the accommodation of extended time on a high-stakes license exam, despite the fact that she was provided extended time as an accommodation at her college. Testing agencies often provide elaborate documentation guidelines; however, their practices for determining eligibility for accommodations are more often than not absent from their policies.

As a result of concern over a lack of clarity as to what testing agencies can require examinees to provide as documentation, in a Notice of Proposed Rule Making on June 4, 2008, the U.S. Department of Justice specifically addressed the nature of the documentation that standardized testing organizations may require to substantiate a disability:

> Section 309 of the ADA is intended to fill the gap that is created when licensing, certification, and other testing authorities are not covered by section 504 or Title II of the ADA, and to ensure that individuals with disabilities are not excluded from educational, professional, or trade opportunities because examinations or courses are offered in a place or manner that is not accessible. See 42 U.S.C. 12189. Through its enforcement efforts, the Department has discovered that the requests made by testing entities for documentation regarding the existence of an individual's disability and her or his need for a modification or an auxiliary aid or service are often inappropriate or burdensome. The proposed rule attempts to address this problem.
>
> Section 36.309(b) as revised states that while it is appropriate for a testing entity to require that an applicant document the existence of a disability in order to establish that he or she is entitled to testing modifications or aids, the request for documentation must be appropriate and reasonable. *Requested documentation should be narrowly tailored so that the testing entity can ascertain the nature of the disability and the individual's need for the requested modification or auxiliary aid. Generally, a testing entity should accept without further inquiry documentation provided by a qualified professional who has made an individualized assessment of the applicant. Appropriate documentation may include a letter from a qualified professional or evidence of a prior diagnosis, accommodation, or classification, such as eligibility for a special education program.* When an applicant's documentation is recent and demonstrates a consistent history of a diagnosis, there is no need for further inquiry into the nature of the disability. A testing entity should consider an applicant's past use of a particular auxiliary aid or service.
>
> Finally, a private entity should respond in a timely manner to requests and should provide applicants with a reasonable opportunity to supplement their requests with additional information, if necessary. Failure by the testing entity to act in a timely manner and making requests of unnecessary magnitude could result in the sort of delay that amounts to a denial of equal opportunity or equal treatment.
>
> [D]ocumentation must be reasonable and limited to the need for the modification or aid requested. Appropriate documentation might include *a letter from a physician or other professional, or evidence of a prior diagnosis or accommodation, such as eligibility for a special education program.* (28 C.F.R. 36.309, emphasis added, *www.ada/gov/NPRM2008/titleiii.htm*)

Who Is the "Average Person" in the "General Population"?

One of the most debated legal issues pertaining to the diagnosis of the adolescent and adult populations with LD and ADHD centers on the term used in the ADA and Section 504 to refer to the comparison group for determining severity. By law, a person with a disability must be compared to "the average person." Some professionals believe that consideration of an individual's literacy level, background experiences, and educational level should be irrelevant in the decision making for determining severity; they define a functional limitation as a cutoff score below the 16th percentile, regardless of age or life experiences (Dombrowski et al., 2004; Flanagan & Mascolo, 2005; Kamphaus, 2005). They propose that norms used on academic measures not be adjusted for academic attainment. Other professionals suggest that the eligibility criteria used to identify LD or ADHD in the adolescent and adult population should be robust yet flexible enough to account for individual experiences, education, and abilities (Barkley, 2006; Gregg, Coleman, Lindstrom, & Lee, 2007; Shaywitz, 2003).

Imagine, for example, Kathy, who demonstrates a large discrepancy (2 *SD*) between her estimated verbal reasoning and basic reading skills. She is interested in attending law school. Kathy has requested accommodations on the Law School Admission Test (LSAT) as a result of her disabilities. She was identified with LD (dyslexia) in childhood and received accommodations throughout college (alternative media and AT). During her most recent evaluation, she scored in the superior range (~92nd percentile) on the Verbal Comprehension Index of the Wechsler Adult Intelligence Scale—Third Edition (WAIS-III; Wechsler, 1997a) and at the lower end of the average range on tests of basic reading skills (~30th percentile). However, the only norms accepted by the testing agency are the general ones, not the norms adjusted for educational attainment. Because her reading scores are not below average, the testing agency has denied her access to extra time or a read-aloud on the LSAT. Our observation on Jonta's case (Gregg et al., 2007b, p. 267) applies equally well to Kathy's case: "It is difficult to see such a judgment as being equitable, justifiable, or within the spirit of the ADA."

The ADA and Section 504 specify that the "average person" in the "general population" must be used as the benchmark for determining what are functional limitations. Although a great deal of attention is paid to the "normality" of the score or performance of the individual being tested, little attention has been given to how representative the distribution of specific test scores is of the target population. Standardization sampling allows evaluators to compare an individual's performance to that of a normative group. Most test developers use stratification variables in helping them select a representative sample of the national population to use as the comparison group. However, it is essential for clinicians to remember that test norms embody only a sample of performance for a specified group of individuals identified by a test developer. The stratification variables chosen by test developers differ in number, type, and sample size. A clinician must carefully consider how similar the norming sample demographics are to those of the individual being tested. In addition, when an examiner decides to compare the performance of an individual across different measures that were not co-normed, it is important to remember that significant error can thus be introduced into the comparison process, since the tests were normed on entirely different samples of individuals (Kamphaus, 2005).

We know that numerous variables can influence an individual's performance on academic and/or cognitive measures. For instance, socioeconomic status and ethnic/racial factors have been shown to have significant effects on cognitive test scores (Vanderploeg, Schinka, Baum, Tremont, & Mittenberg, 1998). The relationship of educational attainment to the validity of cognitive and/or achievement scores is an extremely important issue for the identification of adolescents and adults with LD or ADHD.

More recently, Heaton, Taylor, and Manly (2003) have discussed the effects of demographic factors on the WAIS-III (Wechsler, 1997a) and the Wechsler Memory Scale—Third Edition (WMS-III; Wechsler, 1997b) scores, and have encouraged the utilization of demographically corrected norms for the identification of disabilities. Analyzing the standardization data, they found that all six cognitive factors were significantly related to education and ethnicity. The largest effects were on the Verbal Comprehension, Perceptual Organization, and Processing Speed Indexes. Heaton and colleagues (2003) concluded that "highly educated people would need to show a much greater decrement in test performance to be correctly classified as 'impaired' using norms that are corrected only for age" (p. 196).

The importance of educational attainment to score interpretation is not peculiar to the WAIS-III and WMS-III (see Heaton & Marcotte, 2000, for an in-depth discussion of this issue). In order to increase the diagnostic accuracy of cognitive, achievement, and behavioral measures across the various segments of the adolescent and adult populations, many test publishers (e.g., Pearson Education, Riverside) have developed norms to adjust for specific demographic variables, particularly for educational attainment. However, some professionals and agencies infer that the ADA's term "most people" precludes the use of demographically adjusted norms. The influence of such practice and/or policy leads to a significant number of false-negative decisions that deny accommodation access to adolescents and adults with LD and ADHD. The equity of this practice is questionable.

The stratification sampling for a test does not ensure that the "average person" is captured; it is simply a means of reflecting estimated percentages of subpopulations within a given society. U.S. Bureau of the Census data are more representative of "most people." Clinicians must be mindful of small sample sizes, restricted stratification variables, and measurement error of test scores when interpreting the performance of adults with LD or ADHD on psychometric assessment tools.

Questions to Consider during the Evaluation Process

Mather and colleagues (2005) point out that "one should not confuse the comparison group with what is being compared—what is being compared is the *condition, manner,* and *duration* in which one performs the activity, not the actual resulting achievement itself" (p. 139, emphasis added). In an attempt to provide a valid and reliable means by which to operationalize the definition of LD and ADHD for the adolescent and adult population, I suggest that an evaluator address the eight questions presented in Figure 2.3. Answers to question 5 (cognitive and linguistic processes) and question 6 (social, emotional, and behavioral processes) may differ in the amount of investigation required by a clinician and the types of behaviors documented across client profiles. These eight questions address the three constructs underlying the ADA definition of disability: *duration, condition,* and *manner* in which one performs the activity of learning. Specific comments on each question follow.

- *Question 1 (best practice).* Professionals should always base their clinical decision making on (a) advanced measurement theory; (b) current cognitive, linguistic, behavioral/emotional, and achievement research with the adult population without disabilities; and (c) recent research investigating the abilities of the adolescent and adult population with LD and ADHD.
- *Question 2 (duration).* A clinician identifies and documents the *duration* of a disability by collecting background information pertaining to the examinee's learning history. This requires the examiner to collect multiple sources of information. Researchers agree that multiple sources of information are essential to diagnostic decision making (Dombrowski et al., 2004; Flanagan & Mascolo, 2005; Gregg & Scott, 2000; Kamphaus, 2005). A clinician must consider the environmental,

QUESTIONS   CONSIDERATIONS

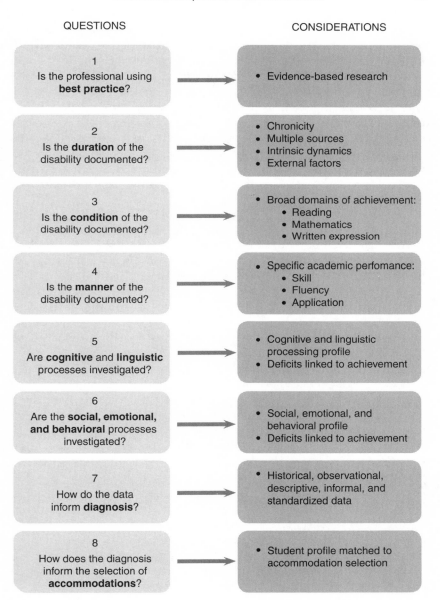

FIGURE 2.3. Questions to support eligibility decision making.

cognitive, language, achievement, and behavioral signs influencing the examinee's ability to learn specific tasks set across specific contexts. Both intrinsic dynamics and extrinsic factors that affect performance should be part of all clinical decision making (Schrank et al., 2005). The critical factors to effective diagnosis are the clinician's expertise and experience in comparing, contrasting, and interpreting the obtained results in light of evidence-based research and best practice.

• *Question 3 (condition)*. The *condition* is first addressed by the examination of both broad domains and domain-specific academic factor scores. Information should be investigated to determine whether the performance can be attributed to factors other than LD or ADHD (exclusionary).

• *Question 4 (manner)*. The *manner* in which the individual performs domain-specific academic tasks should be observed from select data sources that document (a) skill, (b) fluency, and (c) application of skills to tasks or in context. Clinical observations and interview information, historical information, and current functioning should all be used to define the manner of learning. Again, the clinician should determine whether the performance can be attributed to factors other than LD or ADHD (exclusionary).

Documenting the manner of performance is critical to identification of LD and ADHD. For instance, imagine two adults who both read a list of single words at the 30th percentile—a score within the normal range on a bell curve. What would not be evident from a standard score is that an adult with LD might have taken three times longer to read the words (due to halting self-corrections) than the average person. If the test was not timed, the score would not represent the effort. The clinician testing this adult would be observing this reading behavior. Thus it is necessary to consider the manner in which the act of achievement was performed, as well as the standardized scores. The clinician's observations about performance are critical to decision making.

• *Question 5 (cognitive/linguistic ability analysis)*. Essential to determining the existence of the condition or disability is documentation provided by cognitive and linguistic processing factor scores. In addition, there must be evidence-based research to support the relationship of the cognitive/language factor score deficits to the achievement score deficits (e.g., phonemic/orthographic awareness deficits to dyslexia, or executive functioning to ADHD). Once more, information should be reviewed to ensure that performance cannot be attributed to factors other than LD or ADHD (exclusionary).

• *Question 6 (social, emotional, and behavioral analysis)*. Documentation from behavioral and affective measures are also essential in documenting the condition or disability. In addition, there must be evidence-based research to support the relationship of behavioral and affective symptoms to any achievement score deficits.

- *Questions 7 and 8 (clinical judgment)*. The data collected to answer questions 1–6 are used to determine a diagnosis and inform the selection of accommodations.

Clinical Judgment

Clinical judgment is key to reliable and valid identification of adolescents and adults with LD and ADHD. As mentioned previously, the observations of an examiner are what bring insight and meaning to the evaluation of a student's performance during testing. However, according to Brinckerhoff and Banerjee (2007), one difficulty many testing agencies face is that often examiners do not adequately document these observations. In fact, the ETS documentation guidelines (*www.ets.org/portal/site/ets.menuitem*) encourage evaluators to provide "supplemental sources of information" to support the standardized evidence for functional limitations. In addition, ETS provides a list of tips for evaluators providing documentation (*www.ets.org/portal/site/ets.menuitem*).

The application of eligibility criteria to determine functional limitations for individuals with LD and ADHD is dependent upon qualified and experienced clinicians. However, when clinicians do not apply sound measurement theory or do not utilize evidence-based research findings, the validity of observations and decision making is compromised. Although LD and ADHD are considered latent constructs, this does not mean that professionals and agencies can ignore reliable and valid means of making decisions pertaining to severity. The decision-making criteria used to grant or reject accommodation requests should not be magical to the consumers, for whom the difference can be life-altering. Sound eligibility criteria, along with the documentation of clinical observations, provide protection for both individuals with disabilities and the institutions serving them.

Implications for Assessment and Accommodation

✓ *LD and ADHD are developmental disorders*. The idea that fixed symptom thresholds for LD and ADHD can be applied across the lifespan often leads to the use of invalid criteria for the adolescent and adult populations.

✓ *Determining severity*. The two practices most commonly used in determining severity levels have been (1) examination of discrepancies across performance and (2) cutoff standards.

✓ *Statutes supporting the right to accommodations.* The laws protecting the rights of adolescents and adults with LD and ADHD are either entitlement (IDEA 2004) or eligibility (ADA or Section 504) laws.

✓ *IDEA 2004 and LD identification.* Significant changes were made to the identification process for LD in the reauthorization of IDEA 2004.

✓ *ADA and disability.* Under ADA, a "disability" is defined as "a physical or mental impairment that substantially limits one or more of the major life activities of [an] individual."

✓ *Eligibility criteria.* The application of eligibility criteria determines access to modifications and accommodations; therefore, those who apply such criteria are the gatekeepers of services. Eligibility criteria are the methods (discrepancy, cutoff, integrated) by which severity is determined.

✓ *Documentation guidelines.* Documentation guidelines provide the information (e.g., background information, cognitive processing measures, behavior rating scales) necessary for an agency to make decisions pertaining to the provision of accommodations.

✓ *Average person.* Under ADA, a person with a disability must be compared to the "average person" in the general population. Although test scores are often used to define the "average person," clinicians must be mindful of the small sample sizes and restricted stratification variables of many assessment tools.

✓ *Clinical judgment.* Clinical judgment is essential to the identification of LD and ADHD in the adolescent and adult population.

CHAPTER THREE

Broad and Specific Cognitive Processing

Phillip, a 20-year-old European American college sophomore, has sought an evaluation to determine whether he "still has ADD" and whether he may be eligible for extra time on exams and seating in the front of the classroom (accommodations he reports he was granted in high school). Phillip was first diagnosed with ADHD in middle school and continues to take medications to help him focus and sustain his attention. He has described in writing his continued difficulties in sustaining attention during test taking: "I get easily distracted sometimes when listening to someone talk to me. . . . On exams . . . I have trouble going one question at one time, then get stressful [*sic*] when others begin turning in their exams."

Natalie, a 17-year-old European American high school senior, was diagnosed with dyslexia in elementary school. She has sought an evaluation to update her documentation, in order to receive extended time on the SAT. Natalie reports a history of associated symptoms beginning in elementary school (e.g., trouble telling left from right, learning the multiplication tables, reading, writing cursive, learning to tell time).

The atmosphere today in secondary and postsecondary education is extremely litigious, particularly in regard to accommodating students with documented LD or ADHD. The Individuals with Disabilities Education Improvement Act of 2004 (IDEA 2004) and recent postsecondary court cases have ignited a national controversy focusing on the identification of reliable diagnostic methodologies for LD and ADHD. Despite

55

heated debates about the importance of broad and specific cognitive processing abilities for the diagnosis of LD or ADHD, cognitive measures remain significant components of most assessment batteries, and therefore of determining who is qualified to receive accommodations at the adolescent and adult levels (Gordon, Barkley, & Lovett, 2006; Murphy & Gordon, 2006; Gregg et al., 1999). The purpose of this chapter is to present an overview of research related to both broad cognitive processing (general intelligence) and specific cognitive processes as these pertain to supporting the selection of specific accommodations for adolescents and adults with LD or ADHD. The examples of Natalie and Phillip, above, are used in this chapter to illustrate the importance of a comprehensive evaluation in documenting the cognitive disabilities that lend support for specific accommodations.

Research Evidence for LD and ADHD as Neurodevelopmental Disorders

Several years ago, Frith (1999) proposed a three-level framework for integrating the apparent paradoxes of research results pertaining to the neurodevelopmental disorder of LD for professionals. This framework is equally applicable to ADHD. She discusses the importance of considering how the interaction of environmental, biological, cognitive, and behavioral factors influences the ability to learn specific tasks. Frith reminds us that ongoing biological research in the fields of genetics and neuroanatomy provides support for cognitive models generated by research in cognitive psychology, developmental psychology, and neuropsychology. Therefore, I begin by summarizing some significant genetic and neuroanatomical research on adolescents and adults with LD and ADHD, in order to provide a foundation for a better understanding of research from various disciplines (e.g., neuropsychology, neurolinguistics, measurement).

In addition, I encourage us all to reflect at this point on two other important points put forth by Frith (1999). First, there is a formidable distance between brain and behavior, particularly when we consider environmental influences. Second, the language used to describe constructs in this field can be misused. Words and labels "readily become loaded with ideology while the concepts they refer to may be perfectly non-contentious" (p. 193). Terms such as "intelligence," "cognitive processing," "functional limitations," "disorder," or "deficit" at times take on a life of their own. It is critical to remember that performance on behavioral measures should not solely be used to determine causation of disorders. According to Frith (1999), "One danger with cognitive theories is that they can be circular by postulating deficits which are merely restatements of behavioral phenomena" (p. 195). Therefore, professionals should utilize and critically analyze the wealth of available neurological, neuropsychological, and neurolinguistic research. As noted by Berninger and Richards (2002), "It is not clear why so many school psychology trainers [I would add other related professionals] and school psychologists continue to claim that process assessment is not related to academic learning" (p. 787). Through the use of current research findings and advanced assessment measures, professionals are encouraged to augment clinical decision making with empirically based evidence in the selection of accommodations for individuals with LD and/or ADHD.

Neurological and Genetic Evidence for Adolescent and Adult ADHD

Cerebral blood flow studies; studies of brain electrical activity using quantitative electroencephalography (QEEG); neuroimaging studies using positron emission tomography (PET), magnetic resonance imaging (MRI), or functional MRI (fMRI); neurochemical studies; and genetic studies all provide strong evidence that ADHD is a disorder of neurodevelopmental origin (see Barkley, 2006, for an in-depth discussion). QEEG studies indicate that adolescents and adults with ADHD demonstrate reduced arousal to stimulation, diminished sensitivity to reinforcement, increased theta activity (symptoms of drowsiness and poor focus of attention), and decreased beta activity (symptoms of decreased concentration and persistence) (Barkley, 2006; Monastra, Lubar, & Linden, 2001). Although PET technology is more reliable for the adult than the adolescent population, findings for both age groups indicate reduced activation in the insular and hippocampal regions and greater activation in the right anterior cingulate for individuals with ADHD (Barkley, 2006; Schweitzer & Sulzer-Azaroff, 1995; Zametkin et al., 1990).

MRI or fMRI research with the adolescent or adult populations with ADHD is not as extensive as that with children. However, we do know that there are structural or size differences in several brain regions between children demonstrating ADHD and their nondisabled peers. Evidence is available that for younger populations with ADHD, total brain size is smaller, and the brain volume of the anterior frontal lobes, the basal ganglia, and the cerebellar vermis is less dense (Barkley, 2006; Castellanos et al., 2000; Durston et al., 2004; Hynd et al., 1991; Semrud-Clikeman et al., 1992; Semrud-Clikeman, Guy, Griffin, & Hynd, 2000). An especially pertinent finding from brain imaging studies is that the cerebellar volume for individuals with ADHD appears to be less dense. The cerebellum is essential for executive functioning and the aspects of motor functioning that contribute to planning (Barkley, 2006). Research using fMRI provides evidence that typical brain activity in the frontal region, basal ganglia, and cerebellum is different for children with ADHD (Arnsten, Steere, & Hunt, 1996; Barkley, 2006).

Moreover, behavioral and molecular genetic research provides strong evidence for a significant genetic contribution to ADHD (see Faraone, Doyle, Mick, & Biederman, 2001, for a meta-analysis). According to this body of research, 50–95% of the variation in the symptoms associated with ADHD can be accounted for by genetics. In addition, molecular genetic research indicates that more than one gene may account for the expression of the disorder, depending on the type of ADHD (Barr, 2002; DiMaio, Grizenko, & Joober, 2003; Faraone & Doyle, 2001; Fisher et al., 2002; Grady et al., 2003; Willcutt & Gaffney-Brown, 2002; Willcutt et al., 2002).

Therefore, findings from this large and ever-increasing body of research suggest strongly that genetic and neurological factors underlie ADHD symptoms. Past speculation that social factors (e.g., poor parenting, excessive television viewing) cause ADHD is not supported by research (Barkley, 2006). Neurological and genetic studies, combined with neuropsychological and neurolinguistic behavioral research, lend support to the idea that executive functioning and the neurological structures (frontal lobes, basal ganglia, and cerebellum) that govern executive activity are different for individuals with ADHD than for nondisabled individuals.

Neurological and Genetic Evidence for Adolescent and Adult LD

A significant amount of research also provides evidence of genetic and neurological etiologies for different types of LD. Because the type of LD referred to as "dyslexia" (which consists of reading decoding, spelling, and reading comprehension deficits) has received the greatest attention from researchers investigating neurological factors symptomatic of LD, the studies discussed in this section pertain primarily to dyslexia.

Researchers using technologies such as PET, MRI, fMRI, and magnetoencephalography (MEG) confirm that adolescents and adults with dyslexia either underactivate or overactivate specific brain regions, in comparison to their normally achieving peers (see Serafini et al., 2001, for an in-depth review of the literature). The pattern frequently validated across this literature suggests that in individuals with dyslexia, the left posterior regions are underactivated and the left frontal regions are overactivated (Pugh et al., 2000). Results from MEG studies also indicate that individuals with dyslexia differ from their normally achieving peers in temporal processing within the auditory, visual, and higher-level comprehension systems (Berninger & Richards, 2002; Nagarajan et al., 1999).

Differences among subgroups of poor readers have also been identified by brain imaging researchers studying dyslexia. As an example, Shaywitz and colleagues (2003), using fMRI technology. investigated three groups of young adult readers—compensatory readers, who were accurate but not fluent; persistently poor readers; and nonimpaired readers—as they read real words and pseudowords. They found that the compensatory readers demonstrated underactivation in posterior neural systems (left parietotemporal and occipitotemporal regions) for reading. In contrast, the persistently poor readers activated posterior reading systems, but engaged them differently by relying more on memory-based than on analytic word identification strategies. In comparison to the persistently poor readers, the compensatory readers activated the right superior frontal and right middle temporal gyri, as well as the left anterior cingulate gyrus. The compensatory readers appeared to rely more on other neural systems to counterbalance less efficient functional brain regions. The authors attribute some of these differences to the superior cognitive abilities of the compensatory group. The findings from this study support the suggestion made by Berninger and Richards (2002) that "the brain is both an independent (causal) variable and a dependent (outcome) variable" (p. 10). Although the brain provides access to learning, it can also be influenced by learning opportunities.

The phonological deficit theory proposed to explain the etiology of developmental dyslexia has received substantial support from brain imaging researchers investigating the reading performance of individuals across the lifespan (Ramus et al., 2003). However, some of these researchers suggest that in addition to possible phonological deficits, some of these learners demonstrate visual processing deficits, such as unstable binocular fixations and poor vergence (Cornelissen, Munro, Fowler, & Stein, 1993; Eden et al., 1996). In addition, a limited number of brain imaging studies provide evidence of anatomical, metabolic, and activation differences in the cerebellum between individuals with dyslexia and nondisabled readers (Brown et al., 2001; Leonard et al., 2001; Nicolson et al., 1999). Researchers have also shown magnocellular abnormalities in the medial and lateral geniculate nucleus of the brains of individuals with dyslexia (Livingstone, Rosen, Drislane, & Galaburda, 1991), of persons with dyslexia in the tactile domain (Stoodley, Talcott, Carter, Witton, & Stein, 2000), and of persons with mixed visual and auditory problems (Van Ingelghem et al., 2001). Although brain imaging studies provide the strongest evidence for the phonological deficit theory, Ramus and colleagues (2003) suggest that further research is needed to better understand why sensory and motor disorders are frequently associated with phonological deficits.

Behavioral and molecular genetic research in the area of dyslexia provides professionals with a better understanding of the role of the environment versus genetics in reading performance (see Olson, 2007, and Pennington & Olson, 2005, for in-depth reviews). Certainly we can conclude from a vast amount of behavioral genetic research on twins (identical or fraternal) and adopted children, as well as from molecular genetic findings, that there is a strong relationship between reading ability and genetic variation. Recently researchers have been able to demonstrate a strong genetic influence not just on word identification performance, but also on reading comprehension and spelling scores, and they have concluded that the same genes influence all three types of academic abilities (Byrne et al., 2006). Interestingly, these same researchers found that individual measures of memory and learning were less affected by genes. They have concluded that the heritability of dyslexia is between .50 and .70, depending on the phenotype and variability in reading ability across the normal range. Researchers have also tested the hypothesis that the etiologies of reading difficulties may differ for males and females in more severely impaired samples. The results from recent research in this area suggests that there is no evidence for such differences as a result of gender (Hawke, Wadsworth, Olson, & DeFries, 2006).

As we know, individuals with LD are at significantly higher risk than the general population for demonstrating ADHD (Rucklidge & Tannock, 2002). In fact, Willcutt and Gaffney-Brown (2002) found that 60% of children and adolescents between 8 and 18 years of age with reading disorders also met criteria for at least one additional emotional or behavioral disorder. Molecular genetic researchers suggest that dyslexia and ADHD are at least partly attributable to common genetic influences in preschool, elementary, and adolescent populations (Light, Pennington, Gilger, & DeFries, 1995; Stevenson, Pennington, Gilger, DeFries, & Gillis, 1993; Willcutt et al., 2007). However, the significantly strong genetic relationship between LD and ADHD has been supported only for inattentive symptoms of ADHD, not for hyperactive–impulsive symptoms. Although behavioral and molecular genetic studies are at too early a stage to provide conclusive findings, Olson (2007) notes that "The combination of behavior-genetic and molecular-genetic research holds the promise of linking genetic and environmental influences on reading behavior in population studies with twins to specific genes, brain function, and behavior in individuals" (p. 10).

A Process-Oriented View of Cognition

Understanding how specific abilities influence learning across the lifespan is enhanced by taking a "process-oriented" approach to cognitive development. A process-oriented view implies that different networks of cognitive processes are configured in response to different functional demands, and that a given cognitive process may contribute directly or indirectly to several functions (Berninger & Richards, 2002; Kane, Conway, Hambrick, & Engle, 2007). For years, researchers depended on serial hierarchical processing models to describe the relationship of cognitive processes to each other. As professionals recognized that these models inadequately captured the complexities of learning, they were replaced by theories proposing neural networking, or approaches that take into consideration multiple cognitive and language variables operating interdependently in systems rather than in isolation (Gallagher & Appenzeller, 1999).

The multidimensionality and multiplicity of cognitive processes are illustrated when we consider the processes involved with simply reading single words. We know that verbal working memory, cognitive fluency, and word knowledge are all important to reading performance. Many students with dyslexia perform poorly on independent measures of these constructs. However, an examiner may wonder whether the difficulties in reading words are due to inadequate word knowledge or to low verbal working memory and slow processing speed. Certainly there is a vast amount of literature suggesting that word knowledge facilitates performance on oral and reading comprehension measures, as well as on memory tasks (Evans, Floyd, McGrew, & Leforgee, 2002; Recht & Leslie, 1988). Therefore, for some readers word knowledge and working memory may have multiplicative effects, since integrating new information into preexisting knowledge structures depends on the ability to maintain that information for a period of time in an activated state. As Hambrick and Engle (2002) found when they examined the effects of domain knowledge on reading performance, participants with lower levels of working memory capacity (WMC) derived less benefit from domain knowledge.

The implications of the multiplicity of cognitive and language processes for accommodation selection are critical. Although a student might perform poorly on a WMC task, word knowledge deficits could also be contributing significantly to memory performance. In such a situation, a professional would need to consider both memory and vocabulary accommodation options. Selection of accommodations requires sensitivity to the multiple processes involved in learning, so that the most effective choices can be made.

Cattell–Horn–Carroll Theory

Currently, the most comprehensive and empirically based system of cognitive abilities is the Cattell–Horn–Carroll (CHC) theory (McGrew, 2005; McGrew & Flanagan, 1998; Woodcock, McGrew, & Mather, 2001b). The CHC model is most strongly characterized by its structural focus— that is, by its separation of cognitive, language, and achievement abilities into distinct components with different attributes and functions (see Figure 3.1). CHC theory is a synthesis of the Cattell–Horn *Gf-Gc* theory (Horn & Noll, 1997) and the Carroll three-stratum theory of cognitive abilities (Carroll, 1993, 2005). The CHC theory describes a hierarchical framework of cognitive abilities: narrow abilities (stratum I), broad abilities (stratum II), and *g* (stratum III). Narrow abilities include 69 abilities that are limited in scope and generally marked by specific test methods and standard response processes. Broad abilities include fluid reasoning, crystallized intelligence, short-term memory, visual processing, auditory processing, long-term retrieval, processing speed, reading and writing, quantitative knowledge, and reaction time. At the apex of this hierarchical model is general intelligence, or *g*.

Recent and ongoing research is using the CHC model in efforts to construct meaningful and diagnostically valid profiles (Flanagan & Ortiz, 2001). The CHC cross-battery approach (McGrew & Flanagan, 1998) is a subtest selection method that is currently receiving a great deal of attention. Although the cross-battery method is based on a strong theoretical foundation (CHC theory), validity and reliability for the first pillar (stratum I, subtest comparison) and second pillar (stratrum II, factor comparison) of this method face criticism. In essence, the stratrum II factors appear to have strong internal validity but weak external validity—particularly criterion-related validity. As noted by Kamphaus (2005), "the relationship between stratum II abilities and many achievement measures is either unknown or preliminary in nature, requiring further validation. The criterion-related validity problem is even more acute for shared subtests hypotheses" (p. 474).

WMC Models

The specific cognitive processes found to be strongly correlated with different realms of learning (reading, writing, and mathematics) are discussed throughout Chapters Five, Six, and Seven of this book. However, to clarify the relationship of specific cognitive processes to each other and to broader cognitive abilities, two models of WMC are discussed in this section. WMC refers to the limited amount of "information that one can hold in mind, attend to, or technically speaking, maintain in a rap-

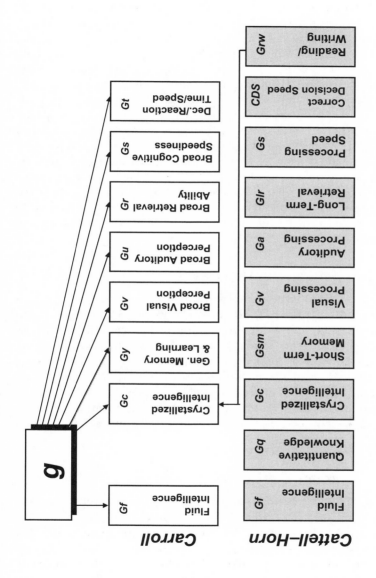

FIGURE 3.1. Carroll and Cattell–Horn model comparison. Not shown are the stratum I abilities—69 narrow abilities found in data sets analyzed by Carroll (1993), as suggested by McGrew (1997) and McGrew and Flanagan (1998). From McGrew (2005). Reprinted by permission of the author.

63

idly accessible state at one time" (Cowan, 2005, p. 1). It has been found to be an important mechanism of general cognitive ability (Baddeley, 2000, 2007; Baddeley & Hitch, 1974; Cowan, 2005; Kane et al., 2007). Certainly, there is strong empirical evidence that WMC and fluid reasoning share substantial variance (Conway, Kane, & Engle, 2003; Engle, Tuholski, Laughlin, & Conway, 1999). Some suggest that general intelligence represents a domain-general working memory system fueling academic performance. For instance, we need WMC during the process of understanding or composing text, to retain information in previous passages in order to integrate it with text processed later. In arithmetic, we need WMC to retain information while calculating results. Two models of WMC that are based on strong empirical evidence have been selected to provide the reader with a better understanding of cognitive processing. These models are Baddeley's (2007) "multiple-component" model and Cowan's (2005) "embedded-processes" model. These WMC models represent the demands on our cognitive processing systems to balance memory storage and ongoing mental activity across different domains of learning.

The Multiple-Component WMC Model

Baddeley's model has undergone several revisions over the years (Baddeley, 2000, 2007; Baddeley & Hitch, 1974). Figure 3.2 illustrates Baddeley's current model of WMC. According to his research, WMC has four subcomponents: the "central executive" (attention functions); the "visuospatial sketchpad" (visual and spatial short-term information); the "episodic buffer" (short-term episodic memory); and the "phonological loop" (speech-based short-term information). In this revised model of his former work, Baddeley also includes representational links to the crystallized processes of long-term memory, visual semantics, and language.

Embedded-Processes WMC Model

Cowan (1997, 2005) proposes a WMC model that embeds attention within activated memory, rather than suggesting the separate storage devices of the Baddeley model. Therefore, the emphasis in this WMC model is more on fluid cognitive activation (Kane et al., 2007). Cowan views working memory as an integrated memory and attentional system consisting of long-term memory, short-term memory coding processes, and executive attentional processes. Although there are certainly differences in the structure and function of specific cognitive processes across the CHC framework, Baddeley's multiple-components WMC

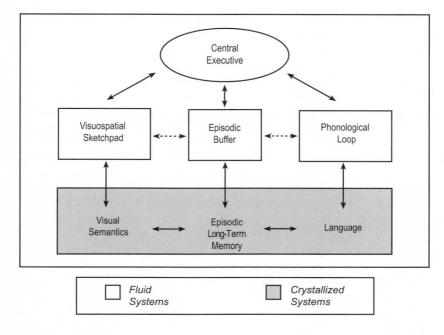

FIGURE 3.2. Multiple-component model. From Baddeley (2007). Copyright 2007 by Oxford University Press. Adapted with permission.

model, and Cowan's embedded-processes WMC model, the importance of the working memory system (i.e., focused attention, short-term storage, WMC, executive control) to cognitive functioning is central to all three of these models.

As noted by Baddeley (2007), "The capacity to direct and focus attention is perhaps the most crucial feature of working memory" (p. 124). The central executive in both the Cowan and Baddeley models is described as an attentional control (focus) system that coordinates cognitive and linguistic processes performed in working memory. One important role attention plays is to enable an individual to focus on (pay attention to) new information across different stages of learning. Therefore, attention can play the role of a gatekeeper that allows specific information to be stored in short- and long-term memory (Awh, Vogel, & Oh, 2006). Researchers have recently identified "executive" attentional processes that manipulate and update information stored in working memory, illustrating the interaction of attention, WMC, and executive functions (Awh et al., 2006).

Adolescents and adults with ADHD most frequently demonstrate problems with nonverbal visual–spatial working memory, nonverbal sequential working memory, and verbal working memory tasks (Barkley, 2006). Swanson and Siegel (2001) suggest that LD is fundamentally the result of both general and specific working memory deficits. They provide strong evidence that for individuals with LD, working memory deficits manifest themselves as domain-specific constraints (e.g., phonemic awareness) or a domain-general constraint (controlled attentional processing). According to Swanson and Sachse-Lee (2001), students with LD (ages 9–15) demonstrate significant working memory deficits that appear to be better attributed to limitations with capacity rather than to processing inefficiency.

The relationship of attention, WMC, short-term memory, long-term memory, and executive processing to the ability to process information and use working memory has certainly received a great deal of attention in the literature (Baddeley, 2007; Cowan, 1997, 2005; Engle, Cantor, & Carullo 1992; Just & Carpenter, 1992; Postle, 2006; Repovs & Baddeley, 2006). As noted by Jarrold and Towse (2006), "Knowledge about working memory has blossomed to such an extent that a comprehensive review of the relevant literature is all but impossible" (p. 39). However, we can conclude from research findings that variation in the working memory system is certainly influenced by independent but intersecting sources that include (but are not limited to) attention, storage capacity, processing efficiency, and executive processing (Cowan, 1997, 2005; Jarrold & Towse, 2006).

Influence of Development

An element missing from some cognitive models is consideration of the developmental trajectories of ability acquisition, and of the constraints these impose on learning across the lifespan (Paris, 2005). As Horn and Blankson (2005) note, researchers discuss age differences more often than they do the findings of change with age. In a thorough review of the conceptual, developmental, and methodological problems inherent in a vast amount of research, Paris (2005) encourages a reinterpretation of research related to the development of abilities. His critique focuses on reading research, but the same points can be made across learning domains. He suggests that many reading models (I would add cognitive models generally) are deficit-driven and have been primarily constructed upon asymmetrical frameworks in which codependent constructs enable one another. According to Paris, an examination of the differences between "constrained" reading skills (learned quickly and completely mastered, such as phonemic awareness) and "unconstrained" reading skills (never completely mastered, such as vocabulary or comprehension) is essential to a better understanding of reading performance. Constrained and unconstrained reading skills differ in their scope and developmental trajectories, and these differences are critical for the interpretation of predictors of reading comprehension performance across the lifespan. Researchers have consistently cautioned that the contribution of any skill to later achievement depends upon the level of development at the time of testing (Adams, 1990; Stanovich, 2000). Unfortunately, despite this knowledge, many professionals continue to allot equal validity to specific cognitive abilities, regardless of the learner's age, skill level, or experience.

Researchers investigating the cognitive abilities of adults have long been concerned that intelligence theories and assessment tools do not adequately measure cognitive performance for this age group. Horn and Blankson (2005) note that as individuals enter adolescence and adulthood, they "continue to think and solve problems, but usually (to an ever-larger extent as development proceeds) this thinking is directed to solving novel problems in fields of work" (p. 56). Therefore, "expertise models" are proposed as being more accurate descriptions of intelligence for the adult population. According to a large body of work, "experts" use more deductive reasoning, apply schemes to organize and evaluate work quickly, and access "expertise wide-span memory" abilities (Charness, 1991; Ericsson, 1996, 1997; Ericsson & Kintsch, 1995; Horn & Blankson, 2005; Walsh & Hershey, 1993). These "experts" make relatively less use of short-term memory, verbal working memory, inferencing, and processing speed/scanning abilities. The implications of this research for the adolescent and adult populations with LD and ADHD have much potential for advancing our understanding of these populations.

Measurement Issues
Influencing Clinical Decision Making

Basic measurement principles must guide the professional decision making that is essential to the identification of LD or ADHD. Lack of sensitivity to these principles has led to significant variability across identification practices, causing many adolescents and adults with LD or ADHD to be denied access to accommodations. First, it is imperative to underscore that evidence of validity is critical to specificity and reliability for all clinical decision making. Diagnostic decisions made by a clinician are dependent on the examination of strong validity evidence. Messick's (1995) assertion that validity is actually a unitary concept and that there are not different types of validity, only different types of validity evidence, is similar to the view stressed in the *Standards for Educational and Psychological Testing* (American Educational Research Association [AERA], American Psychological Association, & National Council on Measurement in Education, 1999; see also Benson, 1998). Although there is considerable interest in separating several of the constructs associated with validity, the unified version of it is still part of the *Standards* (Lissitz & Samuelsen, 2007). As a means of organizing our thinking about specific measurement practices influencing the diagnosis of LD or ADHD, four measurement issues are discussed here: subtest score interpretation, factor score interpretation, confidence levels, and measurement invariance. Careful consideration of how these measurement features influence score distributions for adolescents and adults with LD and ADHD is critical to equitable and ethical practice.

Subtest Score Interpretation

Unfortunately, examination of isolated subtest scores is too often the primary source of evidence upon which professionals base clinical decisions in the diagnosis of LD or ADHD (Gregg, Coleman, Lindstrom, & Lee, 2007). Far too many examiners investigate the magnitude of an individual's subtest score differences on cognitive, behavioral, and/or achievement measures, with little consideration of a norm-based interpretation. As Lovett and Lewandowski (2006) point out, this practice is questionable, due to the high incidence of "extreme scatter" and measurement error across assessment tools. Extreme scatter can be significant but not diagnostically useful (Glutting, Watkins, Konold, & McDermott, 2006).

Subtest score interpretation is a frequently used method for arguing that an adolescent or adult is not "functionally limited" in learning if his or her scores on any one or two subareas of an academic domain (e.g., reading fluency, reading comprehension) fall within the average range. Failure to integrate single subtest scores with other external sources (e.g., test scores, behavioral observations, background information) can lead a professional to make false-negative decisions that result in denied access to accommodations for adolescents or adults with LD or ADHD.

Profile analysis is a variation of subtest score examination. However, rather than examining any subtest scatter, the examiner identifies specific subtests/clusters a priori as "diagnostic." It is an old practice and closely related to analyses of subtest scatter (e.g., the so-called "ACID" pattern—impairment on the Arithmetic, Coding, Information, and Digit Span subtests of the Wechsler Intelligence Scale for Children

[WISC]). Although Kaufman (1979) referred to this practice as the "shared abilities" hypothesis, its validity has been called into question (Kamphaus, 1993, 2005). Like subtest scatter analysis methods, profile analysis is dependent upon individual subtests—the reliability and validity of which are often much lower than those of factor or full scale scores (see Watkins, Glutting, & Youngstrom, 2005, for an in-depth discussion).

Factor Score Interpretation

Factor (index) scores provide more reliable measures of abilities than do subtest scores, since larger samples of behavior are more likely to have greater reliability. However, a professional must also ensure that the factor scores are valid measures of a construct (specific ability), since reliability does not guarantee validity. In fact, Glutting and colleagues (2006) argue against the incremental validity of examining factor scores as opposed to full scale intelligence test scores. Others challenge this assumption in relation to the adolescent and adult population (Bowden et al., 2008). As an essential step in determining the validity of factor scores, professionals should carefully examine the technical manual of a test to determine the reliability and construct validity of its factors. In addition, it is important to examine the research investigating the predictive validity and measurement invariance of factors for specific populations. For instance, the Wechsler Adult Intelligence Scale (WAIS-III; Wechsler, 1997a) is derived from a factor structure different from that used in creating the original WAIS and the WAIS-R. Confirmatory factor analysis (CFA) studies of the WAIS-III have consistently found the four Indexes and the general composite score (Full Scale score) to be the strongest factors. Using reliable-component analysis, Caruso and Cliff (1999) determined that the two most reliable, orthogonal components from the WAIS-III would be measures of Gf (fluid intelligence) and Gc (crystallized intelligence), not the hypothesized main component of the Verbal–Performance model.

Measurement Invariance

Most widely used cognitive, language, and achievement measures are built upon theory and factor-analytic studies (Kamphaus, 2005). Professionals must retain a healthy degree of skepticism that the inferences drawn from test batteries are equivalent across populations with and without disabilities, since very little measurement invariance research investigating test constructs for individuals with disabilities is available. Accurate identification of LD or ADHD requires explicit evaluation of the assumption of measurement invariance. Examination of measurement equivalence provides a direct test of the hypothesis that the same set of latent variables underlies a set of test scores in different groups, and that the metric relationships between observed scores and the corresponding latent variables are the same (Bowden et al., 2008). Unfortunately, the lack of data regarding measurement invariance in the assessment of the adult populations with LD and ADHD has led to a significant number of untested assumptions about cognitive and achievement abilities (Bowden, Cook, Bardenhagen, Shores, & Carstairs, 2004; Vandenberg & Lance, 2000).

Confidence Intervals

The popularity of subtest selection and profile analysis methods has contributed to an environment in which professionals focus primarily on single subtest scores and give little attention to standard errors of measurement or confidence intervals (CIs) (Gregg, Coleman, Lindstrom, & Lee, 2007). When cutoff methods are applied to determine functional limitation in learning, the standard of the 16th percentile is often seen as a single demarcation point when, given the error implicit in assessment, a range of scores would be more appropriate.

A CI reflects the probability that a particular score represents a true score. According to the American Psychological Association (2001), CIs are "in general, the best reporting strategy. The use of confidence intervals is therefore strongly recommended" (p. 22). Although they are related to standard errors, CIs also include the critical value of the relevant test statistic (see Thompson, 2006, and Cumming & Finch, 2005, for in-depth discussions). However, Thompson (2006) warns clinicians not to "fall in love with your point estimate, at least when [the standard error] is large" (p. 205). Accordingly, wider CIs imply less precise estimates of performance. Fortunately, modern software for most advanced assessment batteries computes CIs for an examiner.

Cognitive Ability Measures and the Assessment of LD and ADHD

Current debates about the validity of using broad cognitive measures in the assessment of individuals with possible LD or ADHD afford us all an opportunity to reevaluate past practices within the context of new research. As discussed in Chapter Two, concern has been voiced about the validity and efficacy of including broad and specific cognitive processing measures as central components of the eligibility criteria for these disorders (Barkley, 2006; Gordon et al., 2006; Hale, Kaufman, Naglieri, & Kavale, 2006; Hale, Naglieri, Kaufman, & Kavale, 2004; Mather & Gregg, 2006; Mather et al., 2005; Murphy & Gordon, 2006). In order to demonstrate the importance of cognitive and language processing in accommodation selection, Natalie's and Phillip's profiles are used as examples.

Natalie and Phillip have both been administered a broad cognitive ability test (the WAIS-III; Wechsler, 1997a) and other cognitive, language, and achievement measures as part of their evaluation. Figure 3.3 is a visual summary of Phillip's performance on these cognitive, language, and achievement measures. Phillip's WAIS-III Full Scale CI band places him in the average range of broad cognitive ability. However, his Full Scale score does not appear as reflective of his overall ability. (This determination has also been influenced by the examiner's observations that Phillip's difficulties with attention and impulsivity have negatively influenced his effort.) Within the context of broad cognitive ability, Phillip demonstrates significant problems on tasks requiring executive functioning and motor skills. In particular, Phillip is challenged by tasks that involved selective and sustained attention, organization, planning, self-monitoring, and cognitive flexibility (working memory system). Obviously, a diagnosis should never be based on just one cognitive, language, or achievement test score, or one behavior rating scale. However, Phillip's performance on the WAIS-III has provided the clinician with an opportunity to observe his performance across verbal–nonverbal tasks, timed–untimed tasks, tasks involving different sensory modalities (auditory, visual, motor), and constrained–unconstrained tasks. In other words, the full WAIS-III battery simulates the different types of learning that influence academic performance.

Natalie's assessment profile is illustrated in Figure 3.4. On the WAIS-III, Natalie's Index CI bands range from below average (Perceptual Speed, Working Memory) to average (Verbal Comprehension) to superior (Perceptual Organization). Natalie's nonverbal abilities (including analysis, construction, and problem solving with visual–spatial information such as shapes, patterns, and pictures) are superior to her cognitive processing speed and verbal working memory abilities as measured by the WAIS-III. This pattern has also been noted across other specific measures of cognitive and linguistic abilities, to be discussed in later sections of this chapter. Interestingly, Natalie was administered the Woodcock–Johnson III Tests of Cognitive Abilities (WJ III COG; Woodcock et al., 2001b) 3 years before the evaluation results reported in this chapter. Her WJ III General Intellectual Ability (GIA) score was 10 points below her current WAIS-III Full Scale standard score. The difference between these two general intelligence scores is important

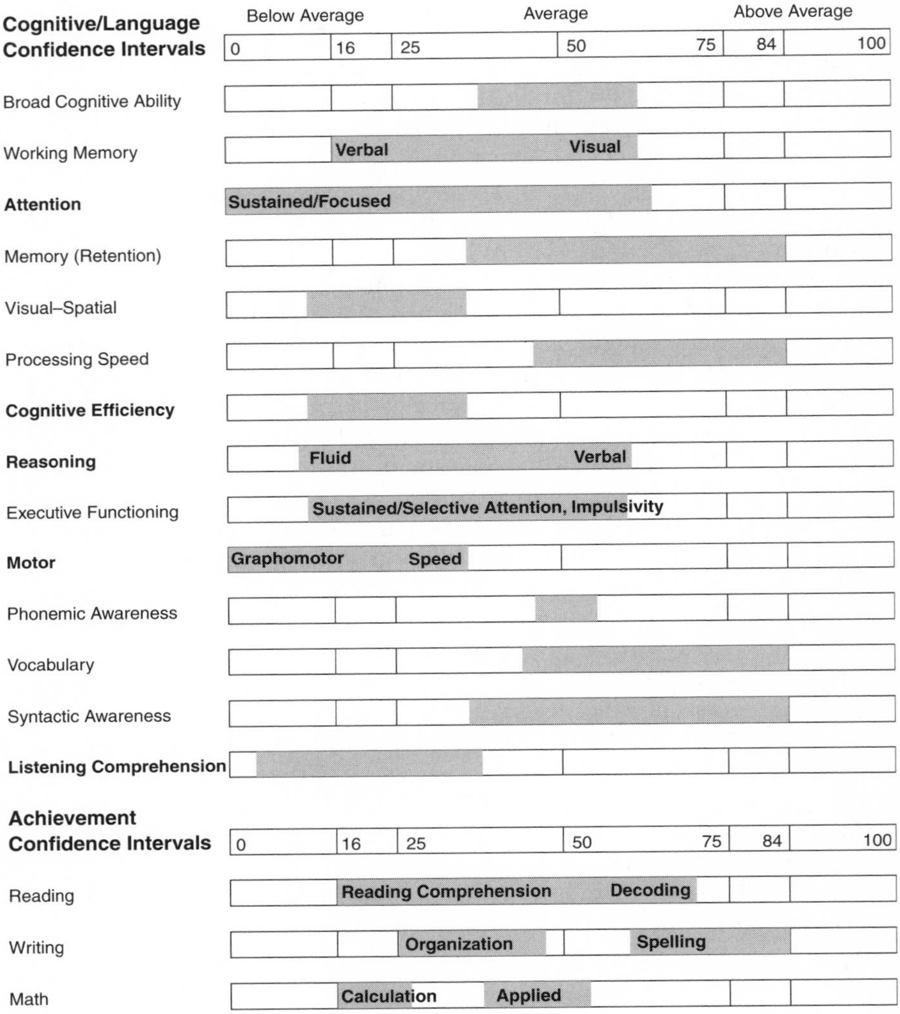

Cognitive/Language Confidence Intervals

	Below Average		Average		Above Average	
	0	16	25	50	75	84	100

Broad Cognitive Ability

Working Memory — **Verbal**, **Visual**

Attention — **Sustained/Focused**

Memory (Retention)

Visual–Spatial

Processing Speed

Cognitive Efficiency

Reasoning — **Fluid**, **Verbal**

Executive Functioning — **Sustained/Selective Attention, Impulsivity**

Motor — **Graphomotor**, **Speed**

Phonemic Awareness

Vocabulary

Syntactic Awareness

Listening Comprehension

Achievement Confidence Intervals

	0	16	25	50	75	84	100

Reading — **Reading Comprehension**, **Decoding**

Writing — **Organization**, **Spelling**

Math — **Calculation**, **Applied**

FIGURE 3.3. Assessment profile for Phillip, a student with ADHD (combined type).

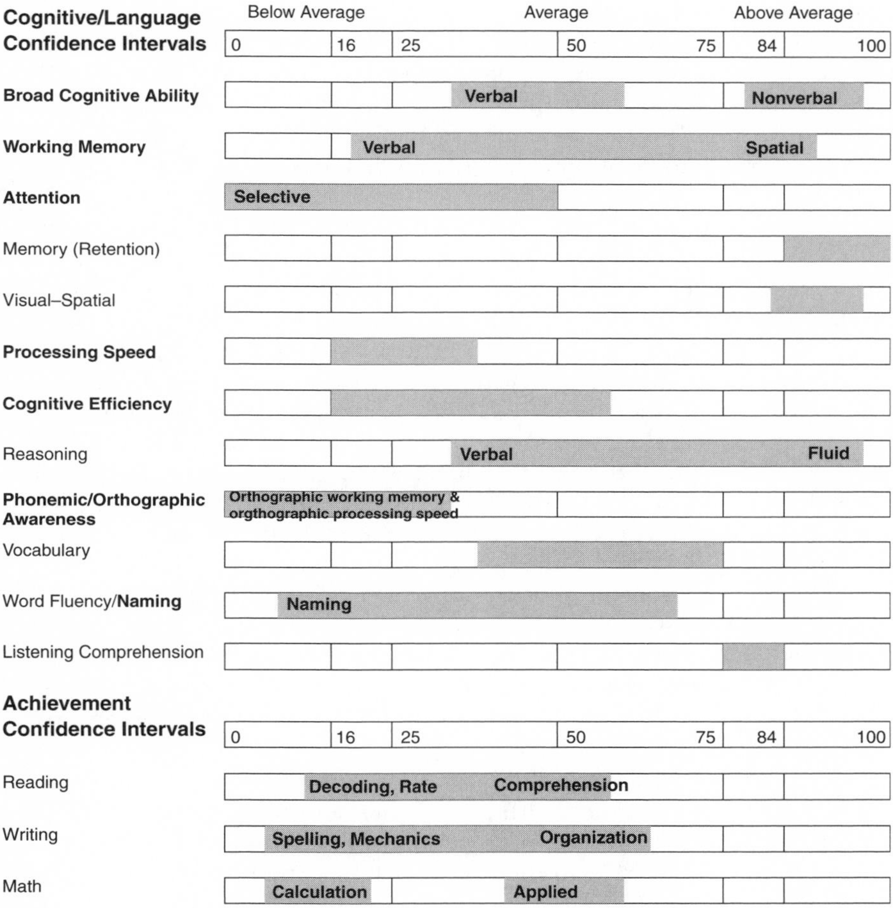

Cognitive/Language Confidence Intervals	Below Average			Average		Above Average	
	0	16	25	50	75	84	100
Broad Cognitive Ability			Verbal			Nonverbal	
Working Memory		Verbal				Spatial	
Attention	Selective						
Memory (Retention)							
Visual–Spatial							
Processing Speed							
Cognitive Efficiency							
Reasoning			Verbal			Fluid	
Phonemic/Orthographic Awareness	Orthographic working memory & orgthographic processing speed						
Vocabulary							
Word Fluency/**Naming**	Naming						
Listening Comprehension							

Achievement Confidence Intervals							
	0	16	25	50	75	84	100
Reading		Decoding, Rate	Comprehension				
Writing		Spelling, Mechanics	Organization				
Math		Calculation	Applied				

FIGURE 3.4. Assessment profile for Natalie, a student with LD (dyslexia).

to address. First, it points out, as discussed earlier in this chapter, the importance of using a CI rather than a single score for describing abilities. However, even more importantly, it illustrates that an individual's performance can vary significantly across different measures of broad cognitive ability. If the possibility of such variations in performance is not factored into decision making, an individual can easily be misdiagnosed.

The magnitude of difference across broad cognitive ability scores (e.g., WAIS-III Full Scale, WJ III GIA) for the adolescent and adult population has been a matter of concern to professionals (Floyd, Clark, & Shadish, 2008). In particular, my colleagues and I (Gregg, Coleman, Davis, Lindstrom, & Hartwig, 2006) found that this magnitude was more significant for young adults with LD than for their normally achieving peers: The students with LD demonstrated a 12-point difference between their WAIS-III Full Scale and WJ III GIA scores. Such a finding may appear confusing to professionals when the technical manuals for these measures provide strong evidence for internal-consistency coefficients, test–retest reliability, and correlation coefficients across instruments of broad ability. Although the correlations between intelligence measures are often psychometrically strong, a significant percentage of the variance still remains unexplained. Perhaps the answer rests in the fact that broad ability batteries differ substantially in the abilities assessed by their subtests. Therefore, scores on the different measures would naturally vary, contributing to the variability in scores for individuals.

Differences in broad ability composite scores can also partially be attributed to the manner in which each measure converts subtest scores into composite scores. For instance, the composite scores for the quotients and Indexes of both the Reynolds Intellectual Assessment Scales (RIAS; Reynolds & Kamphaus, 2003) and the WAIS-III (Wechsler, 1997a) are computed by using equal weights—that is, by allotting each subtest equal influence on the total score. However, on the WJ III (Woodcock, McGrew, & Mather, 2001a, 2001b), principal-component analysis was used to determine the composite scores by finding the best weighted combination of tests that accounted for the largest portion of the variance in each age group (McGrew & Woodcock, 2001). Use of reliable-component analysis, or the weighting of subtests that make up factor (index, cluster) and composite intelligence scores, appears to lead to a lower correlation with g (the composite intelligence score) and with other subtests, "including more potential incremental and discriminant validity and more reliable difference scores, resulting in more precise confidence intervals" (Caruso & Cliff, 1999, p. 205). The use of reliable-component analysis thus provides strong empirical confirmation contributing to the validation of a psychometric definition of intelligence, and it will apparently be a critical tool in the construction of future psychometric intelligence measures.

Another factor influencing the differences between and within groups across intelligence measures may be more sociological. The study of broad cognitive ability in the general population has led to a better understanding of the influence of schooling and many other environmental factors on this ability (Gustafsson, 2001). It has been documented that broad ability scores do not remain constant over time. The steady worldwide rise in broad ability scores is often referred to as the "Flynn effect" (Flynn, 1984, 1987). The average gain is about 3 points per decade (Neisser et al., 1996) and about 3 points per additional year of schooling (Gustafsson, 2001). The influence of intelligence score shifts over time is critical for professionals reviewing the histories of students with documented disabilities. This has significant implications, since under IDEA 2004, many individuals will come to postsecondary institutions with outdated assessment information. As Kanaya, Ceci, and Scullin (2003) note, the average intelligence score of referred students "depends greatly on the year tested and test norms used" (p. 462). Past psychological scores for an individual should never be interpreted as if they were computed according to the same metric as the same person's present scores.

Cognitive Measures
Commonly Used with Adolescents and Adults

Critical to any psychometric measure is the degree to which empirical research and theory support the validity of sources. The *Standards for Educational and Psychological Testing* volume (AERA et al., 1999) identifies substantive, internal, and external validity as imperative to determining construct validity. Benson (1998) states that a strong psychological theory enhances substantive (content) validity through the identification of a well-bounded construct domain as a guide for developing measures in the empirical domain. The ways in which broad and specific cognitive abilities are defined and operationalized often differ across psychometric instruments, as noted above. Investigation of these different theoretical and measurement (empirical) constructs, and especially of how they affect the assessment of adolescents and adults with LD or ADHD, deserves serious attention from clinicians and researchers. Several of the intelligence measures commonly used in psychological assessments of these populations are reviewed below (for more in-depth critiques of these instruments, see Flanagan & Harrison, 2005).

Wechsler Adult Intelligence Scale—Third Edition

The WAIS-III (Wechsler, 1997a) was normed on individuals between
the ages of 16 and 89 years (normative sample composed of 2,450 adolescents and adults). Three broad cognitive scores are provided: Performance (5 subtests), Verbal (6 subtests), and Full Scale (11 subtests).
Four Index scores were derived from both exploratory factor analysis
and CFA (i.e., Verbal Comprehension, Perceptual Organization, Working Memory, and Processing Speed).

Average reliability coefficients for most WAIS-III subtests range
from .82 to .93. The Picture Arrangement, Symbol Search, and Object
Assembly subtests have somewhat lower reliability coefficients. Reliability coefficients of the Full Scale, Verbal, and Performance scores (as well
as the Indexes) range from .88 to .97. See the WAIS-III and Wechsler
Memory Scale—Third Edition (WMS-III) technical manuals (Wechsler,
1997a, 1997b) for in-depth descriptions of the psychometric characteristics of these instruments.

As noted earlier, the WAIS-III is derived from a factor structure different from that used in creating the WAIS and WAIS-R. The inclusion
of four broad first-order factors (i.e., the Verbal Comprehension, Perceptual Organization, Working Memory, and Processing Speed Indexes) is
more closely aligned with CHC theory than is the use of Verbal and
Performance composite scores. Indeed, as described earlier, Caruso and
Cliff (1999) found that the two most reliable, orthogonal components
from the WAIS-III would be measures of *Gf* and *Gc*, not the hypothesized main component of the Verbal–Performance model. However, to
assess *Gf* and *Gc* on the WAIS-III would require differentially weighted
subtests, which are not part of the normal scoring procedures.

The Wechsler scales' Verbal–Performance model of intelligence has
been criticized in the literature for lacking empirical evidence (Flanagan, McGrew, & Ortiz, 2000). Supporting this hypothesis, Caruso and
Cliff (1999) determined that on the WAIS-III, the Performance scale
score was indistinguishable from psychometric *g.* Thus practitioners
should be cautious in interpreting Verbal–Performance IQ differences
(which may be statistically but not practically significant). The four-
factor model (the four Indexes) discussed in the WAIS-III technical
manual should be the theoretical basis for informed clinical decisions
(Arnau & Thompson, 2001; Caruso & Cliff, 1999).

The use of measurement invariance research to make inferences
from assessment tools is essential for informed diagnostic decision making. We (Bowden et al., 2008) investigated the WAIS-III/WMS-III profiles of three groups of young adults—one with LD, one with ADHD,
and the age norm group. We found that the numerical relationships
underlying inferences of deficit on the one hand, and underlying the

interpretation of convergent and divergent validity relationships on the other, did not differ across these groups (i.e., there was measurement invariance). These findings are of particular relevance to the assessment of adolescents and adults with LD and ADHD, because there has been so much debate about the most appropriate model of intelligence for these conditions (Kaufman & Lichtenberger, 2006).

Wechsler Adult Intelligence Scale—Fourth Edition

At this writing, the fourth edition of the WAIS (WAIS-IV; Wechsler, 2008) was scheduled for release to the public during the fall of 2008. Therefore, although studies of special groups (persons with mild cognitive impairment, borderline intellectual functioning, anxiety, etc.) will be provided in the test manual, external studies investigating the reliability and validity of this measure are not yet available. Several new features of the WAIS-IV should enhance its effectiveness with the adult population. For instance, as with the WISC-IV, the Index score structure (Verbal Comprehension, Perceptual Organization, Working Memory, and Processing Speed) is used to interpret ability, rather than Verbal–Performance IQ scores. In addition, new measures of fluid intelligence, perceptual organization, working memory, and processing reflect current research.

Woodcock–Johnson III Tests of Cognitive Abilities

The WJ III COG (Woodcock et al., 2001b) was normed on individuals between the ages of 2 and 90+ years (normative sample composed of 8,818 participants). It was co-normed with the WJ III Tests of Achievement (ACH; Woodcock et al., 2001a). The WJ III COG consists of a Standard Battery (tests 1–10) and an Extended Battery (tests 11–20). The WJ III COG GIA score is a measure of *g* or general intelligence. It is based on a differentially weighted combination of tests of seven broad CHC abilities; the weightings were derived from the first principal-components analysis of tests 1–7 (McGrew & Woodcock, 2001).

Content validity for the WJ III COG is based on the CHC model of intelligence (McGrew, 2005). During 1985–1986, Woodcock and McGrew independently applied CFA methods to the original (1977) WJ battery, while Horn and Carroll independently factor-analyzed the same data (McGrew, 2005). These four analyses became the blueprint for the WJ-R (McGrew, 2005). During the development of the WJ III COG, it was decided that the WJ-R *Gf-Gc* cognitive clusters were too narrow. This decision was informed by the seminal publication *Human Cognitive Abilities* (Carroll, 1993), which advanced theory in factor structure. Revisions for the WJ III COG were based on integrating the Horn–Cattell theory with Carroll's work. Reliability for all WJ III COG clusters is reported to be .90 or higher, and all individual tests have a reliability of .80 or higher. One WJ III COG measurement invariance study for the adolescent and adult populations with LD is available at this time; it supports invariance for adults with LD as compared to the matched age norm on the WJ III (Bandalos & Gregg, 2008).

Reynolds Intellectual Assessment Scales

The RIAS (Reynolds & Kamphaus, 2003) is a relatively new intelligence measure for ages 3 through 94 years that also includes a co-normed supplemental measure of memory. The RIAS provides a Composite Intelligence Index (CIX), a Verbal Intelligence Index (VIX), and a Nonverbal Intelligence Index (NIX). Reliability estimates of the RIAS Indexes have median values across ages that equal or exceed .94, and the estimate for each RIAS subtest across age equals or exceeds .90 (Reynolds & Kamphaus, 2003).

Although the authors indicate that the works of Carroll (1993) and Cattell and Horn (Horn & Blankson, 2005) were used as guides in the development of the test, they state that the primary theoretical framework is a verbal–nonverbal model of intelligence. Two subtests each make up the VIX and the NIX. However, Nelson, Denis, Canivez, and Hatt (2007) conducted a hierarchical CFA on RIAS data using a school-age population. Their data suggests more interpretive weight be placed on the total RIAS IQ score than the verbal–nonverbal scales. They also suggest the RIAS be used as a screener than a comprehensive measure of intelligence. One of the authors' goals was to develop a measure of intelligence that would eliminate the need for motor coordination and visual–motor speed. Nelson, Canivez, Lindstrom, and Hatt (2007) suggest that the RIAS is a weaker measure of general intelligence. They found that only two of the four subtests had good g loadings, suggesting that the measure might be seen better as a screener.

Administration of the entire four-subtest measure is approximately 20–25 minutes. The Composite Memory Index (CMS) derived from the two supplementary subtests requires an additional 10–15 minutes for administration. However, Nelson, Denis, and colleagues (2007), using a larger population ($N = 1,163$) than the norm sample, independent samples of referred students (ages 6–18), and more rigorous factor extraction criteria, suggest that the CMS is not a distinct factor and should therefore not be interpreted. The research findings by Nelson and colleagues and Bracken (2005) indicate that the most valid use of the RIAS is as a brief estimate of general intelligence. No RIAS measurement invariance studies for the adolescent and adult populations with LD or ADHD are available at this time. Unfortunately, the Nelson and colleagues study investigated a school-age population of LD across a large age span.

Differential Ability Scales–II

The Differential Ability Scales–II (DAS-II; Elliott, 2007), the newly revised edition of the DAS (Elliott, 1990), is an assessment tool designed to measure the cognitive assessment of children and adolescents (2½ to 17 years of age). The DAS-II has 20 cognitive subtests, including 17 subtests from the original DAS. During the revision of the DAS, four new subtests were added (Recall of Sequential Order, Rapid Naming, Phonological Processing, and Recall of Digits—Backward). The DAS-II now offers a working memory composite, a processing speed composite, and (for younger children) a school readiness composite.

As with the DAS, it is difficult to decide whether to place the DAS-II within the CHC or a verbal–nonverbal framework of learning. When discussing the DAS, Elliott (1990, p. 54) describes his theoretical framework as "eclectic," contending that it "may be interpreted from a number of theoretical perspectives having used the work of Cattell, Horn, Das, Jensen, Thurstone, Vernon, and Spearman." Certainly, following CHC theory, one could surmise that the composites and scales tap *Gc* (Verbal), *Gf* (Nonverbal Reasoning), *Gv* (Spatial), *Glr* and *Gsm* Working Memory), *Gs* (Processing Speed and Rapid Naming), and *Ga* (Phonological Processing). The DAS-II has dropped the three achievement screening tests that were included in the DAS, but the DAS-II is co-normed with the Wechsler Individual Achievement Test—Second Edition (WIAT-II; Wechsler, 2001). In addition, the manual offers evidence for a comparison between the DAS-II and the WJ III. No DAS-II measurement invariance studies for the adolescent population with LD or ADHD are available at this time.

Kaufman Adolescent and Adult Intelligence Test

The Kaufman Adolescent and Adult Intelligence Test (KAIT; Kaufman & Kaufman, 1993) was normed on individuals between the ages of 11 and 94 years of age (normative sample composed of 2,000 adolescents and adults). Three intelligence scores are provided: Fluid (three subtests), Crystallized (three subtests), and Composite (six subtests). The Expanded Battery includes two supplementary subtests and two measures of delayed recall.

Content validity was drawn from three major theories, including Piaget's (Inhelder & Piaget, 1958; Piaget, 1972) formal operations, Luria's (1980) planning ability, and Horn–Cattell theory (Kaufman & Kaufman,

1997). However, content validity was derived mainly from "broader, more general and correlated versions of the *Gf* and *Gc*" (Kaufman & Kaufman, 1997, p. 210) of the Horn–Cattell theory. The mean split-half reliability coefficients for the total normative sample were .95 for Crystallized, .95 for Fluid, and .97 for Composite (Kaufman & Kaufman, 1993, Table 8.1). Factor analysis results provided evidence for the construct validity of the Fluid and Crystallized Scales and the inclusion of subtests within scales. Kaufman and Kaufman (1997) provided the oblimin factor loadings from exploratory factor analysis of KAIT subtests on the *Gc* and *Gf* factors. No KAIT measurement invariance studies for the adolescent and adult populations with LD or ADHD are available at this time.

Stanford–Binet Intelligence Scales, Fifth Edition

The Stanford–Binet Intelligence Scales, Fifth Edition (SB5; Roid, 2003) is a cognitive battery normed for the ages of 2 to 85+ years. The composite score is derived from scores on five hierarchical factors: Fluid Reasoning, Knowledge, Quantitative Reasoning, Visual–Spatial Processing, and Working Memory (Verbal and Nonverbal). The theoretical framework for the SB5 is derived from the work of Carroll (1993), Cattell (1943), and Horn (1994), and from CHC theory (McGrew, 2005).

Internal-consistency reliability ranges from .95 to .98 for the IQ scores and from .90 to .92 for the five factor scores. For the 10 subtests, average reliabilities range from .84 to .89. Item response theory (Rasch, 1980; Wright & Lineacre, 1999) was used to design the routing procedure and levels, and to check the consistency among the items and tasks within each subtest. Rasch modeling was used to verify fit to the unidimensional, underlying cognitive traits (Roid & Pomplun, 2005; Wright & Lineacre, 1999). The factor structure of the SB5 was extensively studied and is summarized by Roid (2003). CFA studies were also conducted across the SB5 and the WJ III, supporting the SB5 five-factor model (Roid & Pomplun, 2005). However, no SB5 measurement invariance studies for the adolescent and adult populations with LD or ADHD are available at this time.

Validity of a Process-Oriented View of Cognition

The validity of using cognitive processing ability measures as critical components of the diagnostic methodology for LD or ADHD has recently been challenged. For example, Fletcher and Reschly (2005) argue that, at best, "meager evidence" (p. 17) exists to support the assessment of cognitive processes for LD identification or intervention with children. However, this view has been contradicted by other professionals working with the K–12 population (Evans et al., 2002; Flanagan & Kaufman, 2004; Hale, Fiorello, Kavanagh, Hoeppner, & Gaitherer, 2001). Research pertaining to the concurrent or predictive validity of specific cognitive processing measures for the adolescent and adult populations with LD or ADHD is surely pertinent to this ongoing debate.

First, evidence is available that young adults with LD and ADHD can be differentiated from their normally achieving peers on the basis of specific cognitive processing measures (Bowden et al., 2008; Gregg et al., 2006). In addition, results from current research show that the predictive relationships of cognitive processes to learning are influenced by diagnostic category (Gregg et al., 2005). This pattern is best illustrated by data provided in Table 3.1, in which the functional cognitive processing factor differences between adults with and without LD on the WAIS-III Indexes and the WJ III COG Clusters are documented. As can be noted, the normally achieving adults' performance of many tasks (language-based or otherwise) appears to be significantly related to word knowledge. By contrast, for the adults with LD, working memory capacity and processing speed abilities are most predictive of performance. These patterns suggest underlying group differences that are (1) detectable without the use of achievement tests, and (2) reflective of differential neurological functioning. If critics such as Dombrowski and colleagues (2004) were correct in assuming that LD is a developmental delay, we should see differences between adults with and without LD only on measures of achievement, and not on measures of cognitive and linguistic processing. Table 3.1 illustrates not only that there are differences in functional processing between the groups, but that the adults with LD appear to use less efficient cognitive and linguistic processes than do their peers without disabilities.

Some professionals might argue that the reason for the group differences illustrated in Table 3.1 is simply differential ability. Using this logic, one would assume that it is impossible to differentiate the cognitive or linguistic processes influencing performance for adults with ADHD from those for individuals with LD. However, researchers have provided evidence that adults with ADHD appear to present a different profile of cognitive and/or linguistic processes from that of either their peers with LD or their peers with no disabilities (Bowden et al., 2008; Gregg, Coleman, Stennett, Davis, Nielsen, et al., 2002). Investigating the dimensionality of phonemic and orthographic tasks for college students with and without dyslexia and ADHD, we (Gregg, Bandalos, et al., 2007) found that the populations with ADHD, LD, and no disabilities showed significantly different task correlations, significantly influencing factor structures. Again, if cognitive and linguistic processes had little construct validity in the diagnosis of these disorders, there would have been no differences among these groups of adults.

TABLE 3.1. Correlations for WAIS-III Indexes and WJ III COG Clusters for Normally Achieving Adults and Adults with Dyslexia

	WAIS-III Verbal Comprehension		WAIS-III Perceptual Organization		WAIS-III Working Memory		WAIS-III Processing Speed	
	Nondyslexic	Dyslexic	Nondyslexic	Dyslexic	Nondyslexic	Dyslexic	Nondyslexic	Dyslexic
WJ III Verbal Ability	.75**	.57**	.56**	.46**	.54**	.15	.12	.15
WJ III Long-Term Retrieval	.36	.13	.34	.37**	.18	.38**	.21	.18
WJ III Visual–Spatial Thinking	.52**	.15	.40*	.57**	.09	.15	.13	.13
WJ III Auditory Processing	.30	.13	.31	.21	.38*	.27*	.19	.26
WJ III Fluid Reasoning	.50**	.51**	.55**	.56**	.26	.35*	.29	.06
WJ III Processing Speed	.03	.08	.22	.28*	.17	.26	.36	.55**
WJ III Short-Term Memory	.21	.11	.20	.18	.38*	.62**	.17	.06
WJ III Working Memory	.26	.16	.28	.29*	.41*	.67**	.22	.08
WJ III Cognitive Fluency	.34	-.00	.33	.15	.11	.22	.38*	.51**
WJ III Cognitive Efficiency	-.05	.11	.18	.24	.29	.60**	.30	.31*
WJ III Phonemic Awareness	.27	.18	.22	.23	.28	.23	.11	.19

Note. From Gregg, Coleman, Davis, Lindstrom, and Hartwig (2006). Copyright 2006 by John Wiley & Sons, Inc. Reprinted by permission.
*Correlation is significant at the .01 level (two-tailed); **correlation is significant at the .001 level (two-tailed).

Phillip's profile (Figure 3.3) illustrates the importance of using cognitive processing measures as part of diagnostic decision making. Phillip's ability to sustain attention over time is variable, as is his ability to filter out competing information while focusing on the most important aspects of a task. For example, on the Conners' Continuous Performance Test II (Conners & Multi-Health Systems Staff, 2000)—a computerized task of sustained visual attention and selective attention, requiring him to sit at a computer for approximately 14 minutes and press a key in response to alphabetic letters that flashed on a screen—Phillip's indices are within normal limits. In contrast, on the Delis–Kaplan Executive Function System (Delis, Kaplan, & Kramer, 2001) Color–Word Inhibition/Switching Errors task—a task requiring him to look at a page on which the names of colors are printed in ink of a different color (e.g., the word "red" in blue ink) and not to read the color name unless the word is presented inside a box—Phillip has demonstrated significant difficulty in maintaining set, and toward the end of the task has often said the color of the ink rather than the word.

Like many individuals with ADHD, therefore, Phillip demonstrates significant differences on tasks measuring executive functions. In other words, he performs variably on cognitive tasks measuring sustained attention (maintaining attention over time), selective attention (maintaining attention while ignoring potentially distracting stimuli), organization/planning, response inhibition, and maintaining set (the ability to keep in mind the requirements of a task). These deficits contribute to his difficulties in learning unstructured information, efficiently processing information, and retrieving or attending to information consistently. However, Natalie demonstrates some of the central executive processing problems noted in the LD literature: Her problems with inhibition and supervisory attention for switching mental sets are specific to phonemic awareness and orthographic tasks.

The types of tasks used to measure WMC will influence the degree to which scores correlate with other cognitive, language, and achievement measures. Working memory span tasks, such as counting span (Case, Kurland, & Goldberg, 1982), operation span (Turner & Engle, 1989), and reading span (Daneman & Carpenter, 1980), are frequently used in research to measure WMC (Conway et al., 2005). However, the demands of various WMC tasks are different and could prove to be difficult or quite manageable, depending on an individual's profile. On the majority of commonly used standardized tests measuring broad cognitive abilities, working memory span tasks are the norm, but the task demands can be quite different across assessment tools. For instance, the WJ III COG Auditory Working Memory test requires a student to "chunk" and recall individual (real) words and numbers; on the WMS-

III Letter–Number Sequencing task, groups of letters and numbers must be resequenced and recalled; and on the Comprehensive Test of Phonological Processing (Wagner, Torgesen, & Rashotte, 1999), nonwords and numbers are presented for manipulation and recall. Each of these tasks can place different constraints on an examinee. Standardized tests that are designed to measure the verbal working memory demands required for reading a sentence or connected text are currently not available to clinicians.

A strong relationship between phonemic WMC and reading decoding performance has been well documented in the literature. Natalie's profile (Figure 3.4) provides an example of this research finding. On phonemic and orthographic WMC tasks, her scores are below the 16th percentile. As a result, she demonstrates significant underachievement on decoding, spelling, and reading fluency measures. In contrast, Phillip has performed within the average range on all measures of phonemic and orthographic WMC. However, his difficulty with WMC emerges when he has to process connected text (listening comprehension, reading comprehension tasks).

Importance of Speed, Efficiency, Time, and Verbal Ability

Cognitive processing speed, cognitive efficiency, time, and verbal ability are four processes essential to understanding individuals with LD and ADHD. Although they are integrated into the CHC and WMC models discussed earlier, I would like to review their importance to the adolescent and adult population.

Cognitive Processing Speed

Cognitive processing speed, along with WMC, appears to account for a significant amount of the variance on many learning tasks (Hambrick & Engle, 2002; Kwong See & Ryan, 1995; Van der Linden, 1999). However, the relationship between processing speed and academic performance must be put into perspective. Engle and colleagues (1992) found that the correlation between speed and reading comprehension vanished when WMC was covaried. In other words, as processing speed increases, more WMC is available to a learner. "Processing speed" has been defined differently by different researchers and measured with very different types of tools across research studies (McGrew & Flanagan, 1998). Although researchers have documented that many adolescents and adults with LD and ADHD do poorly on timed measures, the types of test items influence performance. In a study investigating the performance of college students with and without LD on speeded cognitive and academic measures, students with LD performed below their peers on all measures (Ofiesh et al., 2005). However, the largest differences were seen on the academic fluency measures (e.g., WJ III Reading Fluency) as compared to general cognitive speed measures (e.g., WJ III Visual Matching). Tasks tapping phonemic and orthographic awareness (letters, numbers) appear to differentiate the adolescent populations with LD and ADHD better than broad cognitive processing measures do (Gregg, Coleman, Stennett, Davis, Nielsen, et al., 2002). Therefore, the fact that an individual performs within the average range on a broad cognitive ability test measuring processing speed does not mean that his or her ability to process print is equal to this score.

Cognitive Efficiency

Cognitive efficiency and cognitive processing speed are distinct variables that, though highly correlated, are not the same construct. Carroll (1993) distinguished the difference between these variables in the following manner: "A speed ability has to do with the rate at which tasks of a specified kind and difficulty are performed, while a level [i.e., cognitive efficiency] has to do with the level of task difficulty at which an individual can perform with a specified amount of accuracy" (p. 506). Often this difference is defined as speed versus accuracy. For instance, some individuals with ADHD can finish a task quickly, but at the cost of accuracy. We (Gregg et al., 2005) compared the performance of young adults with LD to that of their normally achieving peers on the WJ III COG and ACH batteries. We found that the greatest mean difference (12.80) between groups on the cognitive clusters was on the WJ III Cognitive Efficiency—Extended Cluster.

Daneman and Merikle (1996) suggest that an individual's efficiency in executing a variety of symbolic manipulations (i.e., verbal and nonverbal) is strongly related to his or her verbal ability. It may be that, as Daneman and Carpenter (1980) note, the source of individual difference in memory capacity resides less in storage capacity and more in the processes available to maximally utilize limited capacities (i.e., verbal ability and working memory). Cognitive efficiency draws upon attention, working memory, executive processing, short-term memory, and cognitive processing speed. As with other cognitive processes, the task demands strongly influence performance. For instance, a student with LD may perform efficiently if he or she is asked to complete a nonverbal scanning task (pictures), but may score miserably on a speeded task that requires the processing of letters or words. For such individuals, specific phonemic and orthographic awareness deficits constrain the processing speed and efficiency. Natalie's is an excellent example of such a profile. Her scores on cognitive processing speed tasks are average, as compared to her performance on an orthographic processing speed task (see Figure 3.4). Natalie's difficulty in accessing and quickly scanning letters and numbers also interferes with her cognitive efficiency (accuracy scores).

Sense of Time

The sense of time is another multidimensional construct that functions as part of the working memory system. Attention, executive functions, and processing speed are highly correlated with a sense of time. According to Barkley (2006), the dimensions of time most often studied by researchers investigating populations with neurological disorders include time perception, motor timing, time estimation, time production, time reproduction, and routine use of time/time management. Ample evidence is available that of these types of time, individuals with ADHD demonstrate deficits mainly with short-interval time discrimination and with use of time/time management (see Barkley, 2006, for an in-depth discussion). According to Barkley, no differences have been found for individuals with ADHD on tasks measuring time production or reproduction. Difficulties with sense of time for the population with LD are more specific to the subgroup with nonverbal LD (see Chapter Four).

Verbal Ability

LD is a communication disorder affecting the processing of both verbal and nonverbal information. Therefore, detailed observation of an individual's ability to process verbal information at the word, sentence, and text levels is critical for the identification of LD. In addition, the attention, executive, and working memory processing deficits exhibited by adolescents and adults with ADHD influence their verbal communication and achievement performance. As Hunt (2002) has observed, *Gc* (verbal comprehension) has been the "wallflower" (p. 123) of the intellectual trio (i.e., *Gc* [verbal comprehension], *Gf* [fluid reasoning], and *Gv* [visual processing]). Hunt goes on to state that it is time for researchers to "ask *Gc* to put away the horn-rimmed glasses, put on a party dress, and take a turn on the dance floor. Understanding the nature of *Gc* is as important to the study of intelligence as finding Cinderella was to the Prince" (p. 124). During an evaluation, professionals are encouraged to consider both the direct and indirect roles of verbal ability in learning; these roles are discussed throughout this book.

Implications for Assessment and Accommodation

✓ Cognitive measures remain significant components of most assessment batteries, and therefore of determining who is qualified to receive accommodations at the adolescent and adult levels.

✓ Cerebral blood flow studies; studies of brain electrical activity using QEEG; neuroimagining studies using PET, MRI, or fMRI; neurochemical studies; and genetic studies all provide strong evidence that ADHD and LD are disorders of neurodevelopmental origin.

✓ Behavioral and molecular genetic research provides strong evidence for a significant genetic contribution to ADHD and LD.

✓ A process-oriented model of cognition implies that different networks of cognitive processes are configured in response to different functional demands, and that a given cognitive process may contribute directly or indirectly to several functions.

✓ Variation in working memory is certainly influenced by independent but intersecting sources that include (but are not limited to) attention, storage capacity, processing efficiency, and executive processing.

✓ An element missing from some cognitive models is consideration of the developmental trajectories of ability acquisition, and of the constraints these impose on learning across the lifespan.

✓ Failure to integrate single subtest scores with other external sources (e.g., test scores, behavioral observations, background information), in combination with insufficient knowledge of research evidence and theory, leads many clinicians to make false-negative decisions that result in denied access to accommodations.

✓ Factor (index) scores provide more reliable and valid measures of abilities than do subtest scores.

✓ Professionals must retain a healthy degree of skepticism that the inferences drawn from test batteries are equivalent across populations with and without disabilities, since very little measurement invariance research is available.

✓ CIs (rather than single standard scores) should be the data used for diagnostic decision making, as CIs represent "true scores" as opposed to the observed scores.

CHAPTER FOUR

Social, Emotional, and Behavioral Assessment and Accommodation

Tommy is a high school senior who plans to attend a technical college next year to complete a program preparing him to be an emergency medical technician. He was diagnosed with LD and ADHD in fifth grade, and was served by special education from sixth grade through high school. According to Tommy, "My dad tried to help me, but didn't know how," while "my mom just beat me up all the time." His mother was diagnosed with a personality disorder when Tommy was in elementary school. It appears that she received very little treatment to help her cope.

Mary was diagnosed with nonverbal LD (NLD) in high school. In earlier years, she had received several incorrect diagnoses (i.e., autism, schizophrenia, mental retardation). She graduated from high school with a special education diploma and is currently being served by vocational rehabilitation services. Mary is experiencing significant social and academic problems in a job training program.

Chipper is a freshman in college. In second grade, his classroom teacher rubbed his hand with sandpaper, because she thought he was a "smart-aleck for writing backward." Fortunately, the teacher was quickly disciplined by the school system. Chipper was diagnosed with LD (dyslexia) in third grade, and received direct intervention in reading and written language throughout his elementary and secondary programs. He reports his family to "be like the Brady Bunch," and this observation appears quite accurate. Chipper receives a great deal of positive support from both his parents and his brother.

Research on the social and emotional functioning of the adolescent and adult populations with LD and ADHD has produced conflicting and often confounding results. Because this research has been based on very different theoretical perspectives, has used a variety of techniques, and has investigated very different participant profiles, it has often contributed more to professional confusion than to understanding. In addition, many of the tools and research designs used to investigate the well-being of the adolescent and adult populations are somewhat methodologically limited. Throughout the chapters of this book pertaining to academics (reading, writing, mathematics), I point out that the research in these areas is focused primarily on the adolescent and/ or adult populations with LD. In the area of social and emotional functioning, the opposite trend is observed: The majority of this research pertains to the populations with ADHD rather than to those with LD. Such a pattern appears to reflect professional biases related to these two disabilities. In other words, LD is often simply defined by academic underachievement, and ADHD by behavioral manifestations. Unfortunately, this has usually resulted in studying social/emotional well-being and academic competence in isolation, rather than placing them in a more robust model that accounts for the direct and indirect relationships of one to the other.

Researchers interested in the social and emotional well-being of adolescents and adults investigate what Masten (2001) calls either "variable-focused" or "person-focused" variation. Multivariate statistics allow researchers using a variable-focused approach to examine the direct and indirect relationships between individual qualities and environmental stresses. Person-focused designs compare different populations (e.g., individuals with and without an anxiety disorder) to identify what might account for differences in outcomes across groups. Shiner, Tellegen, and Masten (2003) suggest that person-focused approaches often miss interactions that more accurately identify underlying causes for social or emotional outcomes. They state:

> In order to understand why childhood personality predicts later personality and adaptation over such wide swaths of time, we need a more fine-grained understanding of the processes through which children's individual differences shape and are shaped by their day-to-day experiences, as well as the processes through which personality and context transform each other over longer periods of time. (p. 1166).

Understanding the mediating processes underlying risk or protective factors requires that professionals also carefully consider societal and cultural factors in determining what is considered valued and acceptable behavior (Keogh & Weisner, 1993; Masten, 2001; Wong, 2003). Generalizing social or emotional risk or protective factors across populations and cultures (local, national, international) is very risky.

Integrating research results from both variable-focused and person-focused studies contributes to a more sophisticated understanding of individuals' well-being. Unfortunately, a great deal of research investigating the well-being of adolescents or adults with LD or ADHD is based upon designs in which single self-report measures of questionable construct validity are used to predict personality or success outcomes. However, researchers have available to them sophisticated methodologies and statistical tools to introduce greater complexity into their designs. When such methods are used, and when populations and environmental factors are more strictly specified across time, the relationships among the multiple variables influencing the well-being of adolescents and adults with LD and ADHD can be better understood.

Risk and Resilience Model

Many researchers investigating the social and emotional well-being of adolescents and adults with LD or ADHD use a "risk and resilience" framework. The risk and resilience researcher is interested in the multiple factors (both internal and external to a person) that influence the person's outcomes. According to Masten (2001), "Resilience refers to a class of phenomena characterized by *good outcomes in spite of serious threats to adaptation or development*. Research on resilience aims to understand the processes that account for these good outcomes" (p. 228; emphasis in original). Yet it is important to keep in mind that indicators of risk and resilience are arbitrarily labeled, and that often factors are inversely related to each other. For instance, a milder type of ADHD (causal factor) might produce fewer stressful family life events (less risk), provide greater access to higher education (less risk), lead to obtaining better community resources (more assets), and allow for more professional advancements (more assets). Therefore, possible risks can be inversely related as a result of a third causal factor (Jessor, Van Den Bos, Vanderryn, Costa, & Turbin, 1995).

Follow-up and follow-along studies of adults with LD and ADHD provide evidence of the lifelong influence of these disabilities, but also suggest factors of resilience. However, this research has several significant limitations. For instance, the definitions of and eligibility criteria for LD and ADHD used in the childhood identification of these individuals are often not consistent with today's standards. Therefore, in regard to ADHD, Barkley (2006) suggests that there appear to be more positive outcomes for the hyperactive–impulsive than for the inattentive subgroup in the majority of the follow-up studies, and that the initial identification of these individuals took place before the DSM-III (American Psychiatric Association, 1980) consensus on diagnostic criteria for attention-deficit disorder (ADD), as it was then called (August, Stewart, & Holmes, 1983; Cantwell & Baker, 1989; Claude & Firestone, 1995; Lambert, Hartsough, Sassone, & Sandoval, 1987; Schmidt & Moll, 1995; Thorley, 1984; Weiss & Hechtman, 1993). Several other follow-up studies of ADHD, however, have used DSM-III or DSM-IV (American Psychiatric Association, 1994) criteria to diagnose these populations (Barkley, Fischer, Edelbrock, & Smallish, 1990; Biederman et al., 1996). The majority of the follow-up and follow-along studies of populations with ADHD and LD suggest that both these disabilities can be risk factors for negative outcomes, such as high school dropout rates, underemployment, job difficulties, emotional difficulties, and life dissatisfaction (Barkley, 2006; Fourqurean, Meisgeier, Swank, & Williams, 1991; Reiff & Gerber, 1995; Ross-Gordon, 1996).

The follow-up and follow-along studies in the field of LD reflect the same methodological problems as those in the ADHD field (Bruck, 1992; Fink, 1998; Gerber, Ginsberg, & Reiff, 1992; Rogan & Hartman, 1990; Sitlington & Frank, 1990; Spekman, Goldberg, & Herman, 1992; Vogel & Adelman, 1992; Vogel, Hruby, & Adelman, 1993). Unfortunately, many of these early follow-up studies of populations with LD or ADHD sampled primarily European American males, from middle- to upper-middle class families, who were referred to clinics because of learning and behavior problems. Although such studies have provided professionals invaluable and rich observations of individuals with LD and ADHD across the lifespan, caution must be taken in directly generalizing these findings to other populations of adolescents and adults.

Several researchers in the field of LD frame their follow-up research findings around the resilience factors that appear to contribute the most to *success*, as defined by features of emotional, academic, and occupational well-being. For instance, Spekman and colleagues (1992) and R. J. Goldberg, Higgins, Raskind, and Herman (2003) focus on three themes that differentiated successful from unsuccessful adults with LD in data collected through the Frostig Center: Successful adults (1) adapted to life events through self-awareness and acceptance of their LD, were proactive and persevering, and were able to demonstrate emotional stability and the ability to tolerate stress; (2) were able to set appropriate goals and become goal-directed; and (3) were able to establish and use effective support systems.

Gerber and colleagues (1992) conducted a qualitative study of 71 adults with LD whom they identified as "successful." They collected the majority of their data through interviews with these individuals, and they used fairly traditional definitions of "success" (yearly income, educational level, job satisfaction, job classification, and prominence in one's field). One of the major findings of this research was that successful adults with LD were able to acquire control of their lives. Gerber and colleagues measured the ability to obtain control by grouping factors into two categories: "internal decisions" and "external manifestations" (p. 99). Internal decisions involved desire, goal orientation, and reframing; external manifestations were seen as persistence, goodness of fit, learned creativity, and social ecologies. Resilience and success, according to these authors, were the results of a dynamic process rooted in an individual's ability to take control through the interplay of internal and external factors.

Masten (2001) provides empirical evidence from the psychological literature of a set of global factors most directly associated with resilience. She includes the following in this set of factors: positive relationships with competent and caring adults; self-regulation skills and self-efficacy beliefs; positive self-concept; and motivation. These evidence-based factors are used below as a framework to explore outcomes for adolescent and adult individuals with LD and ADHD, based on research with these populations.

Positive Relationships with Caring Adults

The presence of a supportive adult, such as a mentor, appears to be one of the strongest protective factors for an adolescent or adult with LD or ADHD (Gerber et al., 1992; Spekman et al., 1992; Werner, 1993). This mentor need not be, and often is not, a family member. In Werner's (1993) Kauai longitudinal study, such supportive adults "fostered trust and acted as gatekeepers for the future" (p. 32). According to Gerber and Reiff (1991), throughout their interviews with successful adults with LD, individuals emphasized the importance of their "social ecologies" (supportive and helpful people).

Researchers studying the predictive importance of effective parenting and supportive parent–child relationships suggest that these too appear to be protective factors (Fergusson & Lynskey, 1996; Masten et al., 1999; Richters & Martinez, 1993). "Parenting appears to play a key mediating role linking major life stressors to child behavior"

(Masten, 2001, p. 232). Research specific to the LD population suggests that sustained parental emotional support is a strong protective factor and enables these individuals to maintain strong self-concepts (Cosden, Brown, & Elliott, 2002; Reynolds, 1999; Rothman & Cosden, 1995). Additional research evidence indicates that parent–child interactions appear related to an adolescent's or adult's future success with peer interactions (Wong, 2003). Tommy, introduced at the opening of this chapter, did not receive strong, supportive parenting. Therefore, in addition to the risk factors of experiencing two disabilities (LD and ADHD), negative parenting constitutes a third risk factor for Tommy's overall well-being. Accordingly, it is essential that Tommy receive social and emotional support and services.

The follow-up studies with adults demonstrating ADHD suggest that hostility between parents and their children with ADHD is strongly predictive of similar conflicts at the adolescent and adult stage, particularly those involving aggressive behavior (Barkley, 2006). Also, the emotional adjustment of individuals with ADHD and their success with friendships as adults appear to be directly or indirectly related to the emotional climate of their homes, as reflected in the emotional stability of family members (Barkley, 2006). However, no *one* risk factor appears to predict the well-being of adolescents or adults with ADHD or LD. As noted by Barkley (2006), "The combination of child cognitive ability (intelligence) and emotional stability (aggression, low frustration tolerance) with family environment (mental health of family members, SES [socioeconomic status], emotional climate of home) and child-rearing practices provides a considerably more successful prediction of adult outcome" (p. 275). Chipper, also introduced at the opening of this chapter, experienced a traumatic event early in his schooling that had the potential to become a negative influence on his emotional well-being. However, action was quickly taken to prevent such an incident from recurring. In addition, his supportive home environment is an asset that appears to be providing the resilience needed for positive school and social outcomes.

The assumption that LD is a predictor of significant stress for all adolescents or adults with LD has been challenged by Reynolds (1999). She studied three groups of college students: (1) individuals demonstrating LD but not qualifying for a DSM-IV diagnosis of an emotional disorder; (2) students who exhibited emotional disorders as defined by the DSM-IV, but did not demonstrate LD; and (3) students diagnosed with LD who also met criteria for a DSM-IV diagnosis of an emotional disorder. Reynolds found that although demographic variables were strongly correlated with levels of stress, they did not predict high stress. Rather, factors representing strong family support and positive family relations, as well as early diagnosis, appeared to prevent the emergence of an emotional disorder related to high stress. However, I would add that for any adolescent or adult with LD or ADHD, the disability can lead to significant stress if he or she is not supported by family, friends, school professionals, or employers, or is not provided with appropriate accommodations.

Self-Regulation and Self-Efficacy Beliefs

Difficulty in self-regulating behavior and learning appears to be a significant risk factor for many individuals with LD or ADHD. In fact, ADHD is best defined as a self-regulatory disorder. Barkley (2006) provides an in-depth description of his theory of ADHD as a disorder of self-regulation. He proposes that ADHD is a "deficit in the inhibition of behavior that will produce an adverse impact on executive functioning, self-regulation, and the cross-temporal organization of behavior toward the future" (p. 299). His theory describes the primary role of behavioral inhibition; defines "self-regulation"; and identifies four specific executive processes (i.e., nonverbal working memory, internalization of speech [verbal working memory], self-regulation of affect, and reconstitution) that he suggests are related to self-regulatory functioning. As he notes, "ADHD is not a disorder of knowing what to do, but of doing what one knows" (p. 325).

Self-regulation of behavior and learning is also closely linked to individual temperament patterns (Nigg, Goldsmith, & Sacheck, 2004). "Temperament" refers to such personality characteristics as activity level, response intensity, distractibility, mood, flexibility, rhythmicity, and self-centeredness. According to Thomas and Chess (1977), temperament is often conceived of as individual differences in behavioral style. For individuals with ADHD, excessive activity level, impersistence, and demandingness toward others—temperament characteristics often used to describe such individuals—can negatively influence their relationship with others (Barkley, 2006). Less is known about the temperament of adolescents and adults with LD, although one study (McNamara, Willoughby, Chalmers, & Youth Lifestyle Choices–Community University Research Alliance, 2005) compared the temperament characteristics of adolescents with LD and LD + ADHD to those of normally achieving peers. All adolescents were required to fill out a self-report measure in which they were asked to evaluate their own behaviors. McNamara and colleagues (2005) found that the adolescents with LD reported being more fidgety, being less engaged with tasks, and demonstrating a poorer mood than their normally achieving peers. No differences were noted between the group with LD and the comorbid group, however. Whether these characteristics are directly or indirectly related to difficulty with academic tasks needs further investigation. The risk presented by some of these negative temperament characteristics "may set in motion compounded risk factors that put adolescents with LD and comorbid LD/ ADHD at risk for decreased psychosocial adjustment" (McNamara et al., 2005, p. 242).

"Self-efficacy beliefs"— an individual's evaluations of his or her specific competence—are integral to one's ability to self-regulate behavior and learning. Although there also exists a close relationship between self-efficacy beliefs and self-concept, these two constructs are not identical. "Self-concept" is a comparison of self to others, whereas "self-efficacy" is a criterion reference (Bong & Skaalvik, 2003). For instance, a student uses self-efficacy beliefs when he or she poses the question "Can I do this science problem?" Self-concept is observed when a student compares his or her science competency to another person's, thereby revealing positive or negative views of him- or herself.

The two types of efficacy most often discussed throughout the literature are global and specific self-efficacy. "Global self-efficacy" refers to an individual's ability to effectively predict problem-solving solutions and strategies to cope with life changes; these are not domain-specific behaviors (Schwarzer & Born, 1997). However, very little research evidence is available to support the validity of this construct. "Specific self-efficacy" refers to one's confidence about using various strategies in particular life domains. Three types of specific self-efficacy beliefs have been identified by researchers: academic, social, and emotional (Bandura, Barbaranelli, Capara, & Pastorelli, 2001).

"Academic self-efficacy" is an individual's belief in his or her ability to manage and master academic expectations. Academic self-efficacy appears to be acquired through several different routes: (1) past academic success; (2) exposure to effacious models; (3) positive reinforcement; and (4) emotional arousal in the area of task performance (Bandura, 1995). It appears that disability status does not always have a direct effect on academic self-efficacy; rather, it has an indirect effect, in which disability appears to influence the sources of self-efficacy beliefs (Hampton & Mason, 2003).

Klassen (2007) investigated the self-efficacy abilities of a small number of adolescents with and without LD, using self-report measures of general self-efficacy and several areas of academic self-efficacy. He found that the students with LD overestimated their spelling performance by 52% and their writing by 19%, whereas the individuals with no disabilities were much more accurate in evaluating their true academic performance. As Klassen notes, "The students who need to work the hardest end up doing the least work because they fail to recognize their academic short-coming" (p. 185). According to Klassen, self-efficacy influences choice of task, perseverance at task, and degree of success with specific tasks.

Many researchers have documented the overprediction of academic competence by adolescents and adults with LD and ADHD (Hampton & Mason, 2003; Hoza et al., 2004; Hoza, Pelham, Dobbs, Owens, & Pillow, 2002; Hoza, Pelham, Waschbusch, Kipp, & Owens, 2001; Hoza, Waschbusch, Pelham, Molina, & Milich, 2000; Lackaye, Margalit, & Zinman, 2006; McNamara et al., 2005; Rubin, McCoach, McGuire, & Reis, 2003; Stone & May, 2002). Although a few studies do suggest that adolescents with LD may accurately evaluate their academic competence in comparison to that of their nondisabled peers (Bear, Minke, Griffin, & Deemer, 1998; McPhail & Stone, 1995), the bulk of the research indicates that the self-perceptions of adolescents and adults with LD or ADHD may not be in line with their own actual academic skills (Alvarez & Adelman, 1986; Heath, 1995; Meltzer, Roditi, Houser, & Perlman, 1998; Stone, 1997; Stone & May, 2002). I discuss possible reasons for these findings below, but first I briefly define the other two types of specific self-efficacy.

"Social self-efficacy" refers to individuals' belief in their ability to manage and master their social lives, including peer relationships and assertiveness. "Emotional self-efficacy" is belief in the ability to regulate emotions and cope with negative affect. Both social and emotional self-efficacy appear to have a strong influence on academic performance and satisfaction, especially during adolescence and adulthood (Bandura et al., 2001; Lackaye et al., 2006). Researchers provide evidence that persons with ADHD often appear to demonstrate higher levels of irritability, hostility, negative affect, excitability, and emotional hyperresponsiveness to others than their nondisabled peers do (Barkley, 2006). This has led some to suggest that emotional self-control may be difficult for the population with ADHD. However, as Barkley (2006) notes, "These findings merely suggest rather than confirm a link between ADHD and emotional self-regulation, and they tend to imply that the poorest emotion modulation may be within the aggressive subgroup of children with ADHD" (p. 148).

Research findings indicate three possible explanations for why adolescents or adults with LD or ADHD often overestimate their academic abilities: (1) the nature of the reference group, (2) poor metacognitive awareness, and (3) self-protection. In regard to the first explanation, we know that modeling is an effective means of developing an individual's self-efficacy beliefs and academic achievement (Bandura, 1995; Schunk & Zimmerman, 1998). Researchers also suggest that the closer the similarity between the observer's and the target person's profiles, the more effective the modeling (Bandura, 1995; Hampton & Mason, 2003). Usually adolescents and adults with LD or ADHD are asked to evaluate themselves in relation to their nondisabled peers, rather than to successful individuals with similar disabilities. The relative absence of opportunities for them to compare themselves to similar peer models has been suggested by some researchers to have an impact on their self-efficacy beliefs (Hampton & Mason, 2003). In regard to the second explanation, some researchers have suggested a direct link between poor metacognitive awareness and overestimation of ability by adolescents or adults with LD (Butler, 1998; Sliffe, Weiss, & Bell, 1985; Stone & May, 2002), but no evidence of such a link has been provided. However, the third suggestion—namely, that overestimation of academic competence is related to ego protection—has received some promising attention in the literature and illustrates the correlation between self-efficacy and self-concept (Alvarez & Adelman, 1986).

One also has to wonder whether overestimated self-efficacy may actually free an individual to consider possibilities rather than limitations. That is, researchers might begin to ask themselves whether, for many individuals with LD or ADHD, overestimating their abilities may allow them to discover possibilities through nontraditional means of learning. As I discus in Chapters Five and Six, many definitions of academic tasks (e.g., reading, writing) are undergoing huge transformational shifts. Professionals should be open to the possibility that some adolescents and adults with LD or ADHD whose academic self-efficacy appears inflated on traditional measures of this construct may actually be well suited to make effective use of new tools and techniques.

However, there is a large body of research suggesting that many students at risk for learning failure demonstrate problems with academic self-regulation. In particular, adolescents and adults with LD and ADHD often do not appear to make optimal use of effective strategies for learning skills and obtaining knowledge (Lenz & Deshler, 2005; Swanson, 1993). Pintrich (2000) defines self-regulated learning as "an active, constructive process whereby learners set goals for their learning and then attempt to monitor, regulate, and control their cognition, motivation, and behavior, guided and constrained by their goals and the contextual features in the environment" (p. 453). Readers interested in a more indepth discussion of self-regulation theories, research, and interventions should consult other resources (Barkley, 2006; Boekaerts & Niemivirta, 2000; Zimmerman & Schunk, 2001).

Several researchers have identified self-regulatory processes that are necessary for success with academic learning (Pintrich, 2000; Zimmerman & Schunk, 2001). The abilities to manage academic time, practice, master learning methods, set goals, and demonstrate strong self-efficacy are all important in academic self-regulation. Looking at college populations with and without LD, Rubin and colleagues (2003) found that the students with LD differed significantly from students without LD in the relationship between their motivation for, and use of, standard self-regulated academic learning strategies. There is strong evidence in the literature to support the effectiveness of direct instruction that improves academic self-regulatory methods for adolescents with LD and ADHD (Butler, 1998; Deshler & Lenz, 1989; Deshler & Schumaker, 1993; Schumaker & Deshler, 1992). However, Perels, Gurtler, and Schmits (2005) provide data suggesting that a combination of training in self-regulation with problem-solving instruction is more effective in enhancing self-regulation and achievement than is either of these methods in isolation.

Positive Self-Concept

A very significant factor influencing resilience is positive self-concept. Self-concept is a multifaceted and dynamic construct "that is both a structure and a process and that can present the self as both 'known' and 'knower'" (Markus & Wurf, 1987, p. 35). According to Markus and Wurf (1987), "self-concept" refers to what individuals think, feel, and believe about themselves, and they use the term "working self-concept" to refer to the accessible self-concept of the moment. In addition, they suggest that self-concept is a critical variable in the effectiveness and consistency of self-regulatory mechanisms.

Poor self-concept has historically been linked with having LD or ADHD (Kloomok & Cosden, 1994; Vaughn & Elbaum, 1999). However, recent research is challenging this paradigm and certainly providing evidence that the construct referred to as "self-concept" or "self-esteem" is multidimensional. Individuals view themselves differently across different domains, at different times in life, and in different situations (Eccles, 1983; Eccles & Wigfield, 1995; Elbaum & Vaughn, 2003; Wigfield, Eccles, & Pintrich, 1996). The three types of self-concept that are most often investigated in studies of individuals with LD or ADHD are academic, social, and general self-concept. As in the academic self-efficacy studies, the nature of the reference group to which individuals with LD or ADHD compare themselves influences their academic self-concept evaluation results. Researchers have provided evidence that when children or adolescents with LD or ADHD compare themselves to peers with average or high-average achievement, they rate themselves lower on self-concept scales, as compared to higher ratings when they compare themselves to low-achieving peers (Elbaum & Vaughn, 2003; Hager & Vaughn, 1995; Hoza et al., 2002, 2004). However, in two meta-analyses of the research comparing the academic self-concept ratings of children and adolescents with LD to those of their normally achieving peers, the average rating of the populations with LD was only 0.71 to 0.81 of a standard deviation (*SD*) below that of the nondisabled groups (Chapman, 1988; Prout, Marcal, & Marcal, 1992). Although differences were found, their clinical significance needs further investigation. Similar findings have been noted by researchers investigating the academic self-concept of individuals with ADHD (Barkley, 2006; Hoza et al., 2002, 2004).

The term "social self-concept" is used most often in referring to peer acceptance, self-confidence, effective copying, psychosocial well-being, and happiness (Elbaum & Vaughn, 2003). There appears to be conflicting evidence about the social self-concept symptoms of the population with LD (Berndt & Burgy, 1996; Clever, Bear, & Juvonen, 1992; Durant, Cunningham, & Voelker, 1990; Hagborg, 1999). Hoza and colleagues (2002) found that in the area of social and behavioral self-concept, individuals with ADHD appeared to give themselves lower self-ratings than those of their peers.

There is no strong evidence to indicate that adolescents or adults with LD or ADHD display lower global self-concepts than those of their nondisabled peers (Barkley, 2006; Elbaum & Vaughn, 2003; Hoza et al., 2002, 2004). Neither receiving the diagnosis of LD or ADHD nor having attended special education classes as a child appears to have a negative influence on the self-concept of these adolescents or adults (Lewandowski & Arcangelo, 1994). Indeed, some adolescents and adults with LD and ADHD do not appear to experience poor self-concept at all. Many of these individuals often compensate for their disabilities and adjust effectively to their limitations and their environments, despite the fact that their disorders do not dissipate with time. Gerber and Reiff (1991) discuss the successful adults in their study as individuals who were able to recognize, accept, and understand their disabilities; in fact, many of these individuals came to believe that their LD could be turned into a positive experience. However, it should be noted that although an LD or ADHD diagnosis does not *cause* a poor self-concept, these disorders do introduce a stress risk factor. If these individuals are not provided with adequate services and accommodations, significant stress could result in serious psychological disorders (Gleckman, 1992; Reynolds, 1999).

Motivation to Be Effective

The influence of an individual's motivation and engagement on his or her academic and psychological adjustment can constitute a significant risk or protective factor. Researchers provide strong evidence that students whose motivation is more intrinsic engage more deeply in learning activities (Wigfield & Wentzel, 2007). Therefore, motivation appears to have a direct effect on academic and social functioning (Wentzel, 1999; Wigfield, Eccles, Schiefele, Roeser, & Davis-Kean, 2006). Despite evidence that motivation or effort is critical to learning, very little research to date has examined the relationship of motivation to performance for adolescents and adults with LD and ADHD (Lackaye et al., 2006; Meltzer, Katzir, Miller, Reddy, & Roditi, 2004).

Researchers suggest that the theory of intelligence held by an individual is a key belief that is closely associated with academic motivation (Dweck, 2002). In a recent study, researchers explored the role of implicit theories of intelligence in adolescents' mathematics achievement (Blackwell, Trzesniewski, & Dweck, 2007). What these researchers found was that a belief that intelligence is malleable (an incremental theory) predicted an upward trajectory in grades. As they note, "Children's beliefs become the mental 'baggage' they bring to the achievement situation" (p. 259). The implications of this finding for at-risk learners (those with LD or ADHD) are important, as many of these individuals demonstrate negative beliefs about their own learning that have the potential to influence their effort on tasks. Some adolescents and adults with LD and ADHD also maintain preconceived perceptions that others view them as unsuccessful learners. The incremental strategy training used in the Blackwell and colleagues (2007) study is reminiscent of Steele's (1999) seminal work on the stereotype threats felt by many African Americans.

Steele and Aronson (1995), speaking about black students, use the term "stereotype threat"—which they define as a person's belief that he or she is viewed through the lens of negative stereotypes, or the fear that he or she will do something that would inadvertently confirm such a stereotype (p. 616). A stereotype threat is a situational peril causing intense and acute pressure in a person's life (Allport, 1954; Steele, 1999), and as such it may have a negative influence on performance. A great deal of cognitive and emotional energy must be expended to guard oneself against a perceived untrusting environment (e.g., a testing situation). Like many African Americans, many individuals with LD and ADHD may believe that their performance will be judged through the negative stereotypes others may have about their disabilities. The threat to self-esteem is not global, but rather specific to the situation (Crocker & Major, 1989). Many of the African American university students that Steele (1999) observed taking tests appeared to try too hard, by rereading and rechecking too many times: "Stereotype-threatened participants spent more time doing fewer items more inaccurately—probably as a result of alternating their attention between trying to answer the items and trying to assess the self-significance of their frustration"

(Steele & Aronson, 1995, p. 809). The possibility that stereotype threats may interfere with academic and social performance in adolescents and adults with LD and ADHD should not be ignored or underestimated by professionals.

Comorbidity

A diagnosis of LD or ADHD appears to place an individual at a greater risk for other, coexisting psychiatric and/or developmental disorders. Common underlying etiologies (e.g., genetic, neurological, environmental) or artifacts of methodological problems (e.g., referral bias, overlapping symptoms) are but a few of the factors contributing to the high odds of coexisting disabilities (Barkley, 2006). In a meta-analysis of research on the prevalence, causes, and effects of diagnostic comorbidity among groups of child and adolescent psychiatric disorders, Angold, Costello, and Erkanli (1999) provided estimates of such comorbidity. They investigated the relationships between and among the following disorders: ADHD, depression, anxiety, oppositional defiant disorder (ODD), and conduct disorder (CD). From their data, they concluded: "There is little evidence that any one disorder directly causes any other disorder, but it is likely that some homotypic comorbid patterns (depression with dysthymia and ODD with CD) represent developmental sequences of unitary underlying developmental psychopathologic processes (at least in some individuals)" (p. 78). Several disorders were not investigated in their research, such as LD and bipolar I disorder (BPD). Therefore, I provide additional evidence to cover these disorders, as well as to supplement the findings of Angold and colleagues (1999) with empirically based studies specific to the adult population.

Co-Occurrence of LD and ADHD

Figures on adolescents and adults who demonstrate both LD and ADHD are difficult to find, despite clinical observations and suggestions by professionals of a high correlation. There is evidence of high comorbidity between ADHD and LD in the child population; however, the exact prevalence figures depend on the eligibility criteria used by the researchers (see Barkley, 2006, for an in-depth discussion). As discussed in Chapter Two, the controversy surrounding cutoff, discrepancy, and clinical models has led to both over- and underidentification of both LD and ADHD. However, when more rigorous eligibility criteria (i.e., regression or clinical models) are applied, then approximately 8–39% of children with ADHD demonstrate LD (dyslexia), and 12–27% with ADHD dem-

102   Adolescents and Adults with Learning Disabilities and ADHD

onstrate LD (mathematics disorder) (Barkley, 2006; Semrud-Clikeman et al., 1992, 2000). Murphy, Barkley, and Bush (2002) found a greater likelihood of LD among adults with the predominant inattentive type of ADHD than among adults with no disabilities. As Angold and colleagues (1999) learned with the populations they investigated, there is no evidence in either the child or adult populations that ADHD leads to LD or that LD leads to ADHD, as once suggested by researchers (Barkley, 2006; Chadwick, Taylor, Taylor, Hepinstall, & Danckaerts, 1999; McGee & Share, 1988).

Comorbidity of LD and ADHD with Other Disorders

Generalized Anxiety Disorder

The high incidence of anxiety among individuals with LD or ADHD has been noted for some time (Biederman, Newcorn, & Sprich, 1991; Gregg, Hoy, King, Moreland, & Jagota, 1992a; Gregg et al., 1992b; Peterson, Pine, Cohen, & Brook, 2001; Tannock, 2000). According to Angold and colleagues (1999), the odds that children or adolescents with ADHD also demonstrate generalized anxiety disorder (GAD) range from 2.1 to 4.3, with a median of 3.0. Therefore, it appears that an adolescent with ADHD has about a threefold increase in the odds of also having GAD.

The prevalence of GAD in the adolescent and adult population with LD is best understood by reviewing the epidemiological longitudinal data collected through the National Collaborative Perinatal Project (Marin et al., 2007). This project involved the observation and examination of over 50,000 pregnancies in 12 cities across the United States between 1959 and 1966. In 1996, when the participants in the original study were entering middle adulthood (ages 30–37), researchers at one of the cohort sites (Providence, Rhode Island) selected to study a subsample ($n = 1,015$) of these adults with and without LD. They found that the participants with LD were almost twice as likely as their nondisabled peers to meet lifetime criteria for GAD. One of the questions Marin and colleagues (2007) investigated was whether cognitive ability was associated with the development of GAD across the lifespan. The results indicated that a 15-point (1 SD) advantage in cognitive ability was associated with a 50% reduced risk of lifetime GAD, and with an 89% and 57% reduction in risk of GAD in childhood and adolescence, respectively. Interestingly, the results were not affected by behavioral inhibition or LD. However, they do indicate that individuals with LD who demonstrate lower cognitive abilities may not have as many strategies or resources available to them to cope with life stresses. In addition, the fact that adolescents and adults with LD are almost twice as likely as nondisabled persons to experience GAD is very important for clinicians and professionals serving this population to keep in mind. Interventions and accommodations should address the stresses of growing up and living with LD.

Depressive Disorders

Elevated rates of comorbidity for ADHD and depression have been observed by many researchers. There is research evidence that 16–31% of adults with ADHD also have major depressive disorder (MDD) (Barkley, Murphy, & Kwasnik, 1996). A milder form of depression, dysthymic disorder, has also been found in 19–37% of adults with ADHD (Murphy & Barkley, 1996; Murphy et al., 2002). In their meta-analysis of comorbidity studies, Angold and colleagues (1999) found a median odds ratio of 5.5 for the co-occurrence of ADHD and MDD, with a range of 3.5–8.4. However, they also found significantly elevated comorbidity between depression and CD (mean of 6.6, with a range of 4.4–11.0) and between depression and anxiety (mean of 8.2, with a range of 5.8–12.0). Both Barkley (2006) and Fischer and colleagues (2002) raise the possibility that the presence of CD or an anxiety disorder may mediate the relationship between ADHD and MDD. In addition, since MDD and ADHD both demonstrate familial linkage, there is a strong possibility of shared etiological factors (Spencer, 2004).

Since very little research evidence examining the relationship between LD and MDD is available, caution must be taken at this time in drawing any conclusions. In a meta-analysis of the child and adolescent literature, Maag and Reid (2006) did not find strong comorbidity between these disorders. They did suggest that several studies identified *some* depressive symptoms (i.e., loneliness, loss of hope, poor self-concept) commonly demonstrated by the population with LD, but not enough symptoms to warrant a clinical diagnosis of MDD. Maag and Reid conclude that the significant variability across the research related to depression and LD suggests the possible presence of a moderator variable (e.g., age, SES, gender).

Epidemiological evidence is available to suggest that family disruption and low SES in early childhood increase the long-term risk for MDD (Gilman, Kawachi, Fitzmaurice, & Buka, 2003). The significant relationship of SES to the outcomes for adolescents and adults with LD is addressed in Chapter One. Therefore, researchers will need to explore this variable in relation to the occurrence of depression or depressive symptoms in the population with LD. Other researchers suggest that since adolescents with poor reading ability are more likely to experience suicidal ideation or attempts and are more likely to drop out of school than their normally achieving peers, concern over possible moderating variables is warranted (Daniel et al., 2006). However, much more sophisticated design methodologies (i.e., greater population specificity, new instruments, and more advanced statistics) need to be part of the investigation to determine the direct and indirect relationship of the many different mediating variables that have been used in studying the relationship of depression to LD in past research.

For instance, Howard and Tryon (2002) suggest that participation in special education is a risk factor for individuals with LD. However, the variables contributing to stress were examined only through ratings of the perceptions of adolescents with LD and their school guidance counselors. Simple tests of significance were used to draw conclusions about the results. The relationships of many other individual and/or environmental factors went unexamined. The factors that may indirectly or directly predict resilience require examination with more complex methodologies and designs before we can draw conclusions about the overall well-being of entire populations. However, the role of the environment (e.g., school or work placement) cannot be underestimated as a risk factor. For instance, we (Gregg et al., 1992a, 1992b) compared the Minnesota Multiphasic Personality Inventory–2 (MMPI-2) profiles of young adults with LD at a rehabilitation training center to those of a college population with LD. The individuals in the rehabilitation center demonstrated more of some symptoms of depression (i.e., social isolation, poor self-esteem, self-doubt, and restlessness) than did their peers with LD in a college setting. The college population tended to have profiles suggesting more symptoms of anxiety, as well as some other symptoms of depression (i.e., fear, obsessive thoughts, poor self-confidence, and self-criticism). Did the environment contribute directly or directly to the current well-being of these young adults? Did the severity of the disability or social status of these populations contribute directly or indirectly to well-being? Did the measurement tools capture the true feelings of these individuals? All these questions illustrate the complexity of identifying risk and protective factors.

Bipolar I Disorder

The prevalence of BPD in the child population is approximately 1%, and it is fewer than 0.4% in adults (Barkley, 2006; Lewinsohn, Klein, & Seeley, 1995; Spencer, Wilens, Biederman, Wozniak, & Harding-Crawford, 2000). Currently, there is no available research to suggest that the prevalence of BPD in persons with LD is any different from that within the general population. However, the comorbidity of ADHD with BPD is a very controversial topic throughout the psychological literature (Barkley, 2006; Carlson, 1998). Some researchers suggest that ADHD with BPD constitutes a distinct familial subtype of ADHD (Faraone et al., 1997). One of the factors leading to such confusion is that many of the symptoms of ADHD are also included in the DSM-IV-TR criteria for a manic episode. To address the issue of symptom overlap, Milberger, Biederman, Faraone, Murphy, and Tsuang (1995) used a subtraction method to remove the symptom crossover, and found that 47% of the children with both diagnoses retained this diagnosis. Therefore, it appears from this one study that about 6–10% of children with ADHD also demonstrate BPD. The implications of this child research for the adolescent or adult populations must be treated with caution. However, the combined impact of these two disorders on an adolescent or adult can be grave if they go untreated. Wilens (2004) found that those adults with ADHD who also had either CD, antisocial personality disorder, or BPD were at significantly greater risk for substance abuse.

Conduct Disorder and Oppositional Defiant Disorder

A number of child studies provide evidence of about 45–84% comorbidity of ADHD with ODD alone or with CD (Barkley, 2006; Pfiffner et al., 1999). According to Angold and colleagues (1999) in their meta-analysis of comorbidity studies, a median odds ratio of 10.7 (with a range of 7.7–14.8) exists between ADHD and CD/ODD. Some researchers suggest that the combination of ADHD + CD represents a unique disorder, separate from ADHD or CD alone (Barkley, 2006).

Approximately 17–35% of adults with ADHD also demonstrate considerably high comorbidity with ODD or CD (Barkley, 2006; Spencer, 2004). Such a combination appears to put an adolescent or adult at greater risk for substance dependence or abuse (Barkley, 2006; Wilens, 2004). Some researchers have also identified an overrepresentation of adolescents and adults demonstrating both ADHD and antisocial personality disorder in prison populations (Eyestone & Howell, 1994; Rasmussen, Almik, & Levander, 2001). The outcomes for adolescence and adults with combined ADHD and ODD or CD appear to include higher rates of suicide and school dropout, poorer employment records, and overall poorer adaptive functioning (see Barkley, 2006, for an in-depth discussion).

Obsessive–Compulsive Disorder

Peterson and colleagues (2001) suggest a strong comorbidity of ADHD and obsessive–compulsive disorder (OCD) in a study where they followed 976 children into adulthood to examine the relationship among

ADHD, OCD, and tic disorders. According to Barkley (2006), this finding has not been borne out in longitudinal studies of individuals from
childhood into adulthood. He suggests that there is only about a 3–5%
co-occurrence of the two disorders. However, Barkley also concludes
from his review of the literature that the inverse of this finding is different: The available research evidence indicates that 6–33% of children
with OCD may have ADHD (Barkley, 2006; Brown, 2000).

Nonverbal LD and Autism Spectrum Disorders

Adolescents and adults who experience significant difficulties with social
interaction have received the attention of professionals across the disciplines of psychiatry, neurology, neuropsychology, speech/language,
and special education for many years. However, Rourke (1989, 1995)
reminds us that individuals diagnosed with many different psychiatric
and developmental syndromes demonstrate deficits in social cognition.
For instance, individuals with a hydrocephalic condition, lymphocytic
leukemia, acquired right-hemisphere disorders, Turner syndrome, fragile X syndrome, schizoid personality disorder, or Williams syndrome all
demonstrate difficulty in processing nonverbal information that leads
to difficulty with social performance. In recent years, professionals have
directed a great deal of attention to three types of social cognition disorders: high-functioning autism (HFA), Asperger syndrome, and nonverbal LD (NLD). Ongoing investigation of whether a valid distinction
among these three disorders can be supported by empirical research is
very important, particularly in relation to early diagnosis, sensitive diagnostic criteria, interventions, and accommodations.

In a review of the literature, Macintosh and Dissanayake (2004)
provide strong evidence that there are insufficient data to establish the
validity of Asperger syndrome as a disorder distinct from HFA or NLD.
These authors agree with other researchers, however, that even though
no clear consensus or empirical data can separate the groups, it would
be premature to claim that all three represent one disorder (Szatmari,
1998, 2000; Volkmar & Klin, 2000). Determining the overlap and/or
specificity of NLD, Asperger syndrome, HFA, schizoid personality disorder, and semantic–pragmatic disorder—all disorders affecting social
cognition—will require a great deal more research using sophisticated
methodologies to investigate the direct and indirect influence of biological and environmental factors across the lifespan (Gillberg, 1992, 1998;
Gillberg & Ehlers, 1998; Klin, McPartland, & Volkmar, 2005; Macintosh
& Dissanayake, 2004; Szatmari, 1998; Volkmar & Klin, 2000).

Nonverbal Learning Disabilities

Johnson and Myklebust (1967; see also Myklebust, 1975) originally coined the term "NLD" to refer to individuals with LD who demonstrated significant social cognition deficits in addition to academic underachievement, primarily in the areas of spelling and mathematics. Later Rourke (1989) built upon their initial theories and provided empirical research to support the validity of the construct. Since that time, researchers have made several attempts to investigate the characteristics of adolescents and adults with NLD (Gunter, Ghaziuddin, & Ellis, 2002; Klin et al., 2005; Klin, Sparrow, Volkmar, Cicchetti, & Rourke, 1995; Lincoln, Courchesne, Allen, Hanson, & Ene, 1998; Rourke, 1995).

The neuropsychological profile emerging from the available research indicates that individuals with NLD demonstrate difficulty with the following cognitive, social, and achievement abilities: tactile perception; psychomotor skills; adapting to novel information; visual–spatial skills; visual perception; attention; tactile, nonverbal, and visual memory; and orthographic awareness. Moreover, they exhibit a disparity between memory for rote material and memory for complex material and/or material that is not readily coded in a verbal fashion. In addition, significant deficits are observed in executive functioning (i.e., concept formation, problem solving, strategy formation, hypothesis testing, and appreciation of informational feedback). As a result of these cognitive deficits, individuals with NLD are primarily academically limited in the areas of math and written language (spelling and organization). However, several social cognition symptoms (e.g., perspective taking, empathy, and risk taking) appear to seriously limit the overall adaptive functioning of individuals with NLD. This population also appears to be at risk for anxiety, depression, and dissociative disorders. Mary, introduced at the opening of this chapter, is an adult for whom social and work environments are extremely stressful as a result of many of the symptoms specific to the population with NLD.

Individuals with NLD are often described as demonstrating weaknesses with nonverbal communication but strengths with verbal communication. Such a characterization of this population's abilities is inaccurate and often misleading. Over the years, clinicians report that individuals with NLD appear to have an uncommon reliance on language as a primary tool of adaptation, despite the fact that they often use language ineffectively (Johnson & Myklebust, 1967; Myklebust, 1975). Recognition of the interaction between thought and language provides us with a better understanding of the communication abilities of this population. In particular, what influence does language have on the ability of persons with NLD to utilize self-regulation in a problem-solving situation? Barkley's (2006) discussion of the self-regulation deficits that are hallmarks of ADHD provides an excellent framework for thinking about the communication abilities of individuals with NLD: Individuals with ADHD and NLD both demonstrate significant limitations when executive functioning is required.

Observing the dialogic speech patterns of adolescents or adults with NLD provides professionals with an ecologically sound means of examining these individuals' overdependence on language in solving problems and making decisions. Russian psychologist Lev Vygotsky (1962) viewed all forms of higher mental functions as the results of internalized social relationships. Accordingly, Vygotsky believed that interpsychological processes are internalized as intrapsychological processes by means of egocentric speech, leading to inner language. One of the functions of egocentric speech and later inner language, then, is to help humans plan and regulate action. Internal dialogue and often egocentric speech are both effective self-regulative strategies many people use when a problem is difficult or emotionally loaded. For years, cognitive-behavioral researchers recommended the self-regulation strategy of verbal mediation (usually monologic scripts) as a means of helping students with LD or ADHD to solve problems.

However, the real issue for individuals with NLD is not simply verbal mediation, but dialogic rather than monologic speech functions. One of the distinctions made by Vygotsky (1962) between the two language functions (i.e., monologic and dialogic) is the reliance of dialogue on the communicative context through the use of kinetic cues. Vygotsky felt that abbreviation is the semiotic mechanism involved in the transition from interpsychological to intrapsychological functioning. Abbreviation refers to the explicit references reflected in our dialogue. A speaker may use explicit (nonabbreviated) cues if there is concern that the listener shares very little information about a topic. However, if a speaker determines that the listener shares a great deal of knowledge about the topic, very implicit references (abbreviated) may be provided. As less explicit cues are used during a conversation, the level of abstraction rises (Wertsch, 1985). For many adolescents and adults with NLD, the ability to take the perspective of the listener is very difficult, leading to providing too many or too few cues during conversation. Monologue, in turn, depends almost solely on language; therefore, monologue is a limited social tool. Wertsch (1985) quotes another Russian theorist, Yakubinskii, in supporting the restrictions of monologic speech acts: "If everything that we wished to express were enclosed in the formal meanings of the words we used, we would have to use many more words than we in reality use in order to express any thought. We speak only through the use of necessary hints" (p. 87). Theorists suggest that inner language is inherently dialogic (Bibler, 1984; Emerson, 1983; Ivanov, 1977; Wertsch, 1985). Therefore, regulative speech acts initially develop on the interpsychological (social) level and then are mirrored on the intrapsychological plane. It is clear, then, that cognitive and linguistic deficits affecting the acquisition of social skills would lead to difficulties in regulating one's own behavior.

A colleague and I (Gregg & Jackson, 1989) conducted a qualitative study investigating the speech patterns of adults with NLD, particularly their patterns of communicating with others. We found that adults with NLD demonstrated four clearly restricted language patterns: monologic rather than dialogic speech acts; disorganized oral language; overdependence on rehearsed stories; and difficulty in using inner language as a self-regulatory tool. The data provided evidence that for these adults with NLD, constant monologic speech acts served as a problem-solving mechanism.

Dialogic speech requires the use of kinetic cues, abbreviated linguistic codes, and a sensitivity to one's audience. The cognitive processing deficits of persons with NLD appear to have a negative impact on their ability to pick up on or give back kinetic cues, thereby forcing them to depend more on monologic speech patterns. It is possible that automatic sensory–attention deficits could be influencing their communication competency, leading to serious difficulty in regulating behavior or solving problems. Vygotsky (1962) proposed that individual linguistic and cognitive competencies emerge from social interaction. More empirically based research is needed to explore the relationship between social role taking (dialogue) and cognition as it pertains to individuals with NLD, as well as those with Asperger syndrome, and HFA. Certainly the Gregg and Jackson (1989) study provides evidence that the breakdown in social role taking in adults with NLD significantly influences their communicative and problem-solving abilities.

Autism Spectrum Disorders

According to Yeargin-Allsopp and colleagues (2003), the prevalence of autism spectrum disorders (ASD) increased 10-fold since the early 1990s, and from 1 to 6 of every 1,000 Americans suffer from ASD. The Autism Society of America estimates that over $90 billion a year of the U.S. economy is directed toward diagnosis and intervention for the population with ASD. In particular, students with HFA have only recently begun to receive attention, and so there is a general interest in the availability of services, appropriate educational placements, and vocational training for these individuals.

The ASD in general are severe developmental disorders character-ized by major difficulties in social interaction, as well as restricted and unusual patterns of interest and behavior (Shea & Mesibov, 2005). More severe forms of autism, and some other ASD, are accompanied by mental retardation; HFA and Asperger syndrome are the two high-functioning forms of ASD. Adolescents with these high functioning ASD present a special challenge in the general educational milieu, particularly as they enter secondary and postsecondary settings (Howlin, 2003).

The DSM-IV-TR (American Psychological Association, 2000) estab-lishes specific criteria for diagnosing Asperger's disorder and autistic disorder (as Asperger syndrome and autism are termed in the manual), although there is strong evidence that the criteria for Asperger's dis-order will soon need to be revised (Macintosh & Dissanayake, 2004; Szatmari, 2000; Volkmar & Klin, 2000; Wing, 2000). Both disorders, however, involve difficulty with social understanding as the result of neurobiological networks that process information differently from those of normally achieving individuals (Rourke, 1989). Individuals with HFA or Asperger syndrome certainly do not demonstrate a homo-geneous set of characteristics, and the interaction of context, history, and temperament certainly must be examined for each person (Klin et al., 2005). One individual may appear more isolated and introverted, while another may seem more extroverted and eccentric. However, the core impairments in both disorders are in social interaction and reci-procity (Asperger, 1944; Wing, 2000).

The most common characteristics associated with HFA include (1) impairment in social learning, (2) difficulty with the ambiguity and pragmatics of language, (3) rigidity of thinking, (4) preoccupation with special interests or objects, and (5) increased psychological and emo-tional disorders (Wetherby & Prizant, 2001). In contrast to HFA, where preoccupations are more likely to be with objects or parts of objects, in Asperger syndrome the preoccupying interests appear most often to be specific intellectual areas (e.g., obsessive interest in math or history). Communication and cognitive development are often used as markers to distinguish between autism (including HFA) and Asperger syndrome. According to DSM-IV-TR, individuals diagnosed with autistic disorder must show qualitative impairments and/or delays in communication and cognitive delay prior to age 3, whereas this requirement is not made for Asperger's disorder (American Psychiatric Association, 2000). The dis-tinction between HFA and Asperger syndrome becomes more difficult to determine as individuals reach middle and high school, however.

The DSM-IV-TR treats autistic disorder and Asperger's disorder as two distinct syndromes, and does not include separate criteria for HFA. Research using either empirical subgrouping or comparative methodologies has not been able to provide evidence to establish the validity of Asperger syndrome as distinct from HFA, particularly in the adolescent and adult populations (see Macintosh & Dissanayake, 2004, for a meta-analysis of the literature). What does appear to differentiate the two groups across methodologies is the severity rather than the specificity of the disabilities, as well as the level of adaptive functioning (Fein et al., 1999; Klin et al., 2005).

The DSM-IV-TR (American Psychiatric Association, 2000) suggests that specific cognitive, language, social, and adaptive functioning symptoms will provide professionals with evidence to differentiate between Asperger's disorder and autistic disorder. However, while these symptoms are part of the diagnostic criteria, they are not always supported by empirical evidence. According to the research reviews of Macintosh and Dissanayake (2004) and Klin and colleagues (2005), no conclusive evidence is available to differentiate the two groups on comorbidity; language/communication functioning; cognitive and neuropsychological profiles; executive functioning; social-cognitive abilities; motor skills; biological and other etiological factors; epidemiology, onset, and prognosis; restricted and repetitive ritual behaviors and interests; or social behavior. Macintosh and Dissanayake suggest that it appears "that identified differences may be more pronounced during the first years of life than during middle childhood or later" (p. 431). Interestingly, Szatmari (1998, 2000) suggests that Asperger syndrome and HFA may begin as two different developmental trajectories that have the potential to converge as individuals reach adolescence and adulthood.

Regardless of how the Asperger–HFA controversy is eventually resolved, Asperger syndrome, HFA, and NLD are all self-regulatory disorders similar to ADHD. Individuals with all three diagnoses demonstrate problems with self-regulation, pragmatics, executive processing, cognitive flexibility, social perception, processing speed, and academic fluency, although some differences may exist among these disorders. Professionals must be sensitive during the diagnostic process to the possible presence of one of these syndromes, as well as to possible comorbidity with still other disorders.

Assessment of Social, Emotional, and Behavioral Functioning

The assessment of adolescents and adults suspected of demonstrating LD or ADHD requires careful examination of behavioral, social, and emotional functioning. Although an individual may report concern about difficulty with reading, for example, the problem may have many different sources (e.g., lack of instruction, ADHD, LD, motivation, effort). Therefore, a comprehensive evaluation is necessary to consider all factors that might influence learning (e.g., anxiety, depression), as well as to clarify possible comorbidities. Because the ultimate goal of an evaluation for the adolescent and/or adult population is the identification of effective interventions and accommodations, a thorough investigation of cognitive, linguistic, emotional, and achievement abilities is essential to decision making. However, as Barkley and Edwards (2006) note, "The evaluation itself is a process driven by the issues that must be addressed, not necessarily by the methods with which the clinician is most comfortable" (p. 365).

To ensure that all factors are considered in the diagnostic decision making, an examiner should gather information from many different sources. Multiple informants (parents, teachers, significant others, other professionals), multiple sources (interviews, case histories, self-reports, third-party reports, psychological testing), and multiple settings provide the essential information for making accurate decisions. Throughout the chapters of this text that relate to domains of academic learning (Chapters Five through Seven), I suggest gathering specific diagnostic information that is important to a better understanding of the difficulties individuals with LD or ADHD may demonstrate in learning. The purpose of the present section is to review some of the methods and instruments commonly used in the diagnosis of behavioral (e.g., attention), social, and emotional functioning, with a special focus on their strengths and limitations when used with adolescents and adults.

Direct Observation and Interviewing

A structured or semistructured interview is an integral part of a comprehensive evaluation (Barkley & Edwards, 2006). Information from ratings by others, self-report instruments, and observation can be further refined through interviews. Barnett and Zucker (1990) identify three specialized ways in which an assessment interview can be used: as a formal diagnostic technique, as a method to study private experiences, and as a data-gathering technique critical to the assessment–accommodation process. However, clinical interviews have relatively low reliability and validity, compared to norm-referenced measures (Barkley & Edwards, 2006). The low reliability and validity are the results of inherent interviewer bias, due to the interviewer's own values, training orientation, and interviewing skills. Therefore, while very important, the clinical interview is only one piece of information used in decision making. A clinical interview should never be the sole source of data used for a diagnosis of LD or ADHD.

Observation of individual performance across settings, tasks, and examiners provides information that is extremely important for diagnostic decision making. However, observational data are also not solely sufficient for making a diagnosis or for identifying effective accommodations. The purpose of an observation is to confirm the presence of specific behaviors across settings. This might be accomplished by recording occurrence of the behaviors with such techniques as time or event sampling. Careful recording of behaviors and the use of established observational techniques will help make the results more reliable, as well as facilitate communication of the data to other professionals. However, observational information, similar to interviewing data, provides less reliable or valid data than norm-referenced instruments do (Barkley & Edwards, 2006; Hoy & Gregg, 1994).

Self-Report Scales

Self-report instruments are often used during a comprehensive evaluation to investigate symptoms of ADHD, LD, anxiety, depression, substance abuse, eating disorders, CD, or thought disorders. Some self-report measures are designed to be simply screeners, while others are considered comprehensive measures of a construct. It is not the purpose of this chapter to include a critique of all the available social, emotional, and behavioral self-report assessment tools. Rather, a few instruments have been chosen to illustrate some limitations of self-report measures for adolescents or adults with possible LD or ADHD.

Professionals are strongly encouraged to examine the validity and reliability of self-report measures, the number of test items used to measure a construct, the reading demands, the linguistic complexity of item questions, the norm sample, and any available measurement equivalence research specific to the population with LD or ADHD. In addition, very little available measurement invariance research pertaining to social or emotional measures used with adolescents or adults is available to provide examiners the information necessary to interpret test results for the populations with LD and ADHD. Therefore, the scores from these measures should be interpreted cautiously, and information from clinical interviews, case histories, and observations should support results from psychometric scores. See Chapter Three for a review of why professionals should be concerned about measurement equivalence research prior to interpreting test results.

Clinicians must also take great care in reviewing the number and complexity of items on a self-report measure. For individuals with LD, difficulties in reading items can influence their responses, and this can result in invalid measurement of their abilities. Information about the item readability and/or linguistic complexity of items is rarely provided in the technical manuals of ADHD or social/emotional self-report tests. In addition, none of the computer-based self-report measures available to professionals are currently accessible through the use of screen readers. For the adolescent and adult populations with ADHD, a self-report measure such as the MMPI-2 requires the examinees to sustain attention for a very long time; therefore, it is important for the clinician to determine whether the results of such measures may reflect attention problems rather than other types of psychological stress.

Another important issue to consider in using any self-report measure is the instrument's degree of sensitivity (identification of target group) and specificity (avoidance of false positives) for measuring a specific construct (e.g., anxiety, ADHD). A colleague and I (Coleman & Gregg, 2004) investigated two self-report measures—the Adult Reading History Questionnaire (ARHQ; Lefly & Pennington, 2000) and the Adult Version of the Brown Attention-Deficit Disorder (ADD) Scales (Brown, 1996)—to illustrate the importance of examining the sensitivity and specificity of an instrument used for diagnostic decision making.

All of the participants were university students who completed a comprehensive psychological evaluation. The ARHQ and Brown ADD Scales were not part of the evaluation or used in any way to determine diagnoses. Four groups of students were administered the self-report scales: group 1 ($n = 106$) demonstrated LD (dyslexia); group 2 ($n = 83$) demonstrated ADHD; group 3 ($n = 23$) received diagnoses of both LD (dyslexia) and ADHD; and group 4 ($n = 65$) received no diagnosis of either a psychiatric or a developmental disorder.

The ARHQ (Lefly & Pennington, 2000), a revised version of the Reading History Questionnaire (Finucci, Isaacs, Whitehouse, & Childs, 1982), is a self-report questionnaire designed to screen for dyslexia. The total score is based on 23 items presented in a Likert format. The reported characteristics of the measure include reliability of .92–.94 (internal) and .81–.84 (test–retest); sensitivity of 81.8%; and specificity of 77.5%. The authors claim that, along with SES and intelligence (24% of variance), the ARHQ explains 51% of the variance in the reading quotient. Table 4.1 provides the reader with the number and percentage of groups scoring above two cutoffs on the ARHQ: the cutoff score recommended in Lefly and Pennington (2000), and the cutoff score based on our (Coleman & Gregg, 2004) discriminant analysis. Of 231 examinees, 173 scored above the ARHQ cutoff score (only 93 were diagnosed with LD). When the original cutoff score (36.8) was used with the clinic population, the ARHQ provided good sensitivity (84%) but poor

TABLE 4.1. Use of Different Cutoff Scores on the Adult Reading History Questionnaire (ARHQ; Lefly & Pennington, 2000) with Four Groups of Students

| | ARHQ cutoff score | | | |
| | 36.8[a] | | 45.5[b] | |
Group	n	%	n	%
1: Dyslexia (*n* = 92)	75	81.5	59	64.1
2: ADHD (*n* = 69)	52	75.4	32	46.4
3: Dyslexia + ADHD (*n* = 21)	20	95.2	19	90.5
4: No disability (*n* = 49)	26	53.1	10	20.4
1 + 3: All dyslexia (*n* = 113)	95	84.1	78	69.0
2 + 4: All no dyslexia (*n* = 118)	78	66.1	42	35.6

[a]Cutoff score recommended in Lefly and Pennington (2000).
[b]Cutoff score based on Coleman and Gregg (2004) discriminant analysis.

specificity (34%). To increase specificity (to 64%) in a clinical setting of college students, we (Coleman & Gregg, 2004) suggest that professionals use a higher cutoff score (45.5), which corresponds with better sensitivity (69%).

Several researchers suggest that the Brown ADD Scales (Brown, 1996) do not provide strong specificity results (Hatcher, Snowling, & Griffiths, 2002; Rucklidge & Tannock, 2002). In fact, Hatcher and colleagues (2002) state:

> According to the published norms for this test, a total score of above 55 is thought to indicate a diagnosis of `ADD highly probable'. It is interesting to note that the Total scores . . . fell in the clinical range for both our dyslexia (mean score = 72) and a control group (mean score = 60). These data lead us to doubt the appropriateness of the norms for UK [university] students. (p. 21)

The reported characteristics of the measure as provided in the test manual include reliability of .79–.92 (internal) and .87 (test–retest on only an adolescent sample); a norm sample of 285 adults (142 were clinical); sensitivity of 96%; and specificity of 94%.

Table 4.2 provides our (Coleman & Gregg, 2004) findings on the sensitivity and specificity of the Brown ADD Scales for a group of college students. Of 218 subjects, 200 scored in the "ADD probable" or "ADD highly probable" range. However, only 103 participants received a clinical diagnosis of ADHD. When the suggested Brown ADD Scales cutoff score (>54) was used with this group of college students, the instruments provided good sensitivity (80%) but poor specificity (51%). Therefore,

TABLE 4.2. Use of Different Cutoff Scores on the Brown ADD Scales (Brown, 1996) with Four Groups of Students

Group	Brown cutoff score			
	>54[a]		>63[b]	
	n	%	n	%
1: Dyslexia (n = 71)	40	56.3	30	42.3
2: ADHD (n = 81)	64	79.0	53	65.4
3: Dyslexia + ADHD (n = 22)	18	81.9	15	68.2
4: No disability (n = 44)	21	47.7	14	31.8
2 + 3: All ADHD (n = 103)	82	79.6	68	66.0
1 + 4: All no ADHD (n = 125)	61	48.8	44	35.2

[a]Cutoff score recommended in Brown (1996).
[b]Cutoff score based on Coleman and Gregg (2004) discriminant analysis.

both the Brown ADD Scales and the ARHQ provide good sensitivity but poor specificity with a population of 275 college students seeking evaluation for possible LD or ADHD. Professionals are always strongly encouraged to examine the sensitivity, specificity, and norm population of a self-report measure to help in the interpretation of scores. It should be noted that both the Brown ADD Scales and the ARHQ were developed with very small and restricted norm samples.

Third-Party Rating Instruments

A third-party rating instrument is similar in its strengths and weaknesses to the self-report instruments discussed previously. However, on a third-party measure, another adult (parent, teacher, significant other) rates the examinee on specific constructs. Because it is essential in making an ADHD diagnosis to obtain the observations of persons who see an individual in situations outside a clinical setting, third-party rating scales are critical to the identification of specific symptoms. Almost all ADHD measures include both self-report and third-party versions.

The Behavior Assessment System for Children—Second Edition (Reynolds & Kamphaus, 2004) is a commonly used battery of third-party scales for rating a range of child and adolescent behaviors. Another popular third-party behavioral battery is the Achenbach System of Empirically Based Assessment (Achenbach & Rescorla, 2001). Both of these batteries demonstrate strong construct validity across a range of social/emotional and behavioral (e.g., attention) abilities. However, no measurement invariance research is available with either battery specific to adolescents with LD or ADHD.

Cognitive Tests for Assessing ADHD

As with self-report measures, cognitive tests for ADHD often exhibit stronger sensitivity than specificity. An example of this issue is the Conners' Continuous Performance Test II (CPT II; Conners & Multi-Health Systems Staff, 2000), one of the most widely used cognitive tasks for the diagnosis of ADHD (Gordon et al., 2006; Riccio, Reynolds, & Lowe, 2001). Although the CPT II can detect inattention, it cannot specify the cause for the inattention (e.g., illness, medication, ADHD). For an in-depth review of the validity of the CPT II and other related neuropsychological measures in the diagnosis of ADHD, see Riccio and colleagues (2001).

There is much professional debate about the specificity and effectiveness of neuropsychological tools in the diagnosis of ADHD (Barkley & Edwards, 2006; Gordon et al., 2006; Murphy & Gordon, 2006; Riccio et al., 2001). Although cognitive measures should not be used alone in making an ADHD diagnosis, they do provide an examiner with important information related to the examinee's cognitive processing profile. This information can also help the clinician determine whether other comorbid disorders are influencing learning. Interestingly, a recent survey of school psychologists suggests that the majority of these professionals continue to utilize psychological tools (intelligence measures), self-report tests, third-party measures, and interviews in the diagnosis of ADHD, but that they rarely administer neuropsychological measures—particularly those targeting executive functioning (Koone, 2007). There is also significant variability among the methods and instruments used by these psychologists in making ADHD diagnoses. As noted in Chapter Two, to meet the ADHD documentation requirements at the postsecondary level (i.e., colleges, employment), an individual must provide the results from a comprehensive evaluation to support accommodation requests. In addition, as also discussed in Chapter Two, the documentation requirements for ADHD at the secondary level are usually not as comprehensive as those at the postsecondary level, despite the fact that the DSM-IV-TR diagnostic criteria are the eligibility criteria most often cited by psychologists and institutions as their standard for decision making.

Effort: Just What Do the Scores Tell Us?

The assessment of symptom validity or malingered cognitive performance is an area of psychological practice that is problematic from both clinical and measurement perspectives (Boone, 2007; Hartman, 2002;

Hom, 2003; Rogers, 2008). As noted for many of the other measures discussed in this chapter, symptom validity tests may be sensitive to performance, but their specificity to response bias is not as reliable. With the increase in the number of individuals with possible LD or ADHD requesting accommodations on high-stakes tests, some researchers suggest that many of these adolescents and adults are really exaggerating their cognitive problems. Other researchers suggest that problems with the construct validity of many malingering measures, an absence of a consensus criterion measure, and an item bias can overidentify malingering with these populations (Bowden, Shores, & Mathias, 2006; Frederick & Bowden, in press).

A two-alternative, forced-choice procedure is most widely employed for detecting incomplete effort or exaggeration of cognitive impairment (Gervais, Rohling, Green, & Ford, 2004; Iverson & Binder, 2000). Depending on the test, the items may include digit recognition (Allen, Conder, Green, & Cox, 1997), word recognition (Green, Allen, & Astner, 1996), and picture recognition (Tombaugh, 1996). However, Gervais and colleagues (2003) found that tests of recognition memory using digits, pictorial stimuli, or verbal stimuli resulted in very different failure rates for the population of adult claimants referred for disability. They suggest that a clinician should never rely on one measure of effort to determine whether an individual is malingering, since the types of items and the validity of these measures are questionable.

Unfortunately, tests of effort often have very poor reliability and validity (Bowden et al., 2006). In addition, no currently available research has examined the measurement invariance of these tests for the adolescent and adult populations with LD or ADHD. Three commonly used forced-choice measures of effort are the Word Memory Test (Green, 2003), the Test of Memory Malingering (Tombaugh, 1996), and the Word Reading Test (Osmon, Plambeck, Klein, & Mano, 2006). Professionals are encouraged to carefully review the types of items used on these tests, the reliability and validity of the measures, and the norm populations.

Chapters Three, Five, Six, and Seven of this book provide research evidence of the deficits many adolescents and adults with LD and ADHD exhibit in processing speed, orthographic awareness, and working memory. In fact, in Chapter Five, several of the tasks used to measure orthographic awareness are described, as well as evidence from the literature that adolescents and adults with LD and ADHD often demonstrate significant difficulty in completing such tasks. Forced-choice tasks such as Homophone/Pseudohomophone Choice (Olson, Forsberg, & Wise, 1994) or Orthographic Choice (Stanovich, West, & Cunningham, 1991) have been used extensively by researchers and clinicians in identifying

LD (dyslexia). The Colorado Perceptual Speed Test (DeFries & Baker, 1983), an orthographic fluency measure, has also been a strong predictor of dyslexia for the child and adult population. Researchers have provided evidence not only that phonemic and orthographic measures are good predictors of reading difficulties, but also that they discriminate between dyslexia and ADHD (Gregg, Coleman, Davis, Stennett, Nielson, & Knight, 2002; Gregg, Bandalos, et al., 2008). Interestingly, orthographic fluency, as measured by many of these tasks, looks very similar to the verbal forced-choice effort tasks. Although a test of effort can be very helpful during an evaluation, the lack of sensitivity requires evaluators to consider results in light of an individual's overall cognitive and linguistic profile, as well as the validity of the measure and the cutoff criterion used.

Accommodations and Interventions

Accommodations

Accommodation suggestions for specific content areas (i.e., reading, writing, mathematics, science, and foreign languages) are discussed in Chapters Five, Six, and Seven. The purpose of this section of the present chapter is to review the literature pertaining to three broad, non-domain-specific groups of accommodations that have been found to be effective for individuals with LD or ADHD alone, as well as for adolescents and adults experiencing comorbid psychiatric impairments (e.g., LD + anxiety, ADHD + depression). They include accommodations used for time management, general memory, maintaining concentration, and organization/prioritization. However, as yet there is little empirically based research supporting the effectiveness of these accommodations for the adolescent and adult populations with LD and ADHD. A great deal of the information provided here is based on the clinical observations of professionals working with these populations.

Time Management

Adolescents or adults demonstrating ADHD, LD, and comorbid psychiatric or neurological disorders often experience difficulties with time management. The management of time includes sensitivity to the passage of minutes or hours, the ability to gauge the time necessary for tasks, and the ability to anticipate activities that will occur in the future (i.e., weeks, months, years). As discussed throughout this text, difficulties with fluency, cognitive efficiency, and self-regulation often have a negative impact on academic task success for individuals with LD or ADHD.

However, time issues are not just specific to academic content domains; many of these individuals demonstrate difficulty managing time in their daily social and work environments. Professionals are encouraged to work with adolescents and adults with LD and ADHD on developing their own techniques for time management. Some strategies that may be effective include color-coding due dates for work assignments on a syllabus; developing color-coded record systems (e.g., each color representing a task, a file, or even a level of importance); and using electronic calendars (Dendy, 2006; Job Accommodation Network, 2007).

Memory

Adolescents with LD or ADHD alone, and those with comorbid psychiatric disorders, often experience problems with working and long-term memory (see Chapter Three). Such problems may cause difficulties in completing tasks, remembering personal responsibilities, or recalling daily actions or activities. Therefore, accommodations that are appropriate for these individuals include (but are not limited to) providing written instruction, allowing extra time for tasks, allowing the use of a note taker, permitting the audio- or videotaping of class lectures, and providing copies of an instructor's notes or slides. Again, an electronic device such as a voice recorder (e.g., Belcan) used with an iPod or a personal digital assistant can be carried around by an individual as a voice notepad. (See later chapters for additional technology devices effective for memory.)

Maintaining Concentration

Individuals with ADHD alone or with comorbid psychiatric disorders often experience decreased concentration, either visual or auditory, and thus may require specific accommodations for this deficit. To decrease distraction, effective accommodations include (but are not limited to) using noise-canceling headsets, providing white noise machines, relocating workspace away from visual or auditory distractors, and reducing clutter in learning or work environments.

Organization and Prioritization

Adolescents and adults with LD, ADHD, and comorbid psychiatric disorders often demonstrate difficulty with getting and staying organized, as well as with prioritizing activities for school or work. Effective accommodations for this problem might include having individuals develop color-coded record systems, such as those needed for time deficits. In addition, they might be encouraged to develop visual charts to organize activities. Electronic organizers (e.g., Inspiration) that utilize flowcharts or semantic maps are often effective means of organizing and prioritizing activities.

New advances in technology as discussed in later chapters are providing additional electronic accommodations for individuals demonstrating time, memory, and organizational problems. For example, Winnie and Hadwin (1998) developed CoNoteS2, a software system designed to support students' self-regulated academic learning. CoNoteS2 provides a scaffolding of the skills needed for studying a textbook. Embedded text and frames help a student define a task, set goals, plan, and adapt metacognitive strategies. See Winnie (2001) for an in-depth discussion of CoNoteS2.

Other Interventions

Medications

Some individuals with ADHD, or with LD and a comorbid psychiatric disorder, require medications. Central nervous system stimulant medications are the medications most commonly used to treat the symptoms of ADHD (for an in-depth discussion, see Connor, 2006). However, according to researchers, approximately 30% of individuals with ADHD do not adequately respond to these stimulants, and must be put on antidepressants and specific norepinephrine reuptake inhibitors (for an in-depth discussion, see Spencer, 2006). It is always important to remember that medications do not cure ADHD; rather, they are interventions that allow individuals to manage functional life activities (i.e., school, work, social life). An individual taking any type of medication should periodically be monitored by a psychiatrist to ensure that the medication and dosage are providing the most effective treatment.

Therapy

Little currently available research provides evidence of the effectiveness of different types of therapy for adolescents and adults with LD or ADHD. However, there is clinical agreement in the literature that these populations might benefit from nonpharmacological treatments (Barton & Fuhrmann, 1994; Murphy, 2006; Reiff & Gerber, 1995; Reynolds, 1999). Certainly the academic, social, and work frustrations frequently experienced by adolescents or adults with LD or ADHD have the potential to create significant psychological stress. As noted earlier in this chapter, anxiety and depression frequently co-occur with these disorders. In addition, dependency and alienation are experienced by some individuals with LD or ADHD, and therapy may be effective for these (Barton & Fuhrman, 1994; Gregg et al., 1992a, 1992b; Murphy, 2006; Reiff & Gerber, 1995). Research suggests, however, that cognitive-behavioral therapies or social skills training alone have not proven effective for individuals with ADHD (Pfiffner, Barkley, & DuPaul, 2006). Since so little research on effective therapies for the adolescent and adult populations with LD and ADHD is available, professionals need to be cautious in drawing any conclusions about the usefulness of different types of psychological therapies. Moreover, as with medications, counseling or therapy alone is never going to be "the" treatment. Rather, as Murphy (2006) has so aptly stated, "Multimodal treatment that combines medication, education, behavioral/self-management skills, a variety of counseling approaches, coaching, and either academic or workplace accommodations is likely to result in the best outcomes" (p. 702).

Implications for Assessment and Accommodation

✓ The social/emotional well-being and academic competence of individuals with LD and ADHD have often been studied in isolation, rather than placed in a more robust model that accounts for the direct and indirect relationship of one to the other.

✓ Many researchers investigating the social and emotional well-being of adolescents and adults with LD or ADHD use a "risk and resilience" framework.

✓ Follow-up and follow-along studies of adults with LD and ADHD provide evidence of the lifelong influence of these disabilities, but also suggest factors of resilience.

✓ The presence of a supportive adult, such as a mentor, appears to be one of the strongest protective factors for an adolescent or adult with LD or ADHD.

✓ Difficulty in self-regulating behavior and learning appears to be a significant risk factor for many individuals with LD or ADHD.

✓ LD or ADHD does not *cause* a poor self-concept, but these disorders can introduce a stress risk factor. If these individuals are not provided with adequate services and accommodations, significant stress could result in serious psychological disorders.

✓ The influence of an individual's motivation and engagement on his or her academic and psychological adjustment can constitute a significant risk or protective factor.

✓ The diagnosis of ADHD or LD appears to place an individual at a greater risk for other, coexisting psychiatric and/or developmental disorders.

✓ Three types of social cognition disorders (HFA, Asperger syndrome, and NLD) are similar to ADHD in some ways and are receiving a great deal of professional attention.

✓ Multiple informants (parents, teachers, significant others, other professionals), multiple sources (interviews, case histories, self-reports, third-party reports, psychological testing), and multiple settings provide the essential information for making accurate decisions.

✓ Clinicians must take great care in reviewing the number and complexity of items on a self-report measure. For individuals with LD, difficulties in reading items can influence their responses and can result in invalid measurement of their abilities.

✓ A very important issue to consider in using any self-report measure is the instrument's degree of sensitivity (identification of target group) and specificity (avoidance of false positives) for measuring a specific construct (e.g., anxiety, ADHD).

✓ The assessment of symptom validity or malingered cognitive performance is an area of psychological practice that is problematic from both clinical and measurement perspectives.

✓ Many adolescents and adults with LD or ADHD require accommodations for time management, general memory, maintaining concentration, and organization/prioritization.

✓ Some individuals with ADHD, or with LD and a comorbid psychiatric disorder, require medications.

✓ Little currently available research provides evidence of the effectiveness of therapy for adolescents and adults with LD or ADHD.

CHAPTER FIVE

Reading Assessment and Accommodation

Donny, a 19-year-old European American, comes from a rural farming community where he was identified as demonstrating LD in first grade. Four years ago, he was unable to pass the state reading and writing tests that are required for promotion to high school. Therefore, Donny decided to drop out of school and work as a mechanic in his hometown. He recently found out about a new technical institute where he can be trained to be a NASCAR technician. In order to be accepted, he is required to have at least a general equivalency diploma (GED). Therefore, he is going to adult basic education classes to help him prepare for taking the GED test. Vocational rehabilitation services has assisted him in obtaining an evaluation, in order for him to have the documentation required for receiving accommodations on the GED test.

Lawana is a 21-year-old African American student with a history of LD services dating back to second grade. She is currently attending a local community college. Lawana reports that despite significant difficulties with reading, she really enjoys listening to her mother read Shakespeare, the Bible, and Yeats. At no time during her schooling was she encouraged to receive an assistive technology (AT) assessment, and she was never provided alternative media (alt media) and/or AT as an accommodation.

Peter is a 19-year-old African American college freshman who achieved a very high SAT score with the accommodation of extended time. He was diagnosed with ADHD (predominantly inattentive type) in high school, but he is not taking any medications to help him manage the disorder. Currently, he is having a great deal of trouble dealing with the amount of reading required in his social science classes (e.g., history, psychology, sociology). He is seeking an evaluation to determine whether he is eligible for any accommodations that might help him with his reading and writing assignments.

A significant number of adolescent and adults with LD and ADHD demonstrate chronic reading underachievement as a result of their disabilities, influencing both their school and work outcomes (Bruck, 1992; Gregg, Coleman, Stennett, Davis, Nielsen, et al., 2002; Shaywitz, 2003; Shaywitz et al., 2003). As discussed in Chapters Two and Three, epidemiological research provides evidence of the persistence of LD in reading (i.e., dyslexia) across the lifespan, and behavioral and biological research has validated the lack of reading fluency in this population (Shaywitz, 2003). Results from evidence-based research also indicates a moderate to large discrepancy in reading performance between adolescents and adults with ADHD and their normally achieving peers (Barry, Lyman, & Klinger, 2002; Frazier, Youngstrom, Glutting, & Watkins, 2007). The profiles of Danny, Lawana, and Peter are provided to represent the heterogeneous populations of adolescents and adults with LD and ADHD demonstrating underachievement in reading. For such individuals, access to accommodations is essential to their success in today's digital learning and work environments.

Digital Learning and Work Environments

The digital, multinetworked, multitasking, constantly changing world of information and communication is redefining literacy in the 21st century (New Literacies Research Team, 2007). Online reading competencies, such as proficiency with the Internet, are now essential for success in school, social life, and the workplace. The greatest global productivity gains during the past decade in the economics of the world are due to the integration of the Internet into the workplace (Matteucci, O'Mahony, Robinson, & Zwick, 2005; van Ark, Inklaar, & McGuckin, 2003). According to Riley (2003; quoted in Leu et al., 2008, p. 321), "To thrive in the global knowledge economy, it is going to be important to change the whole educational system to ensure a wide base of knowledge workers who understand and use information technologies." However, as the RAND Reading Study Group (2003) has noted, "accessing the Internet makes large demands on individuals' literacy skill; in some cases, this new technology requires readers to have novel literacy skills, and little is known about how to analyze or teach those skills" (p. 4).

With the increasing importance of technology in our school and work environments, the critical need is for more researchers to examine the similarities and differences among the demands of offline reading (traditional reading practices), of online reading (the Internet), and of reading in other digital formats (e.g., electronic text [e-text]). Initial research in this area suggests that there is often very little correlation between offline and online reading proficiency for students with or without disabilities (Coiro & Dobler, in press; Leu & Reinking, 2005; Leu et al., in press).

An individual who is functionally limited in the area of reading standard print is currently referred to as demonstrating a "print disability." However, little consensus exists as to what categories of disabilities meet the criteria for this term. The DAISY Consortium, a group promoting the Digital Accessible Information System (DAISY) for accessible print, defines a print disability as "the inability to access print due to a visual, perceptual, or physical disability. Examples include blindness, learning disabilities, and the inability to hold a book" (DAISY Consortium, 2007, paragraph 6). Bookshare.Org, the leading alt media lender, specifies print disabilities as "visual impairments and blindness, reading disabilities, and physical impairments that make it difficult or impossible to read printed books" (Bookshare.org, 2007, paragraph 2). However, Wolfe and Lee (2007) define a print disability as "the inability to access standard print independently due to deficits in the ability to take in, process, retain, or manipulate printed text" (p. 256). Therefore, they suggest that the functional limitation (i.e., underachievement in reading), rather than any particular disability category, be the criterion used for identifying print disabilities. For instance, an adolescent or adult with ADHD whose executive processing deficits severely limit his or her reading comprehension would be considered to have a print disability under the Wolfe and Lee definition, but not under the DAISY Consortium or Bookshare.org policy. The importance of this distinction to an individual lies in the fact that it may determine whether he or she is granted access to specific accommodations (e.g., alt media, AT). Lawana (see Figure 5.1) and Donny (see Figure 5.2) are two individuals with print disabilities for whom technology has the potential to provide greater access to learning.

Our ability as professionals to serve individuals with print disabilities is going to require us to reassess our definitions of such terms as "reading," "reading assessment," "reading proficiency,"and "reading accommodations." The "new literacies" or "multiliteracies" will require us to broaden our definition of "literacy" to include both traditional print and other media (New London Group, 2000). As Alverman and

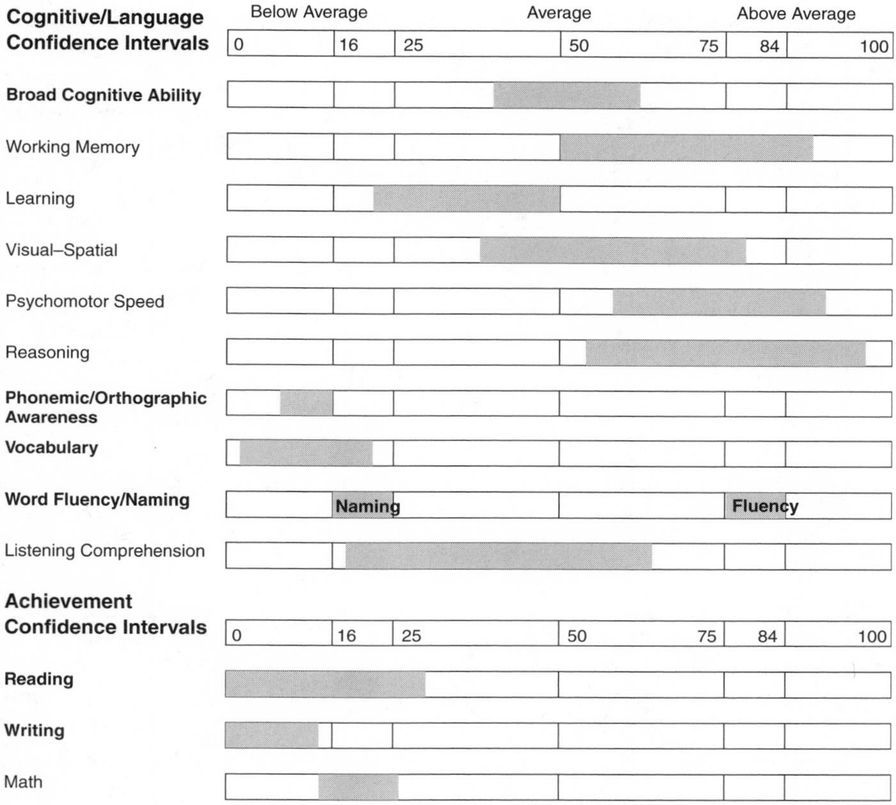

Cognitive/Language Confidence Intervals	Below Average		Average		Above Average	
	0	16	25	50	75	84	100

Broad Cognitive Ability

Working Memory

Learning

Visual–Spatial

Psychomotor Speed

Reasoning

Phonemic/Orthographic Awareness

Vocabulary

Word Fluency/Naming — Naming — Fluency

Listening Comprehension

Achievement Confidence Intervals						
	0	16	25	50	75	84	100

Reading

Writing

Math

FIGURE 5.1. Assessment profile for Lawana, an individual with dyslexia.

Rush (2004) note, the bias toward print-based literacy suggests a possible discomfort on the part of professionals with the multiple literacies (e.g., visual, digital, spatial) that our new generation of learners must utilize to gain knowledge. For adolescents and adults with LD and ADHD, these new literacies have the potential both to redefine their disabilities and to give them new ways of overcoming them.

Some researchers suggest that we "re/mediate" our thinking and practices that surround literacy (Alverman & Rush, 2004; Luke & Elkins, 2000). Reading is an increasingly interactive, nonlinear experience for many adolescents and adults (Reinking, 1998). As noted by Alverman and Rush (2004), "Teaching [and I would add evaluating] with an eye to re/mediation requires letting go of (or at the very least rethinking) some old adages" (p. 211). Unfortunately, many professionals continue to use only traditional thinking and assessment tools to predict the reading competencies needed for success in the classroom or the world of work. Yet the new literacy practices do not always align themselves with the underlying assumptions of traditional measures of assessment. Although federally mandated, standards-based monitoring of students' reading performance often depends on the use of traditional test formats, the assumption that such scores will predict performance in the literacy classroom or the work world of the future is flawed. The assessment of both "online" and "offline" reading skills provides a more valid and ecologically sound means of understanding an individual's reading profile.

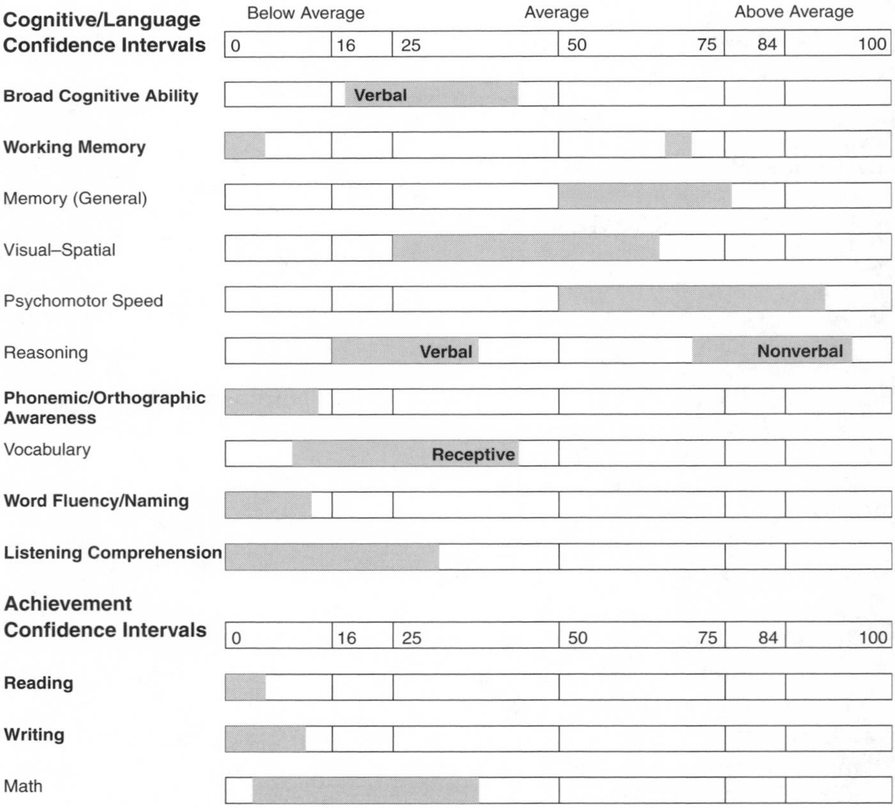

FIGURE 5.2. Assessment profile for Donny, an individual with dyslexia.

Cognitive and Linguistic Processes Influencing Reading Decoding Performance

Knowledge of current research related to the cognitive and linguistic factors influencing the reading performance of adolescents and adults with LD and/or ADHD is critical from the perspectives of both assessment and accommodation. However, the majority of research in this area pertains to individuals with LD in reading (dyslexia). Professionals are left to infer from this research how the deficits in executive functioning, working memory, attention, metacognition, and oral language that are common among the populations with ADHD and with other types of LD may directly or indirectly influence their reading performance. The sources of academic underachievement differ both across and within the populations with LD and ADHD, and this heterogeneity requires careful professional attention during the assessment and accommodation decision-making process. Figure 5.3 provides important questions for an evaluator to answer during the process of selecting effective accommodations for adolescents or adults with LD or ADHD. In-depth discussions of each step, and of methods for assessing and determining appropriate accommodations for individuals with problems at each step, follow in the next few sections of the chapter.

Prior Exposure to Print

A reader's ability to read fluently is influenced by such factors as text purpose, content familiarity, world knowledge, reading experiences, and graphic presentation of the text (Black & Watts, 1993; Just & Carpenter, 1987; Rayner, 1978; Tufte,1990). Prior exposure to print has been shown to significantly predict reading decoding abilities (Stanovich & Cunningham, 1993; Stanovich & West, 1989; West, Stanovich, & Mitchell, 1993). Therefore, a reader's prior exposure to and experiences with print are important factors to consider in investigating reading performance.

Print exposure is sometimes measured by using questionnaires to determine a person's reading habits. For instance, Stanovich and West (1989) developed the Prior Exposure to Print Questionnaires to investigate a reader's familiarity with authors, magazines, and newspapers. According to Stanovich and West, "knowledge of [an] author's name was a proxy for reading activities even though the particular author had not been read" (1989, p. 813). However, a difficulty with many exposure-to-print questionnaires is their bias toward a reader's experiences with conventional prose. Although many adolescents or adults with LD or ADHD are required to read traditional prose in educational settings, they also must be proficient in reading other types of text, particularly

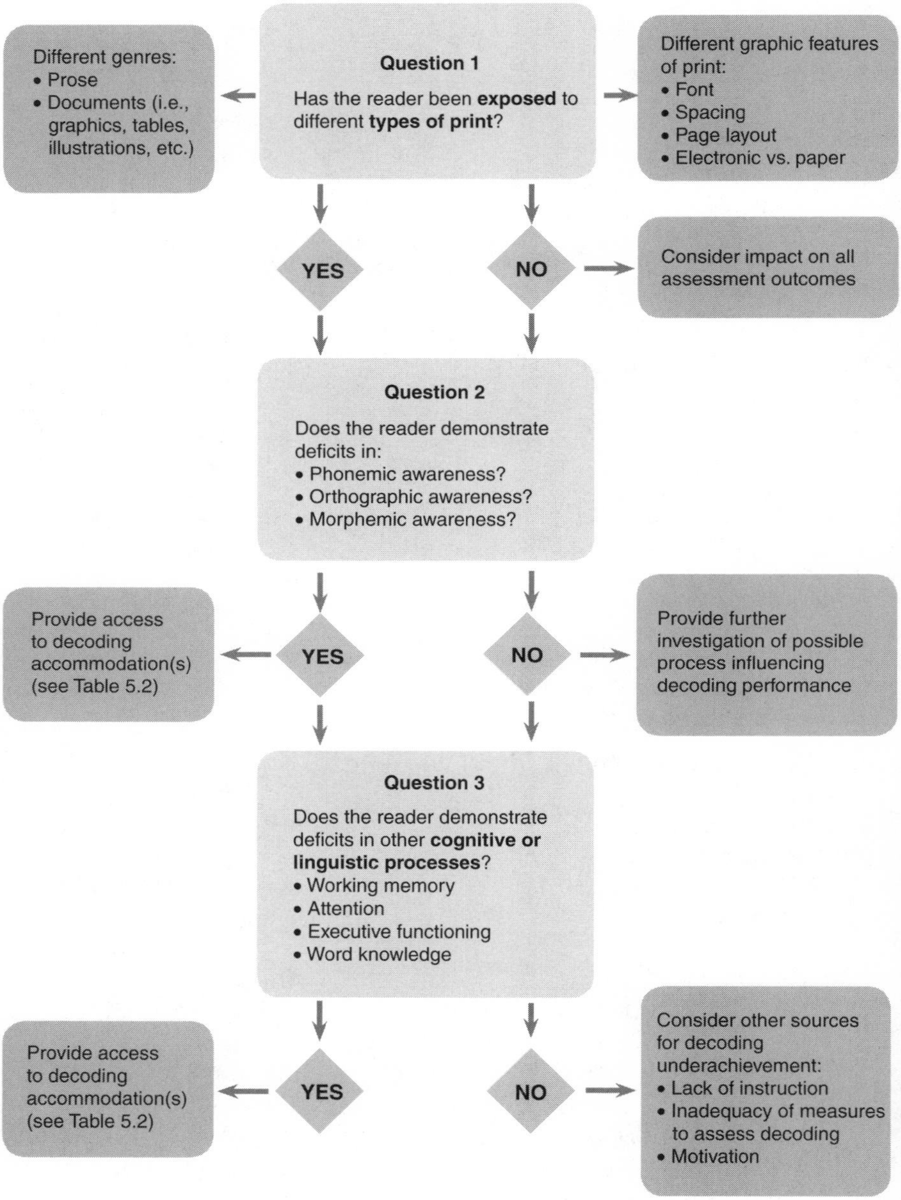

FIGURE 5.3. Questions to support decision making for the accommodation of reading decoding problems.

"documents"—which, in this context, include graphs, tables, illustrations, and the like. According to Guthrie, Weber, and Kimmerly (1993), "Documents distribute information efficiently by presenting information in a format that can be searched without reading the entire content" (p. 189). Such noncontinuous reading is more similar to reading online (i.e., on the Internet). Cohen and Snowden (2008) investigated the document literacy of adult readers by examining the relationships between familiarity and frequency of experiences with, and proficiency in reading, documents. They found that a reader's familiarity and frequency of experiences with documents strongly influenced proficiency. In addition, the Cohen and Snowden study provides evidence that proficiency with the document genre requires familiarity with a different set of strategies from those involved in prose reading. Therefore, an adolescent or adult's success with different types of text (e.g., prose vs. documents) or cybernetic environments requires the flexible use of different literacy strategies.

A reader's exposure to different graphic elements and features of print can also influence reading performance. As Samuels (1982) noted: "In general, physical characteristics of a text can influence speed, comprehension, eye movement, and reading strategies implemented, but these effects are not noticeable with experienced readers who can adopt reading strategies to match design" (p. 231). Stone, Fisher, and Eliot (1999) found that graphic elements had a decided effect on a reader's fluency, accuracy, and choice of strategy. They examined the effects of font, justification (full vs. left), line spacing (single- versus double-space), and mode (paper vs. computer), and found that a reader's prior exposure to different graphic features significantly predicted reading fluency. The importance of graphic print exposure and preference should be considered by professionals working to help adolescents and adults with LD or ADHD access a variety of print and digital text.

Phonemic, Orthographic, and Morphemic Awareness

The persistence of phonemic, orthographic, and morphemic awareness deficits among the adolescent and adult population demonstrating dyslexia has been repeatedly documented in the literature (Berninger et al., 2006; Bruck, 1993; Gregg, Coleman, Stennett, Davis, Nielsen, et al., 2002; Hatcher et al., 2002; Holmes & Castles, 2001). In contrast, researchers have provided scant empirical data about the phonemic, orthographic, and morphemic awareness abilities of adolescents and adults with ADHD. Given the high comorbidity of LD and ADHD, an investigation of the influence of linguistic and attention deficits is critical to a better understanding of reading in both these populations.

Phonemic Awareness

The phonemic awareness performance of adolescents and adults with dyslexia has demonstrated the ability to predict reading decoding performance (Bruck, 1993; Gregg, Coleman, Stennett, Davis, Nielsen, et al., 2002; Hatcher et al., 2002). "Phonemic awareness" has been defined as "the explicit awareness that is needed to segment, identify, and manipulate the phonemes in words" (Westby, 2002, p. 73). Bruck (1993) conducted research investigating the phonemic awareness of young adults with documented dyslexia. As a group, they overrelied on spelling–sound information, syllabic information, and context for word recognition. Bruck's research also documented that phoneme counting (nondigraph items) and phoneme deletion continued to be areas of deficit for this adult population as compared to their peers. The decoding errors demonstrated by individuals with phonemic awareness deficits often represent "phonetically implausible" letter and word choices. These readers often perform very poorly on pseudoword (nonsense-word) reading measures, such as the Woodcock–Johnson III Tests of Achievement (WJ III ACH) Word Attack subtest (Woodcock et al., 2001a).

Adolescents and adults with ADHD appear to present a different profile in relation to the predictive strength of phonemic awareness tasks for reading decoding performance. We (Gregg, Coleman, Stennett, Davis, Nielsen, et al., 2002) found that young adults with ADHD performed significantly better than students with dyslexia on tasks of sound and syllable segmentation, phonemic localization, and phonological segmentation. Moreover, examiners must keep in mind the high demands on attention made by such tasks: Low performance on a phonemic awareness measure for some readers with ADHD might suggest difficulty with attention rather than a linguistic deficit.

Orthographic Awareness

"Orthographic awareness" is defined as "the ability to represent the unique array of letters that define a printed word, as well as the general attributes of the writing system such as segmentation dependencies, structural redundancies, and letter position frequencies" (Vellutino, Scanlon, & Chen, 1994, p. 56). Unfortunately, orthographic awareness has not received the attention that phonemic awareness has in the literature, particularly with the adolescent and adult populations (Berninger, 1994; Foorman, 1994; Roberts & Mather, 1997). Yet researchers provide strong evidence that orthographic awareness significantly influences the ability to decode words (Cunningham & Stanovich, 1990; Kim, Taft, & Davis, 2004; Stanovich & West, 1989). Empirical evidence demonstrates that orthographic processing is a separate latent construct from phonological processing in the adult population (Carr & Posner, 1994; Eviatar, Ganayim, & Ibrahim, 2004; Gregg, Bandalos, et al., 2008; Rumsey, Donohue, Nace, Maisong, & Andreason, 1997). However, as Foorman (1994) notes, "although orthographic and phonological processing can be dissociated statistically, they are conceptually intertwined" (p. 321).

Some individuals with dyslexia demonstrate problems with both phonemic and orthographic awareness. However, the reading decoding errors of individuals demonstrating difficulty specific to orthographic processing are usually "phonetically plausible," meaning that these readers appear to overrely on their phonological abilities. Such readers may accurately represent the sounds in target words that have direct sound–symbol correspondence (e.g., "cat"), but may be unable to recall unusual or irregular sequences of letters that cannot be sounded out (e.g., "yacht"). Readers with stronger phonemic than orthographic awareness often perform better on tests of pseudoword reading (e.g., the WJ III ACH Word Attack subtest, the Wechsler Individual Achievement Test—Second Edition [WIAT-II; Wechsler, 2001] Pseudoword subtest) than on tasks involving the reading of regular words (e.g., the WJ III ACH Letter–Word Identification subtest, the WIAT-II Word Reading subtest). Therefore, an examiner should always administer measures including both pseudoword and regular-single-word reading.

Readers with ADHD often perform significantly better than their peers with dyslexia on phonemic and orthographic awareness tasks, with the exception of tasks tapping orthographic fluency (Gregg, Coleman, Stennett, Davis, Nielsen, et al., 2002). This pattern is well illustrated if we look at Peter's profile (Figure 5.4). His orthographic fluency performance is the only phonemic or orthographic ability that is below average. Peter's reading performance reflects the influence of his difficulties with fluency and cognitive efficiency.

Morphemic Awareness

Vellutino and colleagues (1994) caution that phonemic and orthographic coding are not the only cognitive processes contributing to the ability to decode or spell words. As they note, "printed words not only have phonological and orthographic attributes, but they also have semantic and syntactic attributes that become part of their lexical description, and it is likely that semantic and syntactic coding abilities also contribute significant variance to facility in word identification" (p. 55). "Morphemic awareness" allows the language learner to incorporate semantic and grammatical information at the word and subword

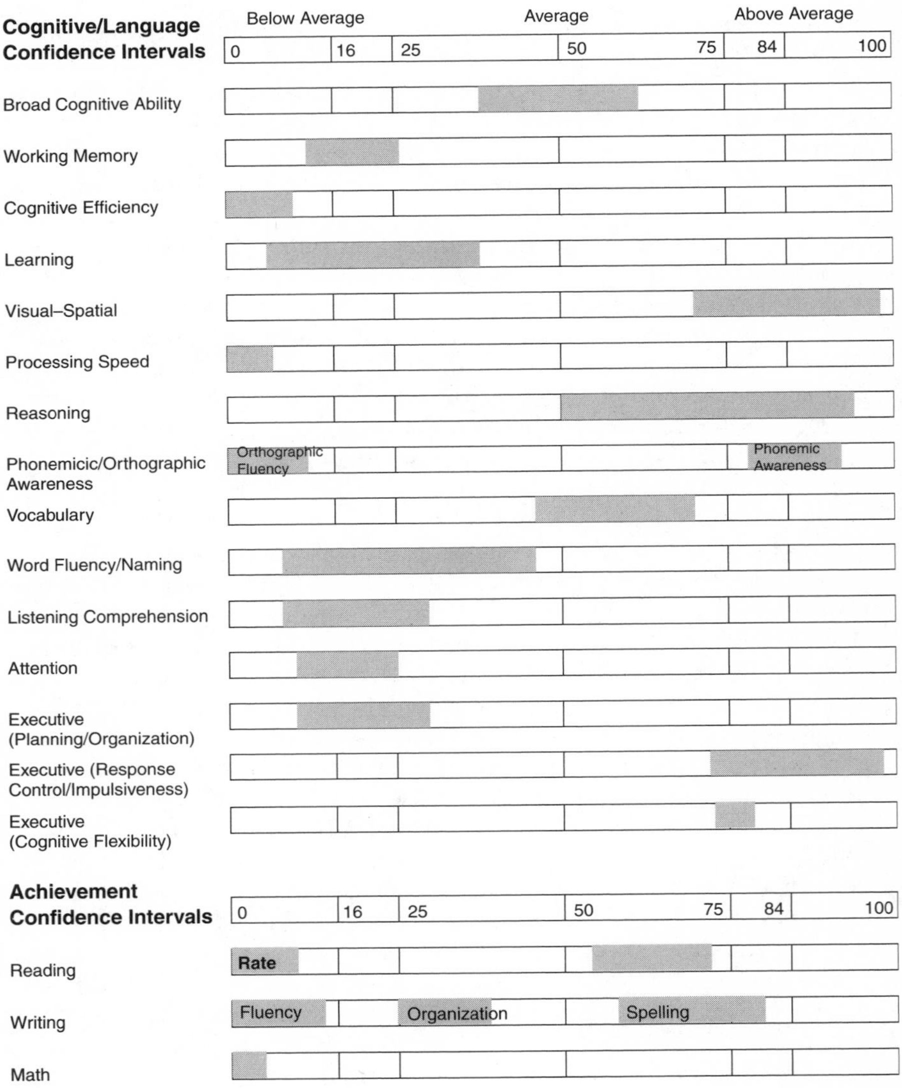

FIGURE 5.4. Assessment profile for Peter, an individual with ADHD.

level. Three types of morphemic features are recognized: inflections, derivations, and compound words. Essential to learning morphemes is the reader's proficiency with phonemic, orthographic, and semantic knowledge (Carlisle, 2004).

A great deal of research supports the significant association between morphemic awareness and word reading (Carlisle, 1995, 2000; Carlisle & Stone, 2003; Nagy, Anderson, Schommer, Scott, & Stallman, 1989). Two recent studies investigating the Hebrew adult population with dyslexia provide evidence that these individuals demonstrate deficits specific to morphemic processing, as well as a general metalinguistic deficiency, neither of which can be accounted for by phonemic processing (Leikin & Hagit, 2006; Schiff & Raveh, 2006). Unfortunately, very little research is available investigating the morphemic processing abilities of English-speaking adolescent or adult populations with LD or ADHD, despite scholars' awareness of the importance of this latent construct to word knowledge.

Assessment of Phonemic, Orthographic, and Morphemic Awareness

The importance of phonemic, orthographic, and morphemic awareness to reading decoding performance has been well documented in the literature, and an assessment of these processes is essential to a comprehensive evaluation of reading. Table 5.1 provides a list of phonemic, orthographic, and morphemic awareness tasks commonly used by researchers to measure these constructs. However, standardized measures normed for the adolescent and adult populations in general, or those with LD and ADHD in particular, are unavailable for many of these constructs. Therefore, professionals might consider developing informal measures to assess specific orthographic and morphemic awareness features, based on the research tasks described in Table 5.1.

A few adolescent and adult standardized measures of phonemic awareness are available, but they are plagued by measurement issues (e.g., norming restrictions, construct validity). For instance, the WJ III Tests of Cognitive Abilities (COG) and the WJ III ACH (Woodcock et al., 2001a, 2001b) provide several measures that professionals can use to investigate aspects of phonological processing (e.g., Sound Awareness, Phoneme–Grapheme Knowledge Cluster, Auditory Processing Cluster, Phonemic Awareness Cluster). However, my colleagues and I (Gregg, Coleman, & Knight, 2003) would caution evaluators that a drawback of these WJ III measures is their exclusive use of real words

TABLE 5.1. Evidence-Based Phonemic, Orthographic, and Morphemic Awareness Tasks

Task	Description of task
	Phonemic awareness
General Rhyming (Johnson & Blalock, 1987)	Stimulus items are presented orally. Examinee is required to generate words that rhyme with stimulus word.
Segmenting by Syllables (Johnson & Blalock, 1987)	Stimulus items are presented orally. Examinee is required to segment each word into its constituent syllables.
Number of Syllables (Johnson & Blalock, 1987)	High-frequency stimulus items are presented orally. Examinee is required to identify number of syllables in each stimulus word.
Segmenting by Sounds (Johnson & Blalock, 1987)	High-frequency stimulus items are presented orally. Examinee is required to segment stimulus word into its constituent phonemes.
Phonemic Localization (Vellutino, Scanlon, & Chen, 1994)	Pairs of one-syllable words/pseudowords are presented orally. Examinee is required to identify relative location of phoneme difference in each word pair (beginning, middle, or end).
Phonemic Segmentation (Berninger, 1994)	Multisyllabic pseudowords are presented orally. Examinee is required to (1) repeat stimulus word, and (2) delete certain phonemes according to examiner instructions.
	Orthographic awareness
Orthographic Expressive Coding (Berninger & Abbott, 1994)	Pseudowords are presented for 1 second apiece. After each exposure, examinee is required to write the item in its entirety or specified letters from it.
Orthographic Choice (Stanovich, West, & Cunningham, 1991)	Timed measure in which a series of stimulus questions with two homophonic answers is presented. Examinee is required to circle the best answer.
Homophone/ Pseudohomophone Choice (Olson, Forsberg, & Wise, 1994)	Timed measure (3 minutes) in which examinee must select the correct spelling from pairs of orthographically plausible spellings.
Colorado Perceptual Speed Test, Trials I and II (DeFries & Baker, 1983)	Timed measures in which examinee is given 1 minute to scan rows of letter–number clusters and circle the cluster identical to the stimulus item presented at the beginning of each row (four choices). Clusters do not resemble pronounceable words.

(continued)

TABLE 5.1. *(continued)*

Task	Description of task
Orthographic awareness (continued)	
Colorado Perceptual Speed Test, Trial III (DeFries & Baker, 1983)	Timed measure in which examinee is given 1 minute to scan rows of letter clusters and circle the cluster identical to the stimulus item presented at the beginning of each row (four choices). Clusters are mostly one-syllable pseudowords.
Morphemic awareness	
Carlisle Decomposition Task (Carlisle, 2000)	Stimulus items are presented orally. Examinee is provided a target word such as "farmer," and is asked to delete a word part to make it fit the blank in a sentence context (e.g., "The plowed fields are on the _____").
Carlisle Derivation Task (Carlisle, 2000)	Stimulus items are presented orally. Examinee is given a target word such as "farm" and is asked to transform the word by adding a part to it to fit the blank in a sentence (e.g., "The _____ is plowing his fields").
University of Washington Morphological Signals Task (Berninger et al., 2006)	Stimulus items are presented orally. Examinee is asked to select one of four morphological word forms (real words or pseudomorphs) containing an inflectional or derivational suffix that fits a sentence context.
Comes From Task (Nagy, Berninger, Abbott, Vaughn, & Vermeulen, 2003)	Stimulus items are presented orally. Examinee is asked to judge whether a word is derived from a base word (e.g., "Does 'baker' come from 'bake'?").

rather than pseudowords. Adolescents and adults with well-developed vocabularies and strong reasoning abilities may be able to perform well on such tasks (e.g., the WJ III COG Incomplete Words subtest) by using these resources, thus masking underlying problems related to phonology.

Pseudowords provide a better means for investigating underlying phonemic, orthographic, or morphemic processes, since an individual does not usually have an established mental representation for the target words. In contrast, the reading of real words is strongly influenced by literacy exposure and vocabulary competency. Regardless of the specific measurement tool, examiners must be sensitive to the standard deviations (*SD*s) of test score distributions when interpreting any reading subtest, cluster, or index score. If a test has a very small *SD* for a particular age group, the spread of ability within that population is so narrow that even small differences in performance can move an individual substantially away from the median.

One of the most popular standardized measures of phonemic awareness is the Comprehensive Test of Phonological Processing (CTOPP; Wagner et al., 1999). Evaluators are always advised to use composites or indexes (Phonological Awareness, Phonological Memory, and Rapid Picture Naming) rather than an individual subtest score (see Chapter Three). Unlike the corresponding tests on the WJ III, the Phonological Awareness items on the CTOPP are measured with both regular words and pseudowords. Unfortunately, the norms for the CTOPP only go through age 24 years, 11 months. In addition, the adult sample is not as representative of the broad spectrum of reading and phonological ability as are the school-age samples. About 82% of the adult samples were from the southern United States, and all of these individuals were drawn from only two postsecondary schools in Florida (i.e., one public university and one community college) (J. K. Torgesen, personal communication, 1999). Therefore, evaluators must take care in interpreting scores from the CTOPP with adult populations.

Individuals with poor orthographic awareness struggle to quickly encode and decode the visual symbols (i.e., printed letters, numbers, and letter clusters) used to represent spoken sounds and words. Unfortunately, standardized measures of orthographic awareness are unavailable for the adolescent and adult populations. A measure such as the WJ III COG Visual Matching subtest, in which an individual must quickly scan number patterns, could indicate possible orthographic abilities. However, the fact that an adolescent or adult can scan and identify numbers or geometric patterns does not necessarily predict success on other orthographic measures. If letters or words were the stimuli rather than numbers or geometric designs, a very different level of performance might be observed. Clinicians are encouraged to supplement their assessment batteries with orthographic processing tasks such as DeFries and Baker's (1983) Colorado Perceptual Speed Test (see Table 5.1). Local norms can be established to provide clinicians with a comparison group.

The tasks listed in the final section of Table 5.1 are commonly used by researchers to measure morphemic awareness. However, the reliability and construct validity of these measures for adolescents and adults are questionable. Clinicians are encouraged to use the task formats described by Carlisle (2000), Berninger and colleagues (2006), and Nagy, Berninger, Abbott, Vaughan, and Vermeulen (2003) to create local norms and/or tasks appropriate for the adolescent and adult populations, since standardized measures of morphemic awareness are not available for this age group.

Working Memory, Executive, and Attention Processes

Ample evidence supports the critical role of verbal working memory in reading decoding performance, and indicates that many adolescents and adults with LD and ADHD experience problems on working memory tasks (Barkley, 2006; Berninger & Richards, 2002; Berninger et al., 2006; Swanson & Siegel, 2001). Swanson and Siegel (2001) suggest that working memory deficits manifest themselves as domain-specific constraints (i.e., phonological working memory) and/or domain-general constraints (i.e., capacity limitations in controlled attentional processing). "Attention" as it relates to working memory refers to the ability to focus on task-relevant information in the face of distraction or interferences, as illustrated by performance on the Stroop task (Delis et al., 2001). Swanson and Siegel argue that in the domain of reading, adolescents and adults with dyslexia have smaller general working memory capacity that is not entirely specific to their reading abilities.

We (Gregg et al., 2005) investigated the predictive ability of several WJ III COG Clusters for the decoding performance of 100 young adults with dyslexia, as compared to 100 age-matched peers with no disabilities. We found that the second and third largest mean differences between these two groups occurred on the WJ III COG Auditory Processing Cluster (11.80 standard score points) and the WJ III COG Working Memory Cluster (11.15 standard score points), reflecting the phonological, working memory, and attention problems significant among adolescents and adults with dyslexia as discussed by Swanson and Siegel (2001). The strong relationship between attention, working memory, and executive processes on the one hand, and the ability to process verbal information on the other, has been of interest for some time to researchers (Engle et al., 1992).

Cognitive Efficiency

The Gregg and colleagues (2005) investigation of the predictive ability of several WJ III COG Clusters for the decoding performance of young adults with and without dyslexia actually provides a perspective somewhat different from Swanson and Siegel's (2001) conclusion that capacity rather than processing efficiency is the critical problem for dyslexic readers. The greatest mean difference (12.80) between our groups on the WJ III was found on the Cognitive Efficiency Cluster—Extended.

This cluster taps working memory, short-term memory, processing speed, and cognitive efficiency. The subtests in this cluster (i.e., Visual Matching, Numbers Reversed, Decision Speed, Memory for Words) measure both verbal and nonverbal abilities. As Daneman and Carpenter (1980) note, individual differences in memory capacity may reside less in storage capacity and more in the efficient use of processes to maximize limited capacity. Peter's profile (Figure 5.4) highlights the complexity of working memory and cognitive efficiency. Whether these processes are unified, bidirectional, or two distinct constructs continues to be debated. However, evaluators should investigate the influence of both processes (capacity and efficiency) during clinical decision making.

Interestingly, in the Gregg and colleagues (2005) study, the smallest between-group difference (5.97 standard score points) was found on the WJ III COG Fluency Cluster. One of the major limitations of this measure for the adolescent and adult populations appears to be the fact that it combines verbal fluency measures (Retrieval Fluency and Rapid Picture Naming) with Decision Speed, a task that has a stronger *Gs* (processing speed) component. We (Gregg et al., 2005) have suggested the need for further validity studies to determine the cluster's effectiveness, particularly as a gauge of rapid naming abilities in adolescent and adult populations. This issue is critical, since rapid naming abilities have been found to be very important to children's development of age-appropriate literacy skills.

Word Knowledge

Word meaning is strongly influenced by the complexity and ambiguity of word relationships, which also provide the context for the learning of phonemic, orthographic, and morphemic features. Awareness of and automaticity with the meaning and spelling of spoken and written words are referred to as "word knowledge."

Interestingly, we (Gregg et al., 2005) also found that the WJ III COG Clusters accounted for almost twice the variance in predicting reading decoding performance for the population with dyslexia as for their normally achieving peers. It appears that the normally achieving young adults were using their cognitive, language, and general world knowledge for decoding words that were not necessarily represented on the WJ III. The question then arises as to whether the difficulties of students with dyslexia in such cognitive and linguistic processes as working memory, cognitive efficiency, and phonemic awareness are the *results* or the *causes* of deficits in crystallized knowledge. Evaluators are encouraged to consider all these processes carefully, to better understand their direct and indirect influences on reading decoding for an individual reader.

Assessment of Reading Decoding

The difficulty many individuals with dyslexia experience as they attempt to read accurately and fluently has been well documented in the literature (Shaywitz, 2003). Therefore, for any referral in which reading underachievement is suspected, an evaluator is well advised to administer several measures of reading decoding. Investigation of standard print, digital text, and online decoding competencies is essential for a comprehensive evaluation of reading abilities.

Offline Decoding Assessment

The evaluation of offline reading decoding for adolescent and adult populations should always include observations of (1) phonemic, orthographic, and morphemic awareness; (2) pseudoword reading; and (3) regular-word reading. The majority of either pseudoword and regular-word reading tasks require an examinee to read a list of words orally with few or no restrictions on time. When time is not factored into a score, the individual is provided the opportunity to employ various word analysis strategies, one of which is guessing. The Test of Word Reading Efficiency (TOWRE; Torgesen, Wagner, & Rashotte, 1999) is an exception to the majority of these tests, as it does provide a way to investigate the accuracy and fluency of pseudoword and regular-word reading. The TOWRE Sight Word Efficiency subtest measures the number of real printed words that can be accurately identified within 45 seconds, and the Phonetic Decoding Efficiency subtest measures the number of pronounceable printed nonwords that can be accurately decoded within 45 seconds. Unfortunately, as is true of the CTOPP (Wagner et al., 1999), the TOWRE only provides norms up to 24 years, 11 months of age, and the norm population is quite restricted at the adult level.

Regardless of the reading decoding measure used, examiners are always encouraged to record the time that it took an examinee to read each word (rate), as well as the accuracy of pronunciation. The total standard score for a subtest may not reflect a reader's hesitations and self-corrections during the oral decoding of a word. In addition, the word errors should be analyzed to determine whether they appear to be phonemic, orthographic, or morphemic in nature. A reader's performance on the three types of awareness tasks should be compared to his or her reading decoding performance across pseudoword–regular-word and timed–untimed word recall tasks.

Online Decoding Assessment

Researchers have identified several critical skills necessary for online reading decoding, which include (but are not limited to) the following: the ability to locate information quickly by using a search engine; reading search engine results; and reading a web page quickly to locate the best link to information (Coiro, 2003, 2006; Leu et al., in press). Professionals working with adolescent or adult populations with LD or ADHD often observe that some of these individuals do not appear to know how to use or read search engine results efficiently. Instead, such individuals rely on a "click and look" strategy, which is not always effective in locating information (Leu et al., 2007). Difficulty in locating information can create a "bottleneck" that prevents success with online reading (Henry, 2007). According to Leu and colleagues (2007), those who possess the online "skills necessary to locate information can continue to read and solve their problem; those who do not possess these skills cannot" (p. 22).

An adolescent's or adult's proficiency in accessing and decoding information online is best measured by observing the individual working online. Professionals might consider using an observational skills checklist, such as that developed by Leu and colleagues (2008) through the Teaching Internet Comprehension Skills to Adolescents Project, as a reliable and valid means of collecting online reading decoding data. In addition to the skills on such a checklist, professionals might consider the importance of what Anderson-Inman and Horney (2007) call "presentational resources" (i.e., font size and style, text and background color, line and page length, page layout, graphics) to online reading proficiency. An evaluator is also advised to observe when difficulties in decoding printed words prevent an adolescent or adult from developing basic online literacy skills. Matching the information collected from the online and offline assessments will assist the evaluator in providing more effective accommodations.

Reading Fluency

Researchers have provided a great deal of empirical evidence for the critical role reading fluency plays in high-speed word recognition and comprehension of text (National Reading Panel, 2000).Converging scientific data suggests that individuals with dyslexia become increasingly accurate in reading as they progress in school, but continue to demonstrate problems with reading fluency. The longitudinal research of Shaywitz and colleagues (2003) demonstrates that children, university students, and adults with dyslexia exhibit a functional disruption in neural systems responsible for fast, automatic reading.

Recent research pertaining to the neurological underpinnings of the mechanisms controlling speed is providing evidence for the direct and indirect relationship of specific cognitive processes to time-dependent learning tasks. For instance, recent brain imaging technology provides evidence of how the automatic and the cognitively controlled timing systems influence different types of learning (Buhusi & Meck, 2005; Lewis & Miall, 2005, 2006; Lustig, Matell, & Meck, 2005). The automatic timing system regulates discontinuous timing events, such as those required for motor tasks (Buhusi & Meck, 2005). In comparison, the cognitively controlled timing system appears to be intricately linked at both a neuronal and a phenomenological level to working memory and executive processes (Lustig et al., 2005). This compelling evidence demonstrates the strong relationship of executive functions, working memory, and timing processes to the ability to learn quickly and efficiently. In addition, it provides professionals with insight into why fluency is such a significant problem for individuals with LD and ADHD attempting to decode words and comprehend text.

The WJ III ACH Reading Fluency subtest appears to be a reliable and valid measure of reading fluency for the adolescent and adult populations (Gregg et al., 2005; McGrew, Woodcock, & Ford, 2002). However, the fact that an individual is able to perform within the average range on this one measure does not always provide evidence of fluent reading abilities. As mentioned later in the discussion of reading comprehension assessment, a reader with strong metalinguistic or inferential reasoning may be able to guess at the answers for this sentence-level, forced-choice task, but may have significant difficulty quickly reading longer passages, particularly of more dense and abstract text. Other measures, such as the Nelson–Denny Reading Test Rate score, are equally susceptible to this problem and can lead an examiner to make false-negative diagnostic decisions. An examiner is always encouraged to observe the manner in which a reader decodes and comprehends text across situations and tasks, in order to better understand the influence of timing on performance.

Accommodations for Reading Decoding and Reading Fluency Deficits

Accommodations for reading decoding or reading fluency problems are discussed separately from those required for reading comprehension problems. However, several of the recommendations (e.g., extra time, a private room) can be appropriate for functional limitations in either decoding or comprehension. See Table 5.2 for a list of suggested accommodations for individuals demonstrating decoding deficits. However, evaluators are encouraged first to answer the questions provided in Figure 5.3, in order to determine whether an accommodation for decoding underachievement would be effective and/or appropriate for an adolescent or adult with LD or ADHD.

Extra Time and a Private Room

Extra time and a quiet or private testing room are often recommended accommodations for reading decoding and fluency problems (Sireci, Li, & Scarpati, 2003). Because difficulties with phonemic, orthographic,

TABLE 5.2. Accommodations for Enhancing Reading Performance

Decoding	Fluency[a]	Comprehension

• Private room
• Quiet room
• Extended time
• Scheduled breaks
• Reader
• Text-to-speech (TTS) software
• Electronic text (e-text)
• Audio text
• Graphic adjustments
  • Font (size, type)
  • Line spacing (single- vs. double-space)
  • Justification (full, left)
• Embedded e-text supports[b]
  • Presentational
  • Translational
  • Enrichment
  • Notational
• Optical character recognition (OCR) software to convert print text to digital text to download on computers, MP3 players, or phones
	• Extended time
	• Decoding options (see left column)
	• Comprehension options (see right column)
		• Private room
		• Quiet room
		• Extended time
		• Modified language
		• Visualization strategies
		• Concept maps
		• Note taking
		• Marking text
		• Annotating text
		• Think-alouds
		• Reader guides
		• Interpreter
		• Embedded e-text supports[b]
		  • Navigational
		  • Translational
		  • Explanatory
		  • Illustrative
		  • Summarizing
		  • Instructional
		  • Enrichment
		  • Notational
		• e-text and TTS when audio feedback is effective for a reader or whendecoding is also an issue

[a] Fluency accommodations are dependent upon whether the reading underachievement results from decoding or comprehension factors.
[b] Described in Table 5.3.

and morphemic awareness slow down the process of decoding, extra time becomes a critical accommodation for students with dyslexia. A significant amount of research supports the effectiveness of this accommodation for individuals with print disabilities (Shaywitz, 2003). In addition, some individuals with dyslexia report that being permitted to read aloud helps them monitor and attend to what they read; therefore, a private room becomes necessary, so that their oral reading will not bother other students in the classroom. Some readers with print disabilities even use earplugs to block out external sounds that interfere with their attending to and processing printed text (Shaywitz, 2003).

Alt Media Accommodations

As a result of emerging technologies, a fundamental shift in how we define literacy is occurring in the world of school and work. For adolescents and adults with LD and ADHD, these technologies offer opportunities to be better prepared for the schools and workplaces of the 21st century. Various new technologies are being used to accommodate the learning and work environments for these individuals. In the area of reading, alt media and the software to access these are essential accommodations for adolescents and adults with functional limitations in the area of reading decoding. As noted in Chapter One, "alt media" is a broad term referring to several formats into which printed text is converted (e.g., audiotaped text, enlarged print, e-text, Braille). The alt media used most commonly by adolescents or adults with LD demonstrating underachievement in reading are e-text and audio files (Wolfe & Lee, 2007). e-text is text made available in machine-readable or computerized formats. The type of file that e-text is converted into has a significant impact on the types of technologies and tools that can be integrated with it (e.g., ASCII, .html).

Regardless of the alt media format, e-text is not accessible for individuals with LD or ADHD unless it is used in conjunction with AT software. Optical character recognition (OCR) software is first used to convert scanned or bit-mapped images of text into machine-readable form. The text may be saved on magnetic media (e.g., hard drives) or on optical media (e.g., CD-ROMs). Text converted by OCR software is then read by text-to-speech (TTS) software. TTS is a type of speech synthesis application that is used to create a spoken version of e-text on a computer or a hand-held device. TTS can enable the reading of computer display information for an adolescent or adult with LD or ADHD, or it may simply be used to augment the reading of a text message. Anderson-Inman and Horney (2007) prefer the term "supported e-text" to refer to the integration of e-text with assistive software.

Research evidence to support the effectiveness of e-text and TTS software for enhancing the reading abilities of adolescents or adults with LD is currently limited in scope and depth (Anderson-Inman & Horney, 2007; Gregg, 2008; MacArthur, Ferretti, Okolo, & Cavalier, 2001). However, even more disheartening is the fact that much of the TTS software cannot access or be integrated with the various social media tools—from text messaging to blogging—that are essential to success in the school, the social environment, and the workplace. As colleges and universities are posting lectures on YouTube, and many officers and employees of major companies are communicating with one another and with their customers through blogging and web pages, AT software needs to be capable of seamless integration with various forms of social media. The lack of empirically based evidence for effective technologies to assist adolescents and adults with LD and ADHD in reading both online and offline is curious, given the explosion of technology in our society.

To help illustrate why TTS software is an important accommodation for individuals with decoding deficits, I use Lawana's (Figure 5.1) profile. Lawana demonstrates strengths in learning, reasoning, and listening comprehension. Her significant problems in reading appear to be deficits in phonemic awareness, orthographic awareness, and word fluency. Therefore, Lawana's reading decoding problems appear to influence her ability to comprehend text in a timed situation. However, when text is read aloud (e.g., by her mother or by a computer), her strengths help her circumvent her decoding problems. Lawana appears to be an excellent candidate for using a TTS software program (e.g., Dragon Naturally Speaking, Read & Write, ReadPlease). Such software can read the text aloud to Lawana and even simultaneously provide a highlighted synchronization of the text with audio feedback. Lawana may elect to download her e-files onto her iPod. An important feature of alt media is their portability, as digital files can be delivered to students via e-mail or Internet portals and used in a variety of electronic and physical environments. In addition, for a college student like Lawana, the ability to access .pdf files is an extremely critical skill to master. Recent advances in e-text and TTS technology now allow .pdf files to be downloaded easily to a computer or an MP3 player, to be read through specialized TTS software (e.g., for a description of the PDF Equalizer, go to *www.amac. uga.edu/publications/pdf_equalizer.pdf*).

Color Filters

The use of color filters to enhance the reading proficiency of adolescents and adults with LD has not been validated by empirically based research. However, the belief by many professionals that color overlays are effective for this purpose continues to receive attention in the literature (Ray, Fowler, & Stein, 2005; Singleton & Henderson, 2007; Smith & Wilkins, 2007). Researchers first suggested in the late 1980s and early 1990s that color lenses would improve the reading performance of students with dyslexia (Robinson & Conway, 2000; Williams, Lecluyse, & Rock-Fauceux, 1992). However, when such a claim could not be specially validated for the population with dyslexia, the proponents of color overlays turned to suggesting their effectiveness for students with visual stress in reading, referred to as "Meares–Irlen syndrome" or "scotopic sensitivity syndrome" (Kriss & Evans, 2005). However, as normally achieving individuals also demonstrate this syndrome, it appears uncorrelated with reading disorders.

The idea that color filters are useful in treating dyslexia stems from the hypothesis that dyslexia is the result of a deficiency in the magnocellular part of the visual system (Livingstone et al., 1991; Stein & Walsch, 1997). However, empirical evidence to support a strong relationship between dyslexia and magnocellular deficits has not been forthcoming (Ramus, 2001; Roach & Hogben, 2004; Skottun, 2000; Skottun & Skoyles, 2007). Over the years, filters of different colors have been proposed as effective in enhancing the reading fluency of individuals with reading disorders. For instance, earlier researchers advocated the use of red or blue filters (Lehmkuhle, 1993; Solan, Ficarra, Brannan, & Rucker, 1998; Williams et al., 1992). More recently, Ray and colleagues (2005) have suggested the use of yellow filters to increase reading fluency. However, Skottun and Skoyles (2007) provides strong evidence to challenge the hypothesized relationship of color filters to reading performance, and concludes that red, blue, or yellow filters do not enhance magnocellular responses. Therefore, there is no evidence-based research to support the claim that color filters are effective in altering the reading performance of adolescent or adults with reading disorders.

Conceptualizing the Process of Reading Comprehension

Top-Down and Bottom-Up Models

Theories of reading comprehension provide a framework for professionals to utilize as they attempt to interpret the multiple factors contributing to a reader's success in extracting and constructing meaning from written text (Sweet & Snow, 2003). Some scholars propose that the skills needed for reading comprehension are organized in a hierarchy ranging from higher-order to lower-order skills. Such theories of reading comprehension have been categorized as following a continuum from top-down to bottom-up models. Researchers taking a more top-down perspective on the process of reading comprehension closely examine the relationship among the reader, the text, and the activity of reading (Galda & Beach, 2001; Sweet & Snow, 2003). Bottom-up models are used by professionals more interested in the specific lower-order processes that influence the act of comprehending text (Kintsch, 1998; Perfetti, Marron, & Foltz, 1996). Such models purport that the reader extracts meaning from the print only after the basic cognitive and linguistic processes involved in word decoding have been completed. In a recent review of the literature, public policy, and best practices, the RAND Reading Study Group (2003) encourages professionals to utilize both top-down and bottom-up models to better understand how readers do or do not comprehend written text.

Integrative models have been developed to address the inadequacy of strictly top-down or bottom-up approaches. Indeed, research has shown that lower-level and higher-level processes may interact and compensate for one another during reading (Adams, 1990; Rumelhart, 1994). For example, less skilled readers who are provided with text at their relative reading level are able to use context to facilitate word recognition to perform as well as more skilled readers (Stanovich, 1980). This finding dispels the notion that higher-level processes, such as context facilitation, must await the development of lower-level skills such as word recognition, and it highlights the interactive nature of the reading process. Other recent models, such as the convergent skills model (Vellutino, Tunmer, Jaccard, & Chen, 2007), emphasize the importance of both bottom-up and top-down processes in the construction of meaning from text. It seems clear that both types of processes are vital for reading comprehension to take place.

Constrained and Unconstrained Reading Skills

As noted in Chapter Three, an aspect missing from many models of learning—top-down or bottom-up—is consideration of how the developmental trajectories of ability acquisition affect reading comprehension across the lifespan (Paris, 2005). Paris (2005) believes that an awareness of the differences between "constrained" reading skills (i.e., learned quickly and completely mastered, such as phonemic awareness) and "unconstrained" reading skills (i.e., never completely mastered, such as vocabulary or comprehension) is essential to a better understanding of reading performance. Unfortunately, despite this awareness, many professionals continue to allot greater significance to the predictive validity of specific cognitive and linguistic abilities (e.g., phonemic awareness, letter naming), regardless of a reader's age, skill level, or experience with literacy. The next section of this chapter covers these specific cognitive and linguistic processes, but readers should continue to keep the "whole picture" in mind.

Cognitive and Linguistic Processes Influencing Reading Comprehension

Ample empirical evidence is available to suggest the importance of specific cognitive and linguistic processes for adolescents and/or adults to comprehend written text. These include (but are not limited to) word recognition, word form awareness, naming, fluency, memory (long-term, working memory), oral language (word, sentence, text), prior knowledge, and motivation (Berninger et al., 2006; Duke, Pressley, & Hildren, 2004; Goff, Pratt, & Ong, 2005; Kintsch, 1998; Nation, Adams, Bowyer-Crane, & Snowling, 1999; Nation & Snowling, 1998; Swanson & Siegel, 2001). In addition, researchers have identified the importance of domain knowledge, inference generation (reasoning), strategic processing, and comprehension monitoring to reading comprehension performance (Buehl, Alexander, & Murphy, 2002; Graesser, 1993; Magliano, Trabasso, & Graesser, 1999; Norman, Kiemper, & Kynette, 1992). There is solid scientific agreement that the reading comprehension performance of adolescents and adults is directly influenced by the following three skills: fluency (word, sentence, and text), vocabulary, and domain knowledge (Hirsch, 2003).

As we consider the adolescent and adult populations, it is important to remember that "constrained skills appear to have predictably unstable data distributions as readers progress from novices to experts" (Paris, 2005, p. 198). In a recent study, we (Floyd, Gregg, Keith, & Meisinger, 2008) were able to provide strong empirical evidence of the changing influence of specific cognitive and linguistic processes on the ability to comprehend reading across the lifespan. With the Cattell–Horn–Carroll (CHC) theory of cognitive abilities (see Chapter Three) as our starting point, we tested theoretical models specifying effects of cognitive and linguistic abilities and reading aptitudes on reading comprehension performance. Subsamples drawn from the standardization sample of the WJ III (Woodcock et al., 2001a, 2001b), and representing five age levels spanning early childhood, childhood, adolescence, and early adulthood, were employed in our analyses. Using a model including general intelligence, broad cognitive abilities, and reading decoding skills, we found significant direct effects for reading decoding and crystallized knowledge (i.e., word and world knowledge) across all age levels. The magnitude of these effects varied as a function of age. For the adolescent and adult populations, the influence of crystallized knowledge (i.e., word and world knowledge) predicted reading comprehension more than reading decoding abilities did. For younger children, reading decoding was the better predictor of reading comprehension. The implications of these findings are significant for assessment and accommodation decision making for the adolescent and adult population.

General Intelligence

Today many researchers see general intelligence (g) as representing a product of the working memory system, which contributes to all conscious thought (including metacognition) and to the management of information in immediate awareness and in the memory stores (Carroll, 1993; Jensen, 1998; Swanson & Alexander, 1997). For many years, researchers considered general intelligence to account for a large percentage of variance in reading comprehension performance, and viewed more specific abilities as contributing very little additional effect. Recent research is challenging this assumption. For instance, using structural equation modeling we (Floyd et al., 2008) found that when general intelligence was allowed to "compete" equally with the broad abilities and narrow abilities as predictors of reading comprehension, the results indicated that the older supposition was not supported. In our research, general intelligence had large but indirect effects on reading comprehension. We obtained consistent findings of indirect effects of general intelligence on comprehension, and direct effects of broad or narrow abilities on decoding, across the lifespan. Therefore, the idea that general intelligence represents a domain-general working memory system fueling reading comprehension and its enabling abilities appears to be gaining evidence-based support (Floyd et al., 2008).

Working Memory, Executive, and Attention Processes

Several recent studies suggest that working memory capacity plays a significant role in reading comprehension (Berninger et al., 2006; Swanson & Ashbaker, 2000; Swanson, Howard, & Saez, 2007; Swanson & Siegel, 2001). In a study involving adults, Berninger and colleagues (2006) investigated three executive functions involved in working memory (set shifting, inhibition, and monitoring/updating) and three forms of word awareness (phonemic, orthographic, and morphemic) to determine their relationship to reading comprehension performance. The reading comprehension measures used in this study were the WJ III ACH Passage Comprehension subtest (Woodcock et al., 2001a), which is a modified cloze procedure, and the Gray Oral Reading Tests—Fourth Edition (GORT-4; Wiederholt & Bryant, 2001), although the GORT-4 is normed only to 24 years of age. The predictive abilities of phonemic, orthographic, and morphemic awareness and of working memory/executive processes were not consistent across tasks, indicating the importance of task to diagnostic decision making.

Oral Language Comprehension

The relationship between oral language and reading comprehension strengthens as readers mature in both age and ability level. Our recent findings (Floyd et al., 2008) provide strong evidence of the importance of language-based declarative knowledge and higher-order language processes to reading comprehension skills; in addition, they draw attention to the importance of prior knowledge across the lifespan. We have suggested that prior knowledge is likely to trigger processes important for comprehension, such as inference making or comprehension monitoring (Kintsch, 1998; Perfetti et al., 1996). We also found that the effects of listening comprehension on reading comprehension were significant from ages 9 to 19. Use of these language processes is common across completion of listening comprehension and reading comprehension tasks (Perfetti, 2007). This finding is consistent with research indicating that oral language comprehension places an upper limit on reading comprehension performance for children (Stothard & Hulme, 1996).

Some individuals experience difficulty comprehending what they read as the result of poor decoding abilities. However, for other adolescents and adults with LD or ADHD, their problem is not primarily the result of decoding deficits, but rather of a receptive language disorder (Cain & Oakhill, 2007; Catts, Adlof, & Ellis, 2006). Donny's profile (Figure 5.2) is representative of adolescents and/or adults with LD for whom deficits related to the understanding of oral language contribute significantly to their reading comprehension problems. Yet an important point to remember is that not all adolescents or adults with LD or ADHD who demonstrate problems with oral language comprehension will exhibit a similar profile. Some individuals with poor comprehension experience more difficulty at the word or sentence level, while others have more trouble at the text level.

Long-Term Memory

Kintsch's (1998) research suggests that a reader, through an integration of propositions with other knowledge sources, constructs a situational model during the process of listening or reading comprehension.

One of the most critical aspects of Kintsch's theory is the importance attached to long-term working memory in the reader's development of text structure. He provides empirical evidence to support the supposition that the development of the mental model that matches the text being read requires two distinct phases: (1) the "construction" phrase, where propositions in the text are linked to the reader's knowledge; and (2) the "integration" phrase, where a meaningful whole is conceived by constraining types of information. Kintsch has applied this theory to several areas of written language (e.g., word identification, inferential reasoning, comprehension monitoring, and learning from text). Unfortunately, the measures of long-term memory in the majority of cognitive batteries available to professionals do not have strong concurrent or construct validity.

Metacognition

Readers must be able to monitor whether they have comprehended text as intended by the author. This ability to be aware of one's own understanding is referred to as "metacognition." Two abilities essential to the metacognitive process are self-regulation and the use of strategies (McNamara, Ozuru, Best, & O'Reilly, 2007; Schraw & Dennison, 1994). Many individuals with LD or ADHD experience difficulty in making use of contextual information in order to gain meaning from printed text, because of their problems with self-regulation and strategy use (Cain, Oakhill, & Elbro, 2002; Cain, Oakhill, & Lemmon, 2004). Difficulties with strategic use of context cues can be related to such problems as difficulty in using cohesive devices; lack of flexibility in word knowledge (e.g., idioms, ambiguous references); and restricted working memory, executive, processes, and attention.

"Comprehension monitoring" refers to both the skill of evaluating text meaning and the corrective strategies taken by the reader to repair inconsistencies during the process of reading. Some readers with LD and ADHD demonstrate significant difficulty detecting inconsistencies in what they read (Berthiaume, 2006). Researchers suggest that difficulty with comprehension monitoring is often the result of restricted working memory and executive processes. For instance, an examinee may perform poorly on the WJ III ACH Reading Fluency subtest because he or she does not monitor the accuracy of the sentences' meaning. In such a case, the low Reading Fluency score is not due to inadequate basic reading decoding or fluency skills, but rather to the reader's poor comprehension-monitoring abilities. Therefore, just providing such an individual with extra time on a reading task may not be very effective unless the reader is also taught cognitive strategies to enhance comprehension monitoring.

The specific discourse-level abilities that allow readers to infer meaning, use cohesive devices, attend selectively to context, apply comprehension-monitoring strategies, and access relevant knowledge all contribute to success in reading comprehension (Cain & Oakhill, 2007). Unfortunately, the difficulties in these areas that many readers with LD or ADHD experience have received limited attention from researchers (Cain & Oakhill, 2007; Carlisle & Rice, 2002; Lorch, Berthiaume, Milich, & van den Broek, 2007).

Strategic Reading Comprehension

Researchers are currently directing a great deal of attention to better understanding the strategies accessed by readers during the process of reading comprehension. Certain cognitive strategies are utilized by all readers whenever there is a breakdown of understanding during the process of comprehending text. According to Graesser (2007), a reading comprehension strategy is "a cognitive or behavioral action that is enacted under particular contextual conditions, with the goal of improving some aspect of comprehension" (p. 6). He identifies three distinctive strategies as essential to effective reading comprehension performance: the reader's ability to (1) set goals; (2) contract meaning at the local (word/sentence) and global (text) level; and (3) generate explanations for why events occur. Adolescents and adults with LD and ADHD often demonstrate difficulty in using these essential cognitive strategies (Hock & Mellard, 2005).

McNamara and colleagues (2007) propose a framework for classifying reading comprehension strategies, and they provide empirically supported interventions to enhance reading comprehension in each of their categories. Their work grew out of collaboration with the College Board to revise the English and language arts standards for middle school through college-reading high school students. McNamara and colleagues organize the evidence-based strategies essential to monitor reading comprehension within a four-pronged framework, which includes the reader's ability to (1) prepare to read; (2) go beyond the text; (3) organize, restructure, and synthesize the text; and (4) interpret the words, sentences, and ideas in the text. These strategies suggest types of accommodations that many adolescents with LD or ADHD can use to enhance their learning performance. For instance, during a reading comprehension task (e.g., reading a textbook), an individual might use a concept map to help him or her organize and record information during the process of reading. The strategy becomes a means of accommodation for the reader (see Table 5.2 for more strategic accommodations).

To sum up the research findings across theoretical perspectives, it is clear that many different cognitive and linguistic factors may influence an individual's reading comprehension performance. These include (but are not limited to) word recognition and the sublexical processes influencing decoding (phonemic, orthographic, and morphemic awareness); fluency; long-term memory; working memory; oral language comprehension; executive strategies; prior knowledge; and motivation (Duke et al., 2004; Vellutino, 2003). Therefore, during the assessment of reading comprehension, an evaluator should consider the various factors that may directly or indirectly be influencing the examinee's reading performance in order to identify the most effective accommodations..

Assessment of Reading Comprehension

Reading comprehension is a multidimensional construct that has traditionally been assessed in several different ways. As with decoding, an evaluator is strongly encouraged to measure both a reader's online and offline reading comprehension abilities.

Offline Assessment of Reading Comprehension

The three most widely accepted methods for assessing offline reading comprehension are retelling, multiple-choice tasks, and modified cloze procedures. All three formats tap different aspects of the process of reading comprehension and require utilization of different cognitive and language abilities. Interestingly, research findings investigating the correlations between these different task formats are not at all consistent and/or conclusive, particularly across the lifespan (Fuchs, Fuchs, & Maxwell, 1988; Knight, 2000; Paris & Stahl, 2005; Parker, Tindal, & Hasbrouck, 1989; Pearson & Hamm, 2005; Shinn, Good, Knutson, Tilly, & Collins, 1992). It is important for a clinician to recognize that performance in one of these reading comprehension task formats does not predict an examinee's proficiency in another format.

Modified Cloze Formats

The WJ III ACH Passage Comprehension subtest (Woodcock et al., 2001a) is a commonly used modified cloze task where only one word per item is omitted, as compared to the traditional cloze format where every fifth to seventh word is omitted. McGrew and Woodcock (2001) claim in the *WJ III Technical Manual* that the authors omitted words that could not be supplied solely on the basis of local context. Some researchers criticize cloze formats as tests of reading comprehension, since they measure more sentence than text structure (Shanahan, Kamil, & Tobin, 1984). However, others have noted that cloze tasks effectively measure the reader's ability to draw anaphoric references across sentence boundaries—a critical skill in comprehending text (Hagtret, 2003).

Multiple-Choice Formats

Multiple-choice tasks for measuring reading comprehension have been criticized as heavily dependent on the reader's background knowledge (Parker et al., 1989). Scores for adolescents or adults with dyslexia on timed multiple-choice measures of reading comprehension, such as the Comprehension subtests of the Nelson–Denny Reading Test (Brown et al., 1993) and the GORT-4 (Wiederholt & Bryant, 2001), can be very misleading. It is not uncommon for students with dyslexia to demonstrate significant decoding deficits and yet to perform adequately on multiple-choice reading comprehension measures. The validity of several such measures has been challenged in the literature. Katz, Blackburn, and Lautenschlager (1991) found that students could proficiently answer multiple-choice items on the SAT without reading the passages. Recently, Keenan and Betjemann (2006) examined the validity of the GORT-4 Comprehension score, and we (Coleman, Lindstrom, & Gregg, 2007) examined that of the Nelson–Denny Reading Test Comprehension score. Similar findings were obtained in both studies: Students did not need to read the passages to determine correct answers to the comprehension questions. Therefore, students with dyslexia or ADHD who have strong stores of prior knowledge can infer answers without actually reading the passages. The reading comprehension score then represents a sentence-level task (i.e., the reading comprehension question) and measures prior knowledge more than it does reading skills. Although this is important information for a clinician, this single score does not represent a student's reading comprehension abilities or predict the ability to comprehend a textbook.

Text Recall Formats

Oral and written recall tasks have been found to be significantly related to reading proficiency (Fuchs et al., 1988). During a recall measure, the examinee is asked to demonstrate the amount and type of information retained after reading a passage. A reader's performance on a reading recall task should thus give the examiner insight into how information is organized in the reader's memory. Adolescents and adults with ADHD who may perform adequately on a cloze or multiple-choice reading comprehension test often demonstrate difficulty with a reading recall task as a result of their working memory, executive processing, and attention deficits. Although standardized oral recall tasks (e.g., the WJ III ACH Oral Recall subtest) are available, reading recall measures are usually curriculum-based measures that were developed for children. However, an examiner might consider developing an informal measure, using one of an examinee's content area texts. Three types of scoring are most common for recall tasks: word count, content word count, and idea unit count. Professionals are encouraged to compare a reader's performance in listening comprehension and writing organization to his or her reading comprehension performance, as underlying cognitive and linguistic deficits often co-occur across these constructs.

Reading Vocabulary Measures

Sometimes, in an attempt to understand a reader's ability to comprehend text, an evaluator will use a task where an examinee is asked to read a word and provide an appropriate word meaning by supplementing corresponding synonyms, antonyms, and words to complete a verbal analogy (e.g., the WJ III ACH Reading Vocabulary subtest). The choice of such a task is supported by evidence that fluent word recognition and understanding of individual words interact with a reader's prior knowledge as the reader goes through a text (Duke et al., 2004). Baddeley, Logie, and Nimmo-Smith (1985) identified vocabulary as one of three factors explaining reading comprehension. In addition, Stothard and Hulme (1996) suggest that vocabulary helps to explain the relationship between verbal ability and reading comprehension. However, if the examinee has significant decoding problems, such measures are not measuring the individual's knowledge of vocabulary, but simply reflect word-reading proficiency.

Online Assessment of Reading Comprehension

Online comprehension is contextually situated in both the purpose as well as the process of reading. According to this perspective, online reading comprehension is almost always initiated by a question or problem, which includes some form of communication (Leu et al., 2008). Therefore, the *purpose* of the reading task becomes central to the evaluation of online reading comprehension proficiency (Castek et al., 2007, cited in Leu et al., in press; Leu & Reinking, 2005). Leu and colleagues (in press) have identified five major functions of online reading comprehension: identifying important questions, locating information, analyzing information, synthesizing information, and communicating information.

Several methodologies are currently being used by researchers to investigate online reading comprehension, including think-alouds (Leu et al., 2007; Leu & Castek, 2006; New Literacies Research Team, 2007), curriculum-based measures (Leu et al., 2007), and performance-based measures (Coiro, 2006; Leu & Reinking, 2005; New Literacies Research Team, 2007). Leu and colleagues (2008) encourage professionals to utilize multiple-choice and short-answer measures to assess online reading comprehension, as they are more time-efficient but still valid alternatives for evaluating a reader's abilities. One such instrument, the Digital Divide Measurement Scale for Students (DDMS-S; Henry, 2007), is a 14-item forced-response measure developed to assess reading to locate and critically evaluate online information. Unfortunately, this measure is only normed for middle school students. In addition, Leu and colleagues have developed a checklist for observing a reader's abilities to understand and develop questions for an online search, locate information, critically evaluate information found online, synthesize information found online, and communicate information found online. Both the DDMS-S and the Leu and colleagues checklists can guide professionals in creating either local norms or other measures of online reading comprehension.

Accommodations for Reading Comprehension Deficits

Underachievement resulting from reading comprehension disorders is much more difficult to accommodate than that caused by decoding and reading fluency problems. Read-alouds or extended time alone do not always effectively accommodate the learning needs of individuals with LD who are struggling with the meaning of oral or written language. For adolescents and adults with ADHD whose executive processing deficits limit their strategic thinking, organization, and revision, such accommodations may also be limited in their effectiveness. Specific reading comprehension accommodation options are provided in Table 5.2, based on current reading strategies and technology research. However, evaluators are encouraged first to answer the questions provided in Figure 5.5 in determining whether an accommodation for reading comprehension underachievement would be effective for an adolescent or adult with LD or ADHD.

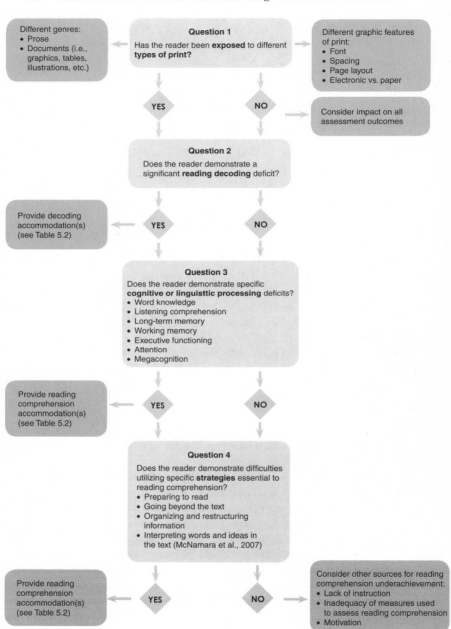

FIGURE 5.5. Questions to support decision making for the accommodation of reading comprehension problems.

Continuing advances in technology are providing professionals with more tools than ever before to help students with language-based or executive functioning deficits to comprehend written text. Anderson-Inman and Horney (2007) have developed a typology that professionals are encouraged to utilize in standardizing decisions about the enhancement and modification of e-text for individuals demonstrating print disabilities. These authors note, however: "We know relatively little about how to construct and present electronic text in ways that have a consistently positive effect on student learning, especially when considering the diverse learning styles and needs of students with disabilities" (p. 155).

Among the most promising technology software accommodations are embedded e-text supports. For example, MacArthur and Haynes (1995) investigated e-text versions of a 10th-grade biology text in which the following embedded supports were evaluated: an online notebook (notational resource); TTS software; and links to definitions, highlighting, and summaries of text. Many of the embedded supports significantly helped readers with reading comprehension problems. Adding other embedded e-text supports to TTS software may be more effective than using e-text or TTS software alone for readers with print disabilities. A growing body of research is providing strong validation for the effectiveness of embedded supports in enhancing reading comprehension for students with print disabilities (Anderson-Inman, 2004; Anderson-Inman & Horney, 2007; Anderson-Inman, Horney, Chen, & Lewin, 1994; Horney & Anderson-Inman, 1994, 1999). Table 5.3 lists the types of supportive e-text features identified by Anderson-Inman and Horney (2008); these may prove to be effective accommodations for adolescents or adults with LD or ADHD who demonstrate significant problems with reading comprehension.

Donny (Figure 5.2) is an individual for whom embedded e-text supports along with TTS software should enhance his ability to comprehend written text. His low working memory, vocabulary, and listening comprehension abilities indicate that processing verbal language is difficult for him. Donny also demonstrates significant problems with decoding as a result of low phonemic and orthographic awareness. Although TTS software will provide the text for him to hear, his difficulty with verbal language will still make understanding what is read to him a problem. Therefore, adding other embedded supports to an e-text file, such as links to definitions, highlighting, and summaries of text (see Table 5.3), will allow him to gain meaning from the printed word. In addition, Donny can download the e-text and supports on his MP3 player, so that he will have immediate access to technical manuals while he is at school or work.

TABLE 5.3. Anderson-Inman and Horney's Typology of e-Text Embedded Supports

Type of embedded support	Purpose	Examples
Presentational	Customizing text and graphics to meet needs of individual readers	Font size Font style Line length Page length Page layout
Navigational	Allowing readers to move within or between documents	Within-document links Across-document links Embedded menus
Translational	Providing equivalent or simplified version of text	Synonyms Definitions Text-to-speech (TTS) software Simplified reading levels
Explanatory	Providing information for clarity	Descriptions or clarification of text
Illustrative	Providing visual (and/or auditory) representation of text	Drawings Photos Videos Music
Summarizing	Summarizing features of text	Tables of contents Concept maps Lists of key ideas Timelines Abstracts
Enrichment	Providing supplementary information	Background information Biographies of authors Bibliographies
Instructional	Providing prompts, questions, strategies to teach some aspect of text	Tutorials Self-monitoring questions Embedded study strategies
Notational	Providing tools for marking or taking notes	Highlighting Bookmarking Post-its Margin notes Outlines
Collaborative	Providing tools for sharing with others or working together	Threaded discussion Online chat Podcasts E-mail links Blogs
Evaluative	Assessing learning	Questions Quizzes Tests Surveys

Note. Based on Anderson-Horney and Inman (2008).

Implications for Assessment and Accommodation

General Ideas

✓ There is very little correlation between offline and online reading proficiency for students with or without disabilities.

✓ A significant number of adolescents and adults with LD and ADHD demonstrate reading underachievement as a result of their disabilities.

✓ The underlying sources of reading underachievement for individuals with LD and those with ADHD are different both across and within the populations.

Assessment

✓ The persistence of phonemic, orthographic, and morphemic awareness deficits among the adolescent and adult populations with LD in reading (i.e., dyslexia) has been repeatedly documented in the literature.

✓ Evidence is available to support the critical role of verbal working memory in reading decoding performance.

✓ Converging scientific evidence suggests that those individuals with dyslexia become more accurate in reading as they grow older, but continue to demonstrate problems with reading fluency.

✓ Individual differences in memory capacity may reside less in storage capacity than in the efficient use of processes.

✓ Word knowledge is significantly related to phonemic, orthographic, and morphemic learning.

✓ An evaluation of reading decoding performance should always include three components: measures of phonemic, orthographic, and morphemic awareness; pseudoword reading; and regular-word reading.

✓ There does appear to be ample scientific agreement that the reading comprehension performance of adolescents and adults is directly influenced by their fluency, vocabulary, and domain knowledge.

✓ Several studies provide evidence of the significant role that working memory capacity plays in reading comprehension.

✓ The relationship between oral language comprehension and reading comprehension strengthens as readers mature in age and ability level.

✓ The three most widely accepted methods for assessing reading comprehension are retelling, multiple-choice, and modified cloze tasks.

✓ Several methodologies have been used to measure reading comprehension, including think-alouds, curriculum-based measures, and performance-based measures.

✓ Identifying the cognitive strategies a reader utilizes to (1) prepare to read; (2) go beyond the text; (3) organize and synthesize information in the text; and (4) interpret language and ideas in the text is essential to determining appropriate reading comprehension accommodations.

Accommodation

✓ Extra time and a quiet or private testing room are often recommended accommodations for reading deficits.

✓ Alt media and AT allowing access to such media are also often recommended accommodations for reading deficits (see Table 5.2).

✓ One promising set of accommodation, embedded e-text supports, appears to have significant potential for enhancing reading comprehension for many adolescents or adults with LD or ADHD (see Table 5.3).

CHAPTER SIX

Writing Assessment
and Accommodation

Juan, a Hispanic high school senior, is very interested in attending a local technical college next year and is concerned about accessing accommodations. He began receiving special education services in the second grade, with an emphasis on reading comprehension and written language interventions. Despite receiving direct instruction and accommodations from his elementary years through high school, Juan still demonstrates significant underachievement in written expression. He reports having experienced very few opportunities to use assistive technology (AT) for reading or writing during his academic career.

Jamilla, a 38-year-old African American student, is currently attending adult basic education classes at her local community college in order to obtain a general equivalency diploma (GED). When she was an adolescent attending an inner-city high school, the expectations for success were low for a female of color demonstrating problems with learning, and the support services were lacking. Therefore, Jamilla dropped out of high school. Recently, her writing instructor has encouraged her to have a psychological evaluation; he has suggested that her significant difficulties with spelling and written syntax appear to be the result of factors other than lack of instruction.

The significance of writing competency for success in the classroom and in the workplace is ever increasing, particularly in today's technology-driven economy. The National Commission on Writing for American's Families, Schools, and Colleges (2003, 2004, 2005) recently provided the U.S. Congress with three important reports outlining the crisis schools and businesses, and governments (state and federal) are facing because of the poor writing skills demonstrated by many adolescents and adults. The 2003 report, *The Neglected "R": The Need for a Writing Revolution*, confirms that teaching and the practice of writing are often shortchanged in our secondary and postsecondary schools. Further evidence of this writing crisis is clearly provided by the 2007 National Assessment of Educational Progress, which indicated that only 31% of 8th graders and 24% of 12th graders performed at or above a proficient level of writing achievement for their grade level (Salahu-Din, Persky, & Miller, 2008).

Business leaders have complained for years that graduating students do not possess the basic writing skills necessary for the world of work. In its 2004 and 2005 reports, the National Commission on Writing stressed the critical role of writing competency in both the public and private business sectors (*Writing: A Ticket to Work . . . or a Ticket Out: A Survey of Business Leaders; Writing: A Powerful Message from State Government*). For instance, according to the Commission, 50–60% of state and federal government promotion decisions are based on an employee's writing competency. Increasingly, workers are asked to produce significant numbers of e-mails, forms, and technical reports, with few or no support staffers available to help edit their products. As noted by the Commission, "Writing today is not a frill for the few, but an essential skill for the many" (2003, p. 2). For students with LD and ADHD, for whom the process of writing can often be challenging, it is essential for professionals to identify evidence-based accommodations that will allow such individuals to demonstrate their knowledge through written expression.

Standards-based reform and federal mandates (the Individuals with Disabilities Education Improvement Act of 2004 and the No Child Left Behind Act of 2001) require that students with writing disorders be included in regular classroom instruction and in all schoolwide assessments. As observed by the National Commission on Writing (2003), the current state of writing instruction for all students is not adequate to ensure that students will be proficient writers at high school graduation. Therefore, simply including writers with disabilities in the regular curriculum does not guarantee adequate instructional opportunities. In addition, students with LD or ADHD need, but are not receiving in their secondary curricula, more intensive and individualized practice than their peers in order to develop fluent writing skills. As my colleagues and I (Gregg, Coleman, Davis, & Chalk, 2007) have noted elsewhere, "Whether one 'writes' with a pencil, word processor, or speech-to-text technology is not the critical point" (p. 316). Rather, the key to success for these writers is giving them authentic opportunities to write text in safe and encouraging environments. Yet professionals (particularly those at the secondary and postsecondary levels) working with students demonstrating written language disorders have very little evidence-based research to guide their assessment, teaching, or accommodation decision making (Cahalan-Laitusis, 2003; Gregg, Coleman, & Lindstrom, 2008; Li & Hamel, 2003).

Individuals with either LD or ADHD often demonstrate difficulties with written expression. Depending on the type of cognitive or language-processing deficits they exhibit, problems can be noted with handwriting, spelling, syntax, organization, fluency, or sense of audience. Unfortunately, very little research has examined the underlying cognitive, language, and affective processes leading to writing underachievement—and such research should inform the selection of specific interventions, strategies, and accommodations for individuals with LD or ADHD (Gregg, Hoy, McAlexander, & Hayes, 1991; Li & Hamel, 2003).

The purpose of this chapter is to provide professionals with an overview of available research to guide written language assessment and accommodation selection for adolescents and adults with LD and ADHD. Six areas of written expression are discussed: graphomotor output (handwriting), spelling, syntax (sentence level), composition (text level), sense of audience, and fluency. Although various types of accommodations (high- and low-technology) are discussed within and across these areas, greater emphasis is placed on the most effective technologies for the school and work environments.

The theoretical model of written expression that provides the framework for the ideas introduced throughout this chapter integrates research from the fields of sociolinguistics, cognitive psychology, and neurolinguistics. Research from neurolinguistics and cognitive psychology informs our understanding of the cognitive and language processes influencing written expression (Berninger & Winn, 2006; McCutchen, 2006; Shanahan, 2006; Torrance & Galbraith, 2006). Understanding how specific processes (e.g., working memory, executive functioning, orthographic awareness, etc.) influence different aspects of written expression performance can provide important information for intervention and accommodation decision making. From the field of cognitive psychology, evidence is also available as to the importance of the strategic aspects of writing. Strategic learning relies not only on the cognitive abilities of writers, but also on their experiences, self-efficacy beliefs, and motivation for writing (Bereiter & Scardamalia, 1985; Graham, 2006; Hayes, 2006; Pajares & Valiante, 2006). Sociolinguistic research affords verification that written expression is influenced by affective, situational, and social variables (Englert, Mariage, & Dunsmore, 2006; Prior, 2006). However, the boundaries among cognitive, linguistic, affective, and social processes are ambiguous. Accurate assessment and effective accommodation decision making are dependent upon a professional's integrating the current research from several theoretical perspectives, each informed by the others.

Multicultural and Multilingual Learning and Work Environments

Today's increasingly global learning and work environments require professionals to carefully consider culturally diverse learners—both what they have to offer and what they need—when identifying best practices in either the assessment or accommodation of writing. Over the years, many seminal studies in literacy provide evidence for the robust relationship between culture and literacy practices (Au, 1998; Ball, 1999; Heath, 1983; Michaels, 1987; Moll, 1990). In particular, researchers have investigated the conflicts faced by many African American students during the process of writing at the phonological, syntactic, semantic, pragmatic, and discourse levels (Ball, 1992, 1996, 1999; Fecho, 2000; Rosaen, 2003).

A recent investigation of African American language (AAL) features and typical speech code errors (SCE) demonstrated several differences in the writing patterns of African American and European American examinees during a high-stakes teaching certification test (Szpara & Wylie, 2007). Speech code errors (SCE) were defined by these authors as spelling, syntactic, or punctuation mistakes that were not considered to be AAL features; such writing errors are common for many inexperienced writers. Table 6.1 summarizes the SCE and AAL features identified across the groups of writers in the Szpara and Wylie (2007) research. This summary of language features can be a useful resource for evaluators involved in assessing the writing of the adolescent and adult populations with LD and ADHD. Both AAL and SCE patterns have the potential to influence diagnostic decision making, as well as to bias the scoring of performance on high-stakes tests. Professionals involved in the assessment of writing performance are encouraged to maintain an ethnosensitive perspective when making judgments about individual writers' proficiency and capability (Ball, 2006). Unfortunately, when we consider the particular needs of African American writers with LD or ADHD, research to support decision making for either writing interventions or accommodations is not available.

Multilingual writers also require special consideration and attention from professionals. In a thorough review of the literature, Fitzgerald (2006) investigated the quantity and quality of available research on multilingual writing in preschool through 12th grade. As she notes,

TABLE 6.1. Summary of Speech Code Errors (SCE) and African American Language (AAL) Codes

SCE (sentence level)	AAL codes (sentence level)
Unnecessary apostrophe in plurals	Regular plural noun, absence of -*s*
No apostrophe in possessive	Possessive noun, absence of -'*s/s*'
Incorrect apostrophe in possessives	Regular verb, simple past tense, absence of -*ed*
Irregular verb, simple past tense, non-EAE[a] form	Regular verb, present/past/future perfect tense, absence of -*ed*
Irregular verb, present/past/future perfect tense, non-EAE form	Regular verbal adjective, absence of -*ed*
Irregular verbal adjective, non-EAE form	Regular passive voice, absence of -*ed*
Irregular passive voice, non-EAE form	Regular third-person singular present tense, absence of -*s*
Irregular third-person singular present tense, non-EAE form	Zero copula
Conjugated "be," non-EAE form	Aspectual or invariant "be"
Subject–verb inversion	Deletion of word-final consonants
Subject–verb discord	
Other non-EAE verb forms	
Other spelling errors	
Missing or incorrect preposition	
Other missing words	
Incorrect use of connecting words	
Noun–pronoun discord	
Pronominal apposition	
Homophones	

Note. From Szpara and Wylie (2007). Copyright 2007 by Oxford University Press. Reprinted by permission.
[a]Non-European American English.

the tendency was toward "low levels of research rigor," and many of the issues addressed "were narrow in scope, resulting in topic clusters that were not deeply researched" (p. 337). As a result, Fitzgerald cautions against making any summary or generalizations about the similarities and differences between monolingual and bilingual writers. Again, for bilingual writers with LD or ADHD, the lack of evidence-based research is even more significant. Because second-language composing will continue to be critical to the success of many adolescents and adults with LD and ADHD, Fitzgerald's advice in regard to improving the state of multilingual research and practice is extremely important for all of us to remember. She states: "Forging solid multilingual writing research agendas that engage investigators and theorists from historically divided disciplines such as linguistics, psychology, sociology, and education is one immediate response to the serious needs of our children [I would add adolescents and adults]" (p. 352).

Luria's Work and Accommodation Selection

One of the many important lessons available to us from the scholarship of the great Russian psychologist Alexander Luria (1980) is the importance of different task formats in the assessment of writing. Luria suggested that an evaluation of a writer's proficiency should always include three different tasks: copying, dictation, and spontaneous writing. Each of these formats calls upon distinctive cognitive and linguistic processes that are discussed throughout this chapter. In addition, as the task demands increase, the integration of cognitive and linguistic processes will change. Accommodation selection should never be based on only one type of writing task (e.g., spelling single words in an untimed situation).

Jamilla's assessment profile (see Figure 6.1) helps to illustrate the importance of task requirements in assessment and accommodation selection. Although Jamilla demonstrates serious deficits in writing, we can note that her graphomotor speed and verbal working memory abilities do not appear to have a negative influence on her writing performance. Therefore, tasks requiring her to copy words, sentences, or even paragraphs will be easier for her than a dictation task. Dictation tasks require an individual to integrate phonemic awareness (sound awareness), orthographic awareness (sound–symbol awareness), and word/sentence structure. For Jamilla, this requires her to utilize cognitive and linguistic processes that appear to be areas of deficit. Therefore, when a professional is selecting accommodations for her, Jamilla's visual and graphomotor abilities are the processes to consider as avenues to enhance her access to learning. For example, an outlining/webbing software program will utilize her strong visual–spatial, motor, and nonverbal reasoning abilities. Verbal mnemonic strategies for writing may not be as effective, since these will require her to recall letters, words, or sentences, which draw more upon her naming or phonemic and orthographic processes. Again, careful consideration of the task demands and of a writer's learning profile helps in the selection of effective accommodations.

Writing Tools

The tool or tools used in writing (e.g., pencil or pen, computer, voice-activated software) are very important to consider in selecting effective accommodations for adolescents or adults with LD or ADHD. Once again, a writer's cognitive and language assessment profile should help

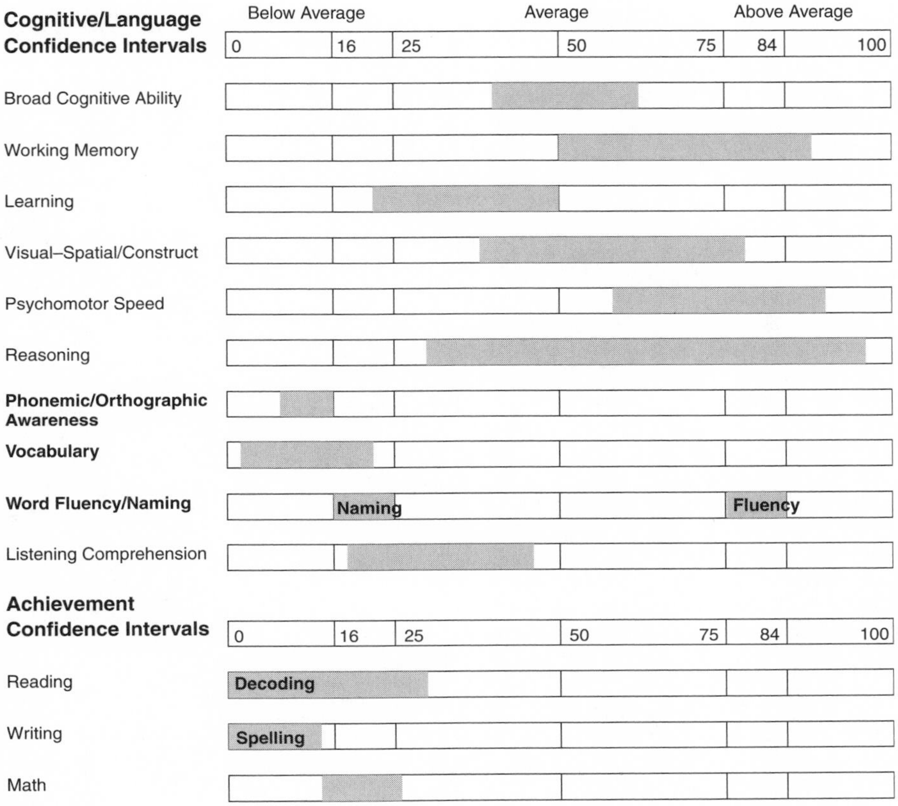

Cognitive/Language Confidence Intervals	Below Average			Average		Above Average	
	0	16	25	50	75	84	100
Broad Cognitive Ability							
Working Memory							
Learning							
Visual–Spatial/Construct							
Psychomotor Speed							
Reasoning							
Phonemic/Orthographic Awareness							
Vocabulary							
Word Fluency/Naming	Naming				Fluency		
Listening Comprehension							

Achievement Confidence Intervals							
	0	16	25	50	75	84	100
Reading	Decoding						
Writing	Spelling						
Math							

FIGURE 6.1. Assessment profile for Jamilla, an individual with dyslexia.

guide decision making—in this case, tool selection. The use of computers for enhancing writing competencies has increased dramatically since the late 1980s (Becker, 1999). The available research evidence suggests that composing with a computer improves writing fluency, editing, and quality of writing for many students with and without writing disorders (MacArthur, 2006; Russell & Cook, 2002). Juan's assessment profile (Figure 6.2) certainly provides strong support for word processing as an appropriate accommodation for enhancing his writing fluency. His problems with graphomotor speed, verbal working memory, sustained attention, and executive functioning make writing very difficult for him. Word processing, Web software, and spell checkers should enhance his writing fluency and accuracy.

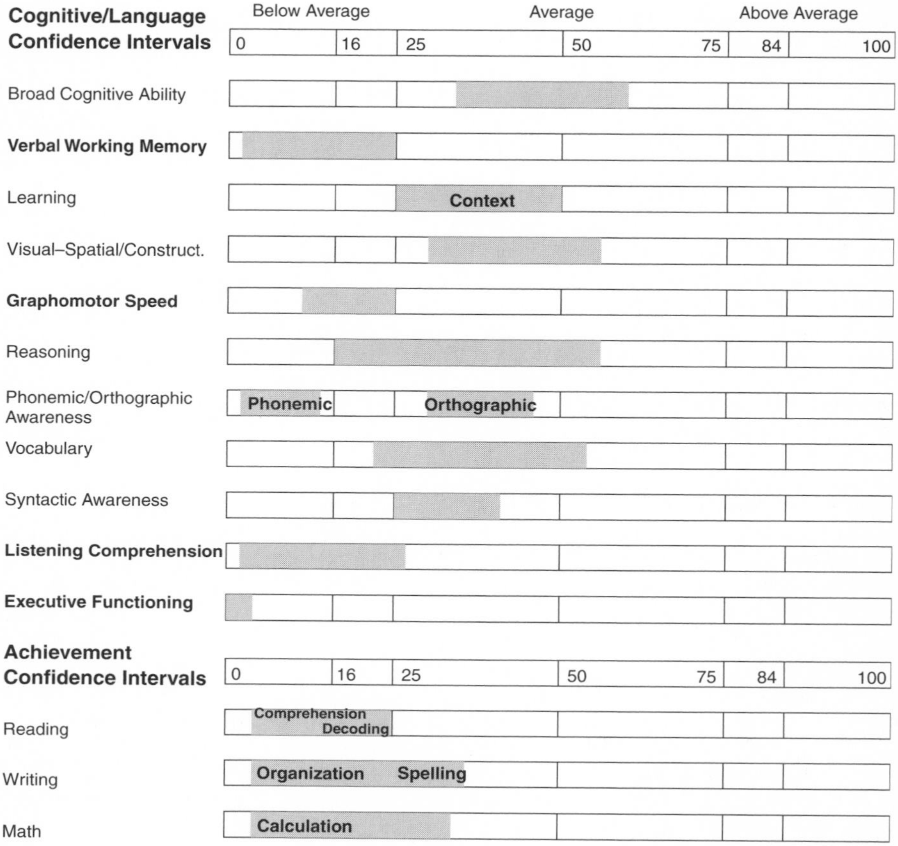

Cognitive/Language Confidence Intervals	Below Average		Average		Above Average	
	0 16	25	50	75	84	100
Broad Cognitive Ability						
Verbal Working Memory						
Learning	**Context**					
Visual–Spatial/Construct.						
Graphomotor Speed						
Reasoning						
Phonemic/Orthographic Awareness	**Phonemic**	**Orthographic**				
Vocabulary						
Syntactic Awareness						
Listening Comprehension						
Executive Functioning						

Achievement Confidence Intervals						
	0 16	25	50	75	84	100
Reading	**Comprehension** **Decoding**					
Writing	**Organization** **Spelling**					
Math	**Calculation**					

FIGURE 6.2. Assessment profile for Juan, an individual with ADHD.

Assessing and Accommodating
Written Expression: General Areas of Concern

Writing underachievement alone does not constitute a written expression disorder. Although there are standardized instruments available to professionals for investigating written expression, the majority of these tests simply screen writing performance, and they often have restricted norms for both age and educational experience (see Gregg & Hartwig, 2005, for an in-depth discussion of the technical aspects of standardized measures of writing). Therefore, professionals working with adolescents and adults who have LD or ADHD are encouraged to develop systematic means of collecting writing observations and informal samples (e.g., classroom writing assignments) for use in accommodation decision making. In addition, the choice of accommodations for written language disorders should reflect the other data collected during a psychological evaluation (e.g., cognitive, language, affective). Finally, an evaluator must take into consideration a writer's exposure to writing instruction; the task demands; the situational context; and the general expectations for writers with similar writing experiences and backgrounds (e.g., cultural, linguistic). Figure 6.3 provides a series of seven questions as a framework to guide professionals involved in the selection of writing accommodations for adolescents and/or adults with LD and ADHD. In addition, Table 6.2 lists different accommodation options that are discussed throughout this chapter for writers demonstrating functional limitations in their writing performance. The remainder of the chapter reviews research on, assessment of, and accommodations for the six areas of written expression noted earlier: handwriting, spelling, syntax, composition, sense of audience, and fluency.

Graphomotor Output (Handwriting)

The graphomotor system is the most relevant of the motor systems for writing, since it is the regulator of finger and hand movements. The graphomotor system monitors the serial motor movements required for handwriting, including the planning, controlling (monitoring/revising), and executing functions (Berninger & Richards, 2002). Many different cognitive and linguistic processes contribute to the efficiency of these functions, depending on the writer's profile and the task demands. Recent brain imaging studies have indicated which brain structures may be responsible for these functions (i.e., supplementary motor area, left premotor cortex, cerebellum, anterior cingulate, primary and secondary motor areas, left fusiform, and left lingual gyri). Berninger and Richards, 2002, provide an in-depth discussion of recent *in vivo* functional imaging studies highlighting the different neural mechanisms underlying graphomotor performance. Neuropsychologists have substantiated that writers with LD and ADHD often demonstrate graphomotor deficits (Berninger, 1996; Deul, 1992). Currently, there is evidence that the three types of graphomotor disorders most prevalent in the adolescent and adult populations with LD and ADHD are symbolic deficits, motor speed deficits, and dyspraxia (Deul, 1992). All three types interfere with a writer's handwriting legibility and writing fluency.

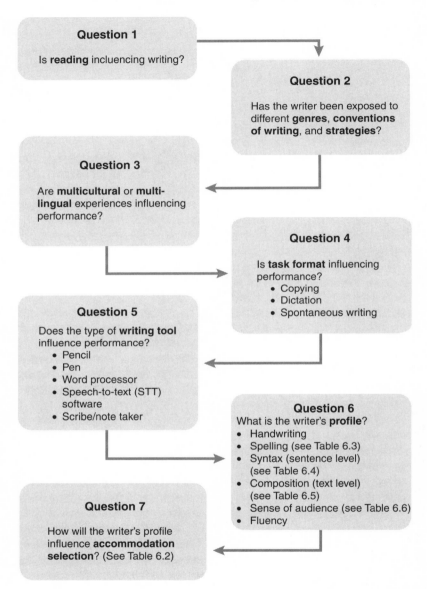

FIGURE 6.3. Questions to support decision making for the accommodation of written language problems.

TABLE 6.2. Written Language Accommodations and Strategies

Handwriting	Spelling	Syntax (sentence level)	Composition (text level)
Extra time	Extra time	Extra time	Extra time
Scribe/note taker	Scribe/note taker	Scribe/note taker	Scribe/note taker
Word processing	Word processing	Word processing	Word processing
Word prediction	Word prediction	Word prediction	Word prediction
Speech-to-text (STT) software	STT software	STT software	STT software
Touch windows	Text-to-speech (TTS) software	TTS software	TTS software
Macro software	Macro software	Embedded e-text supports[a] Translational Explanatory Illustrative Summarizing Instructional Notational	Embedded e-text supports[a] Translational Explanatory Illustrative Summarizing Instructional Notational Collaborative Enrichment
Audio voice recorder	Audio voice recorder		
Audio voice player	Audio voice player	Writing strategies	Writing strategies
Computer	Computer	Graham and Harris (2005)	Graham and Harris (2005)
MP3 player	MP3 player	Deshler et al. (1996)	Deshler et al. (1996)
Phone	Phone		Englert and Mariage (1991)
Mouse options[b]	Spell checkers		Englert Think Sheets (Hallenbeck, 1996)
Double-click speed	Talking dictionary		
Click lock			
Pointer schemes			
Trackball options			
Keyboard options[b]			
Modified keyboards			
Sticky keys			
Filter keys			
Toggle keys			
Mouse keys			

[a]See Table 5.3 in Chapter Five.
[b]See Microsoft Accessibility Resources (*www.microsoft.com/enable*).

Symbolic Deficits

Individuals with "symbolic" graphomotor deficits demonstrate specific phonemic, orthographic, and morphemic awareness deficits that interfere primarily with the planning and controlling functions required of handwriting. As noted by Berninger and Richards (2002), "Letter production requires a precise, complete visual–motor program (kinetic melody; Luria, 1980) for planning and producing each sequentially ordered component stroke: the program must be created, stored, and retrieved on an as-needed basis" (p. 169). Abbott and Berninger (1993) found that the path from orthographic coding to handwriting was direct, but that nonverbal fine motor skills (e.g., copying geometric designs) contributed only indirectly through orthography. Therefore, an adolescent or adult with symbolic graphomotor deficits may produce excellent original drawings (e.g., cartoons), but may not be able to produce legible handwriting. Visual–verbal production (handwriting) draws upon very different neurological systems than visual–nonverbal production (pictures, cartoons) does. Individuals with dyslexia often demonstrate symbolic graphomotor symptoms, resulting in poor handwriting performance. Since it is often difficult for these individuals to recall the letters or words they want to use in order to express their ideas, legibility and writing fluency become problems for them (Berninger, 1996; Myklebust, 1965).

Motor Speed Deficits

Individuals with motor speed deficits demonstrate problems with the timing and temporal aspects of graphomotor tasks that draw upon the planning and execution functions of writing. These individuals are usually capable of legible and accurate handwriting, but they produce the product very slowly (Deul, 1992). Historically, motor speed problems were called "clumsiness" or "limb-kinetic apraxia" (Liepmann, 1900). Individuals with ADHD often demonstrate this type of graphomotor symptom (Deul, 1992).

Dyspraxia

Dyspraxia is often symptomatic of individuals with nonverbal LD (see Chapter Four). According to Deul (1992), "dyspraxia" is the "inability to learn and perform age-appropriate sequences of voluntary movements in the face of preserved coordination, strength, and sensation" (p. 264). Unlike writers with symbolic graphomotor deficits, these individuals demonstrate motor pattern difficulties regardless of whether the symbols are verbal (letters) or nonverbal (pictures). One of the most distinguishing aspects of dyspraxia is the unusual formation of letters and words. These writers will often print in distinct block-like symbols, usually in all capitals. Inaccurate spaces between letters and words, as well as difficulty with letter formation, are noted.

Assessment of Handwriting

Handwriting performance (speed and legibility) continues to be of importance to professionals working with adolescents and adults who have LD and ADHD, as many high-stakes tests (for graduating from high school, entering college, etc.) require the examinee to write a timed impromptu essay by hand. We (Gregg, Coleman, Davis, & Chalk, 2007) studied college students with and without dyslexia who were required to complete a timed impromptu essay. We investigated the influence of handwritten, typed, and typed/edited formats on the writing quality scores of these students. In addition, we examined the contribution of spelling, handwriting, number of words, and vocabulary complexity to these scores. We found that vocabulary complexity, verbosity, spelling, and handwriting ability accounted for more variance in the writing quality scores for the students with dyslexia than for their peers. The significantly negative influence of handwriting on the performance of these young adult writers with dyslexia is consistent with past studies of children and adolescents with LD (e.g., Graham, Harris, & Fink, 2000). Legibility problems can easily influence raters' perceptions of competence, because a writer who is slow and laborious in forming letters and words may write fewer words and sacrifice ideation and planning time (Graham & Weintraub, 1996; Gregg, Coleman, Davis, & Chalk, 2007).

Neuropsychologists often use such tasks as finger tapping, pegboard speed, and hand strength to assess graphomotor abilities. However, the norming restrictions and validity (predictive and construct) of these measures for the adolescent and adult population with LD and ADHD is questionable. Two approaches that have stronger validity in the evaluation of handwriting proficiency for older writers are global and analytic evaluations of legibility (Mather & Woodcock, 2001; Rosenblum, Weiss, & Parush, 2004). Global evaluation measures require a rater to judge handwriting holistically by comparing it to examples of graded handwriting. Analytic scales evaluate legibility by having a rater apply predetermined quantitative criteria. Recent advances in digital technology have provided legibility measures, but currently these devices are not as reliable or valid as global or analytic scales (Rosenblum et al., 2004). However, future advances in digital technologies may provide excellent methods for measuring graphomotor speed and accuracy. Currently, global handwriting measures appear more reliable and valid for children, whereas global and analytic scales appear to be comparable in providing measures of legibility for the adult population (Dennis & Swinthe, 2001; Graham, 1986; Gregg, Coleman, Davis, & Chalk, 2007).

Accommodations for Handwriting Disorders

Very little research evidence is available to provide guidance in choosing accommodations for adolescents with LD or ADHD demonstrating graphomotor disorders. Therefore, professionals are totally dependent upon well-supported clinical observations and assessment data in choosing specific accommodations. Table 6.2 lists several accommodation options for individuals demonstrating poor handwriting. Obviously, for all three types of graphomotor disorders (i.e., symbolic deficits, motor speed deficits, dyspraxia) discussed above, extra time is an essential accommodation. Word processing and various types of AT also provide accommodation options appropriate for the different types of graphomotor disorders. Traditional forms of AT used with more severe motor disorders, such as adapted switches, adapted keyboards, and keyboard overlays, have not been well investigated by researchers for their effectiveness with the adolescent or adult populations with LD or ADHD. A few studies do support the effectiveness of word processing, word prediction software, and voice input (speech-to-text [STT] software) for enhancing the legibility and fluency of these adolescents' and adults' writing (Handley-More, Deitz, Billingsley, & Coggins, 2003; Higgins & Raskind, 1995; MacArthur, 2006). In addition, researchers need to investigate the usefulness of touch windows and macro software for accommodating the writing of adolescents and adults with LD and ADHD, since these recommendations are often suggested by professionals. With the popularity and accessibility of mobile touch devices (e.g., iPod, iPhone), we should be seeing applications of this technology for accommodating graphomotor disorders in the near future.

Spelling

Spelling is a writer's ability to represent words accurately in print. Researchers have provided evidence of the regularities and opacities of the English spelling system itself; the role of morphology in spelling; developmental trajectories; spelling acquisition strategies; cognitive, linguistic, and environmental predictors; the nature of mental representations of words; the role of implicit memory; the relationship between spelling and other academic skills (e.g., decoding); and possible reasons for spelling underachievement (Coleman, Gregg, McLain, & Belair, in press). There is a spectrum of spelling competency that depends on a variety of factors (e.g., exposure to print, reading style) unrelated to cognitive and language abilities. Even among adolescents and adults with average or higher levels of reading proficiency, some may be unexpectedly poor spellers (Frith, 1980; Holmes & Castles, 2001). Table 6.3 provides a summary of several cognitive and linguistic processes that influence spelling competency.

The importance of phonemic awareness to literacy development and spelling achievement has been well documented in the literature for the child population (e.g., Allyn & Burt, 1998; Bruck & Waters, 1990; Burt & Shrubsole, 2000). However, the persistence of spelling problems into adolescence and adulthood for individuals with dyslexia has also been

TABLE 6.3. Cognitive and Linguistic Processes Influencing Spelling Performance

Cognitive and linguistic processes	Relationship to spelling
Graphomotor functioning	Letter formation; legibility
Auditory discrimination and selective attention	Accurate recognition and selective attention to sounds and words
Verbal working memory	Retention/analysis of spoken words during the process of spelling
Phonemic awareness	Appreciation of the concept that words contain phonemes; accurate identification of phonemes
Morphemic awareness	Appreciation of prefixes, affixes, and other morphological forms
Orthographic awareness	Knowledge of phoneme–grapheme correspondences; accurate perception and encoding of symbols; sensitivity to implicit spelling rules
Word knowledge/retrieval	Appreciation and on-demand recall of various aspects of words (pronunciation, spelling, primary–secondary meanings, semantic–syntactic constraints)
Print exposure/instruction	Experience with/exposure to printed words and general patterns related to their spelling and use

Note. From Gregg, Coleman, and Lindstrom (2008). Copyright 2008 by Psychology Press. Adapted by permission.

supported by empirically based evidence (Berninger et al., 2006; Bruck, 1993; Gregg, Coleman, Stennett, & Davis, 2002; Holmes & Malone, 2004). Phonemic awareness involves facility with language sounds—for example, the ability to identify, discriminate, and isolate phonemes; proficiency with rhyming; and the ability to repeat and/or manipulate spoken pseudowords (see Chapter Five for a more in-depth discussion). Some researchers suggest that phonemic awareness problems may be reflected in spelling attempts that lack phonetic plausibility—that is, in attempts that, if decoded according to typical grapheme–phoneme conversion rules, do not sound exactly like the target word (Coleman et al., in press; Holmes & Castles, 2001). Recently, researchers have identified morphemic awareness (sometimes called "morphological awareness" or "morphophonemic awareness"; again, see Chapter Five for more detail) as another strong predictor of spelling (e.g., Allyn & Burt, 1998; Holmes & Castles, 2001; Leong, 1999) and an area of weakness in adolescents and adults with dyslexia (Bruck, 1993; Coleman et al., in press; Deacon, Parrila, & Kirby, 2006; Leong, 1999).

Orthographic awareness, orthographic sensitivity, or orthographic processing (once again, see Chapter Five for a fuller discussion) is likewise very important to spelling performance across the lifespan (e.g., Cunningham, Perry, & Stanovich, 2001; Fischer, Shankweiler, & Liberman, 1985; Foorman, 1994; Roberts & Mather, 1997; Stanovich et al., 1991). As Holmes and Castles (2001) note, "unexpectedly poor spellers are seen to misspell many words, not because of deficient phonological processing, but because their lexical entries contain inadequately specified word-specific information" (p. 321).

Adolescents and adults with ADHD, while often demonstrating problems with spelling, do not demonstrate the number or types of errors characteristic of their peers with dyslexia. In a recent study, a colleague and I (Coleman & Gregg, 2005) counted and categorized spelling mistakes in the impromptu essays composed by 211 young adults. The students without disabilities (n = 90) averaged 2–3 errors per 1,000 words, and about 80% of their incorrect attempts were judged to be plausible (e.g., "airate" for "aerate"). Students with ADHD (n = 44), though they made more errors (about 4 per 1,000 words), achieved a similar plausibility rate. The errors of students with dyslexia (n = 77) were considerably more frequent (7 per 1,000 words) and less plausible (65%).

For examples of writers demonstrating differences in spelling abilities, let's look at the profiles of Jamilla (Figure 6.1) and Juan (Figure 6.2). Jamilla demonstrates significant underachievement in written expression, with her spelling scores constituting the lower end of her written expression confidence band. Her significant problems with phonemic and orthographic awareness appear to be influencing her ability to spell words, either on contrived tasks (spelling tests with either nonsense or regular words) or in her spontaneous writing sample. Although Juan's written expression performance is low, it appears that his problems lie more in the organizational aspects of writing. His orthographic awareness abilities emerge as a foundation for his spelling competency, as compared to Jamilla's profile, where deficits in phonemic and orthographic awareness negatively influence her spelling abilities. The clinician evaluating Juan has reported that his lower scores on phonemic awareness tasks appear to be due to his inability to sustain attention rather than to a linguistic deficit. The types of writing accommodations will differ for these two learners.

Assessment of Spelling

Researcher have shown that spelling tests are effective at discriminating between "good" and "poor" spellers, but not at determining types of spelling errors that may be symptomatic of certain disabilities (Burt & Fury, 2000). This may be because, as Bruck (1993) notes, "[s]tandardized spelling tests usually contain items that are psychometrically rather than theoretically based" (p. 182). Another concern related to traditional spelling assessment is that a dichotomous scoring system (correct–incorrect or 0–1) does not yield distinctions among incorrect attempts of varying plausibility. In an effort to characterize the inaccurate spelling attempts of writers with and without dyslexia, we (Coleman et al., in press) conducted item-level analyses of the spelling errors on a contrived spelling test (i.e., the Wide Range Achievement Test–4 [WRAT4]; Wilkinson with Robertson, 2004) and from spontaneous writing. Among unconstrained (essay) errors, students with dyslexia had much more difficulty than their normally achieving peers with familiar and easy-to-spell words. On a constrained task (spelling dictation, WRAT-4), group differences were noted on the number and types of errors. Students with dyslexia made more errors reflective of phonemic, orthographic, and morphemic awareness problems.

The most widely used format for measuring spelling involves recall of real-word spellings (see Gregg & Hartwig, 2005, for a review of standardized spelling measures). For adolescents and adults whose graphomotor functioning is also compromised, a multiple-choice recognition format (e.g., the Spelling subtest of the Peabody Individualized Achievement Test—Revised/Normative Update; Markwardt, 1997) may be more appropriate. As phonemic and orthographic processes often negatively influence spelling for writers with LD, a measure that assesses spelling by using pseudowords (e.g., the Spelling of Sounds subtest of the Woodcock–Johnson III Tests of Achievement [WJ III ACH] battery; Woodcock et al., 2001a) provides a means to investigate the influence of these processes on word knowledge performance. Evaluators should be encouraged to investigate a writer's spelling abilities across regular-word and pseudoword tasks, as well as in both contrived and spontaneous writing samples.

Accommodations for Spelling Disorders

As noted throughout the literature, underachievement in spelling is a hallmark of writers with dyslexia. Table 6.2 lists the options available to accommodate spelling disorders. Although some research supports the effectiveness of AT in enhancing spelling performance, the number of studies for the adolescent and adult population is limited. As for students with graphomotor disorders, extra time is an appropriate accommodation for students with significant spelling deficits, since they require more time to recall the motor and orthographic patterns necessary to spell words. Word processing also appears to enhance the fluency and spelling of adolescent and young adult writers with LD (Bangert-Drowns, 1993; A. Goldberg, Russell, & Cook, 2003; Hetzroni & Shrieber, 2004; MacArthur, 2006). Research supports the effectiveness of spell checkers and word prediction programs for enhancing the spelling performance of adolescent writers with LD (Handley-More et al., 2003). Speech recognition software for dictation has gained some support as a means to enhance the writing of adolescents and adults with LD demonstrating spelling, handwriting, and fluency problems (Higgins & Raskind, 1995; MacArthur & Cavalier, 2004; Reese & Cummings, 1996). However, as significant a problem as spelling is for writers with LD, it is surprising that researchers have paid relatively little attention to accommodating spelling disabilities.

Syntax (Sentence Level)

The term "syntax" refers to sentence-level language, or the manner in which words are assembled to form sentences. The ability to produce syntactically correct sentence structures involves "semantics" (word usage in context), "grammar" (e.g., subject–verb and pronoun–antecedent agreement), and "mechanics" (e.g., application of punctuation and capitalization rules), all working in unison. Problems with any one of these features can create problems with written syntax. Therefore, during an evaluation, an individual's word usage, grammar, and writing mechanics should all be examined for their influence on syntax. The effect of lexical/grammatical errors on the writing of individuals with LD or ADHD is best illustrated by the following sentences produced by adult writers with these disorders: (1) "Walk into church on a Saturday and you can find two people exchanging rings and vowels." (2) "Kids, that don't have parents, tend to get into trouble." (3) "Being a vet, my dog Pepper was soon healthy & happy & home again." Even when the writing samples of adults with LD have been retyped and corrected for spelling, differences have been noted between their written syntax and that of their peers (Gregg, Coleman, Davis, & Chalk, 2007; Gregg, Coleman, Stennett, & Davis, 2002). Such an outcome is a reminder that the writing underachievement demonstrated by adolescents or adults with LD or ADHD is not only the result of graphomotor or spelling deficits.

Very few investigations of the cognitive and linguistic processes influencing the production of written syntax by adolescents and adults with LD or ADHD have been undertaken to date. Unfortunately, moreover, the majority of researchers investigating written syntax in these populations have relied upon frequency counts, such as number of words, sentence length, or number of sentences. Such indices fail to consider the complex interrelationships among words, syntactic structures, and context. Yet research from the field of linguistics, particularly sociolinguistics, has shown the dramatic relationship between context and function in a language user's application of meaning and structure. The association of word meaning to syntactic structure, and of structure to words, provides information pertinent to our understanding of language and to our ability to design instruction in reading and writing (see Biber, Conrad, & Reppen, 1998, for an in-depth discussion).

We (Gregg, Coleman, Stennett, & Davis, 2002) examined the relationship of words and sentence features in the expository essays of four groups of young adults (writers with LD, writers with ADHD, and normally achieving writers). We found that the writers with LD and ADHD demonstrated less variety and complexity of sentence-level features than did the normally achieving writers. Through his extensive research, Biber (1988) identified several sentence features most associated with increased sentence complexity in written text. Using these complexity indices, we (Gregg & Coleman, 2005) found that among young adults with and without dyslexia, two of Biber's sentence features—"integrated structures" (i.e., nouns, preparations, and attributive adjectives) and "word specificity" (i.e., word length and word types)—differentiated the two groups of writers. The writing of the young adults with dyslexia contained significantly fewer of these features, therefore decreasing the linguistic complexity of their writing samples. Interestingly, we (Gregg & Coleman, 2005) also found that the writers with dyslexia had more difficulty with sentence features having to do with time ("be" as main verb, tense, prepositions, and time adverbials), which could have been due to deficits in the executive and attentional processes of working memory. Another distinct feature of the discourse of these dyslexic writers was their overuse of "hedges" (e.g., "at about," "something like," "more or less," "almost," "maybe," "sort of," "kind of," etc.). Such structures result in less specificity and more ambiguity in the meaning of the text. Underlying word knowledge and word access problems may have been contributing to this overuse of hedges.

As summarized in Table 6.4, development of age-appropriate written syntax skills depends on a number of variables. Foremost among these is oral language development (i.e., receptive and expressive syntax). An adult with an expressive (or receptive–expressive) language

TABLE 6.4. Cognitive and Linguistic Processes Influencing Written Syntax Performance

Cognitive and linguistic processes	Relationship to written syntax
Verbal working memory	Ability to compose (mentally) and write at the same time without making errors (e.g., word omissions, substitutions)
Attention	Ability to selectively attend and sustain attention to specific word choices
Executive functions	Ability to organize ideas; time management; monitoring
Morphemic awareness	Ability to use and sustain grammatical agreement between subjects and verbs, pronouns and antecedents, etc.
Word knowledge/retrieval	Ability to use varied/age-appropriate vocabulary choices
Receptive syntax	Ability to understand spoken sentences; appreciation of structural and internal details
Expressive syntax	Ability to use a variety of sentence structures
Knowledge of conventions/ mechanics	Ability to apply rules related to punctuation, capitalization, etc.
Print exposure/instruction/ reading abilities	Experience with/exposure to different registers/genres (e.g., formal academic writing); reading abilities

Note. From Gregg, Coleman, and Lindstrom (2008). Copyright 2008 by Psychology Press. Adapted by permission.

disorder will struggle to construct written sentences, just as he or she struggles to construct spoken ones. Of course, this is not to imply that intact oral syntax abilities are automatically transferred to the written arena; they are necessary but not sufficient for writing proficiency. Mastery of a formal writing system also requires adequate functioning in other cognitive and social areas, as well as extensive instruction in grammar, punctuation, word usage, and other conventions. Exposure to print is also important, since familiarity and proficiency with different styles and registers (e.g., expository, narrative, technical) depend on it. Again, examiners are encouraged to answer the seven questions posed in Figure 6.3 to guide their interpretation of diagnostic information and their selection of accommodations.

Assessment of Syntax

For the adolescent and adult populations with LD and ADHD, the assessment of syntax is complicated by an increase in the variety and sophistication of language structures typically used as people mature, as well as by a decrease in the standardized assessment tools available (Gregg, Coleman, & Lindstrom, 2008). There are, however, several useful tests normed beyond age 17 that can be effective in evaluating the written syntax competency of adolescents and adults with LD or ADHD. These measures require the generation of individual sentences in response to specific prompts (e.g., composing a sentence that contains the words "would," "time," and "if"). Such a "constrained" format often yields important information about an examinee's mastery of different kinds of sentence structures (e.g., conditionals). Some standardized tests include time constraints (e.g., the WJ III ACH Writing Fluency subtest; Woodcock et al., 2001a), while others do not (e.g., the Written Expression subtest of the Oral and Written Language Scales; Carrow-Woolfolk, 1996). Use of both task types is advised, since, as Mather and Woodcock (2001) note, the evaluator wants to determine "whether the subject work[s] (a) slowly but inaccurately, (b) slowly and accurately, (c) rapidly but inaccurately, or (d) rapidly and accurately" (p. 86).

Impromptu writing tasks also provide qualitative information about written syntax that is invaluable for accommodation decision making. Writers with ADHD, who usually demonstrate poor executive functioning, may generate competent sentences within a constrained (i.e., highly structured) format like that of Writing Samples (Woodcock et al., 2001a), but make monitoring errors (e.g., leaving out words) when faced with the more taxing demands of planning and composing an entire essay (Gregg, Coleman, & Lindstrom, 2008). The unconstrained prose of adolescents and adults with LD and ADHD may vary considerably, depending on the nature and severity of the disorder and the task approach. Some writers with LD or ADHD actually make less frequent errors in essays—when they can simplify or "dumb down" their sentence structures and word choices—than on constrained tasks. Others may make more frequent errors, because higher-level task demands (e.g., organization, idea development) draw critical cognitive resources away from the execution of already weak basic skills (e.g., grammar). We (Gregg, Coleman, & Lindstrom, 2008) suggest that an evaluator consider several aspects of syntax in reviewing qualitative writing samples: number of words and clauses; diversity of sentence structures; variety of word choices; frequency of changes/corrections; and frequency and severity of errors in subskill areas (capitalization, comma usage, apostrophe usage, word usage, agreement, and sentence structure).

Accommodations for Syntax Disorders

The effectiveness of accommodations for adolescent or adult writers with LD or ADHD demonstrating disorders in written syntax has not been well addressed in the literature. Table 6.2 lists commonly suggested accommodations for writing underachievement resulting from syntax disorders. However, professionals are well advised to investigate the cognitive and linguistic deficits underlying individual writers' difficulties in producing sentence structures as their guide for selecting specific accommodations (see Table 6.4). For writers struggling to produce written sentences, extra time and word processing are appropriate accommodations. Students whose verbal working memory deficits are interfering with their written sentence structure may be helped by word prediction and outlining/webbing software. For writers with significant attention and/or executive functioning deficits influencing written syntax production, outlining/webbing and text-to-speech (TTS) software may be a very effective accommodation. Research evidence indicates that TTS software can help some students "hear" word choice errors so that they can make revisions (Higgins & Raskind, 1995; MacArthur, 2006). For students whose difficulty in recalling words influences sentence structure production, word prediction software may be recommended. However, STT software is often not as effective for writers also demonstrating oral expressive syntax disorders; the technology is currently not advanced enough to deal with the oral hesitations and pronunciation errors often demonstrated by these individuals. Grammar checkers have not been supported by strong research evidence to support their effectiveness as an accommodation for individuals with written syntax disorders.

The metacognitive problems discussed in Chapter Five as making reading comprehension difficult for many adolescent and adult readers with LD and ADHD also influence their written language performance at both the sentence and text levels. The metacognitive processes that adolescents and adults with LD or ADHD use to access writing strategies during the process of writing are not well understood by researchers. However, the effectiveness of teaching strategies to enhance writing performance at the sentence and text levels for these populations has been well validated by research (Deshler, Ellis, & Lenz, 1996; Hallenbeck, 1996; Graham & Harris, 2005). These strategies, once learned, can become an effective accommodation during the process of writing at either the sentence or the text level. In addition, some of the embedded e-text supports discussed in Chapter Five can be modified for the writing process (see Table 6.2, and Table 5.3 in Chapter Five).

Composition (Text Level)

"Composition" refers to the organization of ideas in writing at the text level. Word and sentence structures, as well as function (purpose), can be very different, depending on the chosen mode of writing (e.g., narrative, expository, persuasive). The language one uses in written discourse comprises a structure, just as words in a sentence determine a syntactic structure. During the evaluation of an adolescent or adult, one should consider the relationship between the syntax (sentence level) and composition (text level) of written text, as well as the function (purpose) of the writing task (Kintsch, 1998; Van Dijk & Kintsch, 1983). Halliday (1973) has discussed three functions of adult language: "ideational," "interpersonal," and "textual." The ideational function relates to the content or knowledge of what the writer is expressing. Usually, the more knowledge one brings to the writing task, the more fluent the writer. Interpersonal functions involve the writer's relationship to the audience (sense of audience). The textual function of writing incorporates both the ideational and the interpersonal in order to construct meaning for the reader. The writer must use both sentence-level (cohesion) and text-level (coherence) features to create meaningful text. Finally, all the areas of written language (graphomotor abilities, spelling, syntax) discussed previously in this chapter are orchestrated by the writer in composing written text. It is the role of the evaluator to determine the direct and indirect relationships among all these aspects of writing. For instance, does a writer receive low-quality writing scores as a result of numerous spelling and legibility errors, or do difficulties with organization at the sentence and text levels impair the meaning for the reader?

Table 6.5 lists the linguistic and cognitive processes essential to the production of written text that have been supported by empirical evidence. Researchers examining the written text of adolescents with LD note that these writers often demonstrate difficulty with metacognitive strategies, such as planning, monitoring, evaluating, and revising (Englert, 1990; Graham & Harris, 1999). Chapman and colleagues (1992) have also identified several strategies necessary for creating written discourse, which include such abilities as retrieving, selecting, isolating, sorting, reducing, and sequencing information.

The role of working memory in composing text is controversial. Perfetti (1985) and Stanovich (1980) suggest that word spelling contributes to an overload in working memory, leading to text structure difficulties in reading and writing tasks. Other researchers provide evidence that working memory deficits often influence written text underachievement (Berninger & Richards, 2002; McCutchen, 2006). Recently, Vanderberg and Swanson (2007) investigated the relationship of working memory to the macrostructure (planning, text structure, revision) and microstructure (grammar, punctuation) of writing. Although they validated the importance of working memory to both the microstructure

TABLE 6.5. Cognitive and Linguistic Processes Influencing Written Text Production

Text requirements	Processes[a]
Word usage	Spelling processes (Table 6.3) Syntax processes (Table 6.4) Graphomotor processes
Cohesion (relationships between words and phrases)	
Lexical (synonyms, superordinates) Grammar (pronominals, demonstratives) Transistional (phrases, clauses)	Spelling processes (Table 6.3) Syntax processes (Table 6.4)
Coherence (idea development)	
Processes and strategies to retrieve, select, reduce, support, and organize ideas	Reasoning (inferential) Controlled attention Oral language Verbal working memory (text level) Executive functioning Spelling processes (Table 6.3) Syntax processes (Table 6.4)
Sense of audience	Subskills (see Table 6.6)

[a]Each of the text requirements listed is influenced by processes described in other tables.

and macrostructure of written text, they also stressed that the writing process is more intricately tied to the attentional components of working memory. Other researchers suggest that long-term memory plays a greater role in the composing of text than working memory does (Kintsch, 1998). During the evaluation of an adolescent or adult, professionals are encouraged to investigate the relationship of the cognitive and linguistic processes listed in Table 6.5 to determine the potential of these processes for interfering with the composing of text. Juan's profile (Figure 6.2) illustrates how his deficits in verbal working memory, receptive language (listening comprehension), and executive functioning interfere with his abilities to organize and produce written text.

Two linguistic features, "cohesion" and "coherence," are critical to our understanding of composing text. Cohesive ties provide the meaningful connections within and between sentences (Halliday & Hasan, 1976). For instance, in the sentence "John was my friend, and he was the best student in the class," the pronominal "he" refers back to "John." Understanding a writer's meaning can be hindered by inaccurate use of such references in a composition. Three important types of cohesive ties for an evaluator to investigate in a writing sample are "grammar ties" (pronominals, demonstratives), "transitional ties" (ties between phrases and clauses), and "lexical ties" (synonyms, superordinates) (Gregg, 1985). Functionally, a writer's cohesive ties operate to meet the requirement that text must be more than simply a string of unrelated sentences, no matter how syntactically correct the sentences may appear (Gregg, Coleman, & Lindstrom, 2008). An evaluator might begin by exploring the word knowledge of a writer, since use of cohesive ties is dependent on one's sophistication with words (see Gregg, Coleman, & Lindstrom, 2008). Word-finding problems can also lead to inaccurate use of lexical ties. In an early study, I (Gregg, 1985) found that among adult writers, a significant number of apparent lexical tie errors resulted from difficulty with morphological endings and inadvertent omission of entire words.

"Coherence" refers to the blueprint of a composition. However, each genre of writing (e.g., narrative, expository, persuasive, descriptive) uses a somewhat different blueprint to build or develop ideas. In addition, the fluidity and clarity of composition structure are dependent on the appropriate use of cohesive ties. Without cohesion, a writer cannot produce coherent text. Research has supported the idea that both the reading and writing of coherent text are dependent on right frontal brain functioning (Cannito, Jarecki, & Pierce, 1986; Engel-Ortlieb, 1981; Huber, 1989). The demands made on self-regulatory processes by the process of composition are often difficult for adolescents and adults with right frontal damage to meet (Brownell, Carroll, Rehak, & Wingfield, 1992).

Assessment of Composition

The standardized evaluation of the quality of essay writing most often involves a guided procedure for sorting or ranking text, referred to as "holistic" or "impressionistic" scoring (Cooper & Odell, 1977; White, 2001). A rater is guided by a scoring rubric, which describes each feature to be evaluated and identifies high, middle, and low quality levels for each feature. The score a rater assigns to a piece of writing is derived impressionistically, after the rater has practiced the procedure with other raters. Such a scoring procedure has been identified as a very valid and reliable means of scoring large samples of writing (Cooper & Odell, 1999; White, 2001). However, as I (Gregg, 1985) have noted elsewhere, holistic scores tend to distinguish good writers from struggling writers, but do little as a diagnostic measure to distinguish among types of underachieving writers.

Accommodations for Composition Disorders

Table 6.2 lists commonly used accommodations for writers with LD or ADHD who demonstrate significant difficulties in composing text. Certainly, a very important accommodation for writers experiencing such difficulties is extended time (Gregg, Coleman, Davis, & Chalk, 2007). Researchers continue to provide evidence that extended time can give these individuals the opportunity to utilize various strategies and/or technologies for improving their written products. If graphomotor, spelling, and/or syntax abilities are also areas of deficit for a writer, the accommodations previously discussed in this chapter for those areas should also be provided.

Both speech synthesis (TTS) software and speech recognition (STT) software have potential for enhancing the production of written text structure. Although limited research is available on the effectiveness of either type of software for the adolescent and adult populations with LD and ADHD, advances in AT appear promising (MacArthur, 2006). In the future, MP3 players (e.g., iPods) with digital voice recorders will also have the potential to increase the writing proficiency of adolescents and adults with LD and ADHD (Banerjee & Gregg, in press).

The effectiveness of teaching adolescent writers with LD and ADHD cognitive strategies to enhance their composition abilities is well documented in the literature (Deshler et al., 1996; Englert, 1990; Englert et al., 2006; Graham & Harris, 2004; Hallenbeck, 1996). For instance, the Think Sheets advocated by Englert in her Cognitive Strategy Instruction in Writing can provide useful tools to help many of these writers manage the different aspects of writing (planning, organizing, drafting, editing, and author–reader relationship) (Hallenbeck, 1996). However, the research on computerized software that provides strategic planning, organization, and revising prompts to adolescent and adult writers with LD or ADHD during the process of constructing text has not provided conclusive evidence for the effectiveness of this software (Bonk & Reynolds, 1992; Reynolds & Bonk, 1996; Rowley, Carsons, & Miller, 1998; Rowley & Meyer, 2003; Zellermayer, Salomon, Globerson, & Givon, 1991). Interestingly, MacArthur (2006), in a review of AT and writing, states that he identified only one study (Sturm & Rankin-Erikson, 2002) that provided evidence for the effectiveness of concept-mapping software, despite its common use by professionals working with students demonstrating writing disorders. However, this lack of research does not diminish such techniques for enhancing the written text of many students. Rather, it suggests that a professional must ensure that adequate evidence from a comprehensive evaluation provides strong support for the use of concept-mapping software with a particular individual. Further investigation of the use of embedded e-text strategies for enhancing the composition performance of writers with LD and ADHD is encouraged (see Table 6.2, and Table 5.3 in Chapter Five). With the increasing number of empirical studies in the area of hypermedia and computer-mediated communication, it appears that new tools will be available in the future to accommodate adolescents and adult writers demonstrating LD and ADHD—tools that we cannot even conceptualize today.

Sense of Audience

Current thinking about the writing process envisions writing as a problem-solving task that engages the writer in contextual dialogue with the reader. Researchers studying the composing processes of inexperienced or remedial (basic) writers reveal that such students often differ from their higher-achieving cohorts in the degree to which, and manner in which, they consider their audiences (Rubin & Looney, 1990). Studies summarized by Rubin and Looney (1990) show that basic writers have little sense of writing as a rhetorical transaction. That is, such writers seldom view writing as a means of communication or persuasion; rather, they tend to think infrequently of potential readers, and fail to use information about their readers even when it is available to them. The problems basic writers experience in revision and audience awareness are interdependent. Rubin (1984) argues that audience awareness is fundamental to revision; to revise is to step back from the writer's own subjective understanding of a text and experience it with naïve eyes (Murray, 1978).

To investigate a writer's sense of audience requires evaluation of the writer's voice, the writer's perceptions of the audience, and the context in which the writing is occurring (Gregg, Sigalas, Hoy, Weisenbaker, & McKinley, 1996). In the past, audience awareness has been treated as a "monolithic" rather than a "multidimensional" construct (Rubin, 1984). However, writer, audience, and context are all involved in the dynamic creation of text, and this leads to choices regarding concepts, vocabulary, style, and text organization. In an effort to evaluate such variables, researchers have identified a number of linguistic and social cognition subskills required for developing sensitivity to audience in written language, including content, execution, perspective taking, differentiation of voice, and organization of text (Gregg & McAlexander, 1989; Gregg, Sigalas, et al., 1996). Table 6.6 lists the writing requirements for maintaining a sense of audience appropriate to a writing genre.

TABLE 6.6. Cognitive and Linguistic Processes Influencing Sense of Audience

Writing requirements	Processes
Content Actual knowledge of topic and writer's confidence with this knowledge	Oral language Knowledge Reasoning Long-term retrieval Working memory Executive functions
Execution Actual linguistic resources	Graphomotor processes Spelling (Table 6.3) Syntax (Table 6.4) Composition
Perspective taking and sustaining perspective Becoming aware of the reader's perspective and maintaining that perspective	Self-concept Attribution Pragmatic communication Social cognition Reasoning Attention
Differentiation of voice The transfer of the mental image of the audience into communication strategies aiding message delivery	Oral language Reasoning Social cognition Executive processes Working memory Attention

Fluency

Fluency is a critical construct to address in the evaluation of writing. Fluency in relation to writing is often referred to as "verbosity" and measured by the length of a composition or the number of words in a composition. We (Gregg, Coleman, Stennett, & Davis, 2002) investigated the written discourse complexity of young adults with and without dyslexia. We found that number of words, quality, and vocabulary complexity were significantly correlated. In particular, number of words and quality could not be viewed as separate constructs, but were statistically co-occurring functions. In other words, the number of words produced by writers increased their chances for higher quality scores. A critical finding from this study was that vocabulary and fluency proxies—number of words, number of different words, and number of words with more than two syllables—were the best discriminators between young adult writers with and without dyslexia.

Although there are many psychometric measures (in both cognitive and achievement areas) whose names include such terms as "fluency" or "processing speed," research on the predictive value of these measures in the area of written expression has not been conclusive. In interpreting the significance of a fluency index or score, an examiner should take into account the task requirements, as well as the average performance of an examinee's peer group on a similar task. Any interpretation of an adolescent or adult writer's fluency requires knowledge of fluency in a comparable group of peers with a similar level of writing instruction and experience.

Implications for Assessment and Accommodation

General Ideas

✓ The importance of writing competency for success in the classroom and in the workplace is ever increasing, particularly in today's technology-driven economy.

✓ Today's global learning and work environments require professionals to carefully consider culturally diverse learners—both what they have to offer and what they need—when identifying best practices in either the assessment or accommodation of writing.

Assessment

✓ Luria suggested that an evaluation of a writer's proficiency should always include three different tasks: copying, dictation, and spontaneous writing.

✓ The tool or tools used in writing (e.g., pencil/pen, computer, voice-activated software) are important to consider in selecting effective accommodations.

✓ The three types of graphomotor disorders most prevalent in the adolescent and adult populations with LD and ADHD are symbolic deficits, motor speed deficits, and dyspraxia.

✓ Spelling deficits are a hallmark of writers demonstrating dyslexia.

✓ The ability to produce syntactically correct sentence structures involves "semantics" (word usage in context), "grammar" (e.g., subject–verb and pronoun–antecedent agreement), and "mechanics" (e.g., application of punctuation and capitalization rules), all working in unison. Many writers with LD and ADHD demonstrate difficulty in producing text at the sentence level.

✓ "Composition" refers to the organization of ideas in writing at the text level. Researchers examining the written text of adolescents with LD and ADHD note that these writers often demonstrate difficulty with cognitive and metacognitive strategies, such as planning, monitoring, evaluating, and revising.

✓ The writing process is a problem-solving task that engages the writer in contextual dialogue with the reader. The degree to which, and manner in which, a writer considers the reader are referred to as "sense of audience."

✓ Fluency in relation to writing is often measured by the length of a composition or number of words in a composition. Many writers with LD or ADHD demonstrate significantly lower writing fluency scores than their peers.

Accommodation

✓ Extra time is an effective accommodation for many writers with LD and ADHD.

✓ Various forms of AT are proving to be effective accommodations for many writers with LD and ADHD.

✓ Cognitive and metacognitive strategies, once these are taught to writers with LD and ADHD, are effective accommodations during the writing process.

CHAPTER SEVEN

Different Symbol Systems
Mathematics, Science, and Second Languages

Ellie, an English major, is an Asian American sophomore in college who was diagnosed with LD in the third grade. Her LD substantially limits her ability to learn mathematics and specific types of science content. However, Ellie demonstrates strong verbal reasoning and language abilities. She has sought an evaluation to provide the necessary documentation to substitute another course for a required math course in her program of study.

David is a European American student who was diagnosed with LD (dyslexia) and ADHD in first grade. He is currently preparing for his high school graduation test. His vocational rehabilitation counselor and special education teacher are concerned about his ability to pass the math portion of the graduation test. Therefore, the school system is reviewing his documentation to determine what specific accommodations will be most effective for him in the area of mathematics.

Joyce is an African American junior in college majoring in forestry. She is seeking an evaluation to provide support for a foreign language substitution. Joyce was diagnosed with LD (dyslexia) during second grade and received special education throughout her elementary and secondary schooling. She attempted German in high school with accommodations. However, after she failed it twice, the school granted her the option of substituting another course for her foreign language course requirement.

193

Human thought is represented by a diversity of representational codes or symbol systems (e.g., verbal, visual, kinesthetic, emotional, scientific). John-Steiner (1997) refers to this multiplicity of languages as "cognitive pluralism," and she stresses the significant relationship between our internal and external forms of symbolization. The theoretical work of Gardner (1983) also provides a framework for considering the different types of cognitive codes. He states:

> To my way of thinking the mind has the potential to deal with several different kinds of content, but a person's facility with one content has little predictive power about his or her facility with other kinds. In other words, genius (and *a fortiori*, ordinary performance) is likely to be specific to particular contents: human beings have evolved to exhibit several intelligences and not to draw variously on one flexible intelligence. (p. xiv)

Professionals are encouraged to remember that individuals with LD or ADHD show greater strengths in some "intelligences" (to use Gardner's term), or abilities in some symbol systems, than in others. Unfortunately, the verbal language code, which is often not the strongest symbol system for many adolescents or adults with LD or ADHD, receives the greatest weight when many professionals predict future success in learning and work environments.

The reflections of famous scientists and mathematicians on the processes and strategies they apply during the solving of novel problems is one means of better understanding the cognitive processes that influence our abilities to access a variety of symbol systems (see, e.g., Curie, 1923; Darwin, 1887/1958; Einstein, 1970; John-Steiner, 1997). In the area of mathematics, many distinguished scientists suggest that they rely on visual symbols and visual patterns during problem solving. John-Steiner (1997, p. 175) quotes the famous mathematician Reuben Hersh: "I remember looking at the bathroom floor, and observing the different patterns that I could see by combining larger and smaller tiles. I also did arithmetic in my mind, rather obsessively, adding things endlessly, and also looking for patterns in numbers." The role of visual processes and images, and their relationships to higher-level cognition, are important when we think about the processes important to the learning of different symbol systems. Some neuropsychologists contend that "images are probably the main content of our thoughts, regardless of the sensory modality in which they are generated" (Damasio, 1994, p. 5). This chapter focuses on direct and indirect relationships of different cognitive and linguistic processes to the learning of math, science, and foreign languages for adolescents and adults with LD and ADHD, as well as on effective accommodations in these areas.

Mathematics

Adolescents or adults with either LD or ADHD can experience significant problems in learning mathematics, for a variety of reasons. However, researchers studying math disorders have devoted much more
attention to understanding the math competencies of individuals with
LD than of persons with ADHD. Therefore, professionals need to be
somewhat cautious in making inferences from this research for individuals with ADHD.

Professionals often use the term "quantitative literacy" rather than
the term "mathematics" to refer to the quantitative knowledge and skills
necessary for an adult to function adequately in the workplace, home,
and community. Quantitative literacy is systematically evaluated every
few years through several large-scale adult self-report literacy assessments (the National Assessment of Adult Literacy and the International
Adult Literacy and Lifeskills Survey). One goal of these national and
international assessments is to evaluate the quantitative literacy levels
characteristic of the general population. The quantitative domains most
often measured by this research include quantity and number; dimen-
sion and shape; patterns, functions, and relations; and monetary concepts (Curry, Schmitt, & Waldron, 1996; Gal, von Groenestijn, Manly,
Schmitt, & Trout, 2005, McCloskey, 2007; Steen, 2001).

One outcome of these large-scale self-report surveys has been the
recognition of the importance of quantitative competencies for success
in the workplace (Cobin, 2003; McCloskey, 2007; Patton, Cronin, Bassett, & Koppel, 1997). Researchers have provided evidence of a strong
correlation between average or above-average numeracy scores and a
successful employment history (Bynner, 1998; Bynner & Parsons, 1997;
McCloskey, 2007). Functional levels of quantitative literacy are also
essential for adults to manage the real-world statistics they encounter
on a daily basis (Patton et al., 1997). As noted by McCloskey (2007),
"Quantitative literacy is not merely useful but, in fact, vital for success in
21st century life" (p. 425).

More research is needed to provide a better understanding of the
influence of LD and ADHD on adolescents' and adults' learning of mathematics. Researchers need to focus on the quantitative abilities required
by adults with these disorders for success in their social and work environments. Currently, most descriptive, quasi-experimental, and experimental research on math disorders has been done with children rather
than with the adolescent or adult populations. Although no prevalence
figures for adolescents or adults are available, the prevalence of LD
in mathematics (hereafter abbreviated as "math LD" or just "MLD")
among the school-age population in the United States is estimated at

between 5% and 8% (Geary, 2004). This range appears to be consistent with international figures (Gross-Tsur, Manor, & Shalev, 1996; Ramaa & Gowramma, 2002; Shalev, Manor, & Gross-Tsur, 2005).

Investigation of the performance of individuals with MLD (or with "dyscalculia," as many early studies called it) is not new (Badian, 1983; Geary, 1993, 2004, 2007; Johnson & Myklebust, 1967; Kosc, 1974; Padget, 1998; Rourke & Conway, 1997). One of the most consistent findings from these earlier studies is that individuals with dyscalculia or MLD appear to be a heterogeneous group exhibiting several different learning profiles. Table 7.1 provides a list of several math disorder subgroups proposed by researchers over the years in their efforts to define the cognitive, linguistic, and academic profiles demonstrated by individuals with MLD. As I discuss the current research in this area, it will be clear to the reader that the findings from many of these initial investigations of the population with MLD are consistent with the results of more recent and sophisticated cognitive and brain imaging studies.

Two significant limitations of both earlier and more recent research on math disorders involve (1) the different eligibility criteria used to identify populations of individuals with MLD, and (2) the restricted tools employed to measure performance. Researchers usually apply cutoff scores to select their participants with MLD. Murphy, Mazzocco, Hanich, and Early (2007) studied the characteristics of children with MLD as defined by a variety of cutoff metrics and found differences in learning profiles, depending on the severity of the eligibility criteria. They studied three groups of learners: those with no LD; those with MLD < 10th percentile; and those with MLD < 25th percentile). The students with MLD demonstrated less efficient working memory performance than the non-LD students. Differences between the two MLD groups did not appear to be the result of deficits in a single consistent math-related skill. The authors hypothesized that further investigation is needed to determine if the MLD groups could be differentiated on the basis of a math ability required for performing a specific math task.

Murphy and colleagues (2007) also suggest that a significant problem with many math studies pertaining to individuals with MLD is that researchers identified the participants by using only one math achievement measure as the selection tool, such as the Wide Range Achievement Test–3 (WRAT3; Jastak & Wilkinson, 1993) or the Woodcock–Johnson III Tests of Achievement (WJ III ACH) Calculation or Applied Problems subtests (Woodcock et al., 2001a). Two problems arise with such a method: First, these psychometric tools often do not measure the fundamental skills that underlie math performance (e.g., number sense, estimation); second, these tests are usually restricted to only one aspect of mathematical learning (e.g., calculation or problem solving).

TABLE 7.1. MLD Subgroups Identified by Different Researchers

Author(s) (year)	Subgroups

Kosc (1974)	Lexical dyscalculia
	    Deficits in reading math symbols
	    Deficits in reading multidigit numbers
	    Deficits in reading horizontally
	    Co-occurring reading decoding deficits
	Ideational dyscalculia
	    Deficits in understanding of math concepts and calculations
	    Deficits in working memory
	Graphical dyscalculia
	    Deficits in writing math symbols orally presented
	    Deficits in copying math symbols
	    Co-occurring reading/writing disorders
	Operational dyscalculia
	    Deficits in carrying out math operations
	    Deficits in nonverbal reasoning

Padget (1998)	Subgroup 1
	    Co-occurring dyslexia
	    Calculation deficits
	Subgroup 2
	    Co-occurring oral language disorders
	    Verbal reasoning disorders
	Subgroup 3
	    Visual–spatial deficits
	    Nonverbal reasoning deficits

Rourke and Conway (1997)	Subgroup 1: Reading and math deficits Subgroup 2: Nonverbal reasoning deficits Subgroup 3: Oral language deficits

Geary (1993, 2004)	Semantic memory
	    Difficulty in retrieving math facts
	    Co-occurring dyslexia
	    Phonological working memory deficit
	    Inefficient inhibition (attention) deficit
	    Executive processing deficits with verbal information
	    Word retrieval deficits
	    Long-term memory deficit
	Visual–spatial
	    Difficulties in spatially representing numbers
	    Difficulties with place value
	    Difficulties with geometry
	    Spatial working memory deficits
	    Spatial reasoning deficits
	    Executive functioning deficits with visual–spatial information
	    Attentional deficits with visual–spatial information
	Procedural
	    Use of immature math procedures
	    Errors in carrying out procedures
	    Difficulty with multistep procedures
	    Conceptual deficits
	    Executive functioning deficits
	    Working memory deficits

Thus there is a greater chance of under- or overidentifying one type of profile with such a methodology—a critical factor for diagnostic decision making as well as research.

Mazzocco, Murphy, and McCloskey (2007) adopted a methodology for better understanding the neurological pathways interrupted as a result of MLD by studying children with genetic disorders that are known to cause cognitive and linguistic deficits proposed to resemble those in MLD. In particular, they studied children with fragile X syndrome, who often display inefficient verbal working memory systems, and children with Turner syndrome, who characteristically demonstrate long-term memory deficits. According to Mazzocco and colleagues, children with these two disorders demonstrated dissimilar manifestations of MLD. These findings should contribute to a better understanding of the neurological systems involved with mathematical learning.

Primary and Secondary Math Abilities

The capacity to learn mathematical concepts, according to Geary (2007), requires an individual to utilize both primary and secondary cognitive abilities. Geary provides a thorough review of recent research distinguishing between biologically primary and culturally specific, or biologically secondary, forms of math abilities. He suggests that six core primary mathematical abilities provide the foundation for the majority of mathematical competencies: numerosity, ordinality, counting, simple arithmetic, estimation, and geometry (see Table 7.2). Brain imaging and comparative studies provide evidence that areas of the parietal cortex, especially the intraparietal sulcus, are the brain systems responsible for the majority of the primary math abilities identified by Geary (Berninger & Richards, 2002; Geary, 2007).

However, Geary (2007) points out that these primary abilities are restricted in comparison to the quantitative literacy demands of our modern societies; more often, we are required to use biologically secondary math competencies that emerge only through formal schooling. For example, the learning of algebra requires an understanding of such secondary concepts as coordinate plans and graphing functions. Although these skills are built upon the primary construct of number lines, secondary knowledge is essential to mastering algebraic problems. Geary states: "The more complex the secondary mathematics, the more primary systems it draws upon, and the more it is dependent on previous secondary learning, the more potential sources of variation in learning and MLD" (p. 481). A great deal of research currently in progress will provide a better understanding of the similarities and differences across

TABLE 7.2. Geary's Core Primary Mathematical Competencies

- *Numerosity*: The ability to accurately determine the quantity of sets of up to three to four items, or events, without counting.
- *Ordinality*: An implicit understanding of "more than" and "less than" for comparison of sets of three to four items.
- *Counting*: A nonverbal system for enumeration of small sets of items and an implicit knowledge of counting principles (e.g., one-to-one correspondence).
- *Simple arithmetic*: Sensitivity to increase (addition) and decrease (subtraction) in the quantity of small sets of items.
- *Estimation*: The ability to make a reasonably accurate estimation of relative quantity, magnitude, or size.
- *Geometry*: Implicit understanding of shape and spatial relations.

Note. From Geary (2007). Copyright 2007 by Lawrence Erlbaum and Associates. Adapted by permission.

and within cognitive systems required for mastering both primary and secondary quantitative competencies (see Berch & Mazzocco, 2007, for an in-depth presentation of current research in the area of math disorders). According to Geary, "We are not yet at the point where we can decompose these complex secondary mathematical abilities, but we can begin to explore the relation between primary abilities and more elementary secondary abilities" (p. 479).

Mediating Cognitive and Language Processes

The identification of the cognitive and language processes that directly or indirectly influence the learning of primary and secondary quantitative abilities will provide the keys to identifying more effective accommodations for adolescents or adults with LD and ADHD who experience difficulty in learning math. Current theoretical and empirical work related to the neuropsychology of quantitative learning is providing the evidence needed for a better understanding of how LD and ADHD influence the learning of primary and secondary abilities. As noted by Berninger and Richards (2002), the brain draws upon many different codes (e.g., quantitative, visual, motor, verbal) and types of reasoning (e.g., quantitative, verbal, visual–spatial), making it "multilingual in its representational form" (p. 194). The purpose of this section of the chapter is to review recent research indicating which specific cognitive and language systems appear to mediate both primary and secondary mathematical competencies (see Table 7.3). During a psychological evaluation of an individual presenting learning problems, professionals are encouraged to explore how these systems might influence mathematical performance.

**TABLE 7.3. Mediating Cognitive and Linguistic Processes
Influencing Mathematical Performance**

Cognitive and linguistic systems	Select evidence-based research
Verbal working memory system	
Executive processes	Swanson and Jermon (2006)[a]
Procedural processes	Geary (1993, 2000, 2004, 2007)[a]
Controlled attention to verbal information	Fuchs et al. (2006)[a]
Phonological coding	Cirino, Morris, and Morris (2002)[b]
Processing speed and efficiency	Swanson and Sachse-Lee (2001)[a]
Metacognition	Wilson and Swanson (2001)
	Osmon, Smerz, Braun, & Plambeck (2006)[a]
	Garrett, Mazzocco, and Baker (2006)[a]
	Berninger and Richards (2002)[c]
	Busse, Berninger, Smith, and Hildebrand (2001)
Long-term memory system	
Semantic memory	Geary (1993, 2000, 2004, 2007)[a]
Naming	Fuchs et al. (2005)[a]
Orthographic coding	Swanson and Jerman (2006)[a]
	Berninger and Richards (2002)[c]
	Busse et al. (2001)
	Cirino, Morris, and Morris (2002, 2007)[b]
Visual–spatial system	
Visual–spatial working memory	Geary (1993, 2004, 2007)[a]
Visual–spatial reasoning	Osmon et al. (2006)[a]
Executive abilities	
Procedural abilities	Procter, Floyd, and Shaver (2005)
Controlled attention to visual–spatial information	Cirino et al. (2002, 2007)[b]
	Berninger and Richards (2002)[c]
Processing speed	Busse et al. (2001)
Fluid reasoning	
Nonverbal reasoning	Geary (2007)[a]
Fluid reasoning	Fuchs et al. (2005)[a]
	Procter et al. (2005)
Verbal ability system	
Oral language abilities	Geary (1993, 2007)[a]
Verbal reasoning	Procter et al. (2005)
Crystallized knowledge	Fuchs et al. (2006)[a]
	Berninger and Richards (2002)[c]
	Busse et al. (2001)
Graphomotor system	
	Berninger and Richards (2002)[c]
	Busse et al. (2001)
	Fayol, Barrouillet, and Marinthe (1998)[a]

[a]Child study or meta-analysis of child literature specific to MLD.
[b]Adult study specific to MLD.
[c]Brain imaging mathematics studies, primarily with normally achieving adults.

Verbal Working Memory System

Numerous studies provide evidence that individuals with MLD do not perform as well as their peers on tests of verbal working memory capacity (Cirino, Morris, & Morris, 2002, 2007; Geary, 2007; Geary, Hoard, Byrd-Craven, & Desota, 2004; Geary, Hoard, Byrd-Craven, Nugent, & Numtee, 2007; Swanson & Jerman, 2006; Swanson & Sachse-Lee, 2001; Wilson & Swanson, 2001). In a thorough meta-analysis of the child literature, Swanson and Jerman (2006) found that the efficiency of the verbal working memory system most clearly differentiated students with MLD from average achievers. Certainly if verbal working memory capacity is reduced, the solving of more complex mathematics problems could easily be impaired (Geary & Widaman, 1992).

Compromised central executive and attentional processes appear to contribute the most to the verbal working memory deficits demonstrated by many individuals with MLD. Brain imaging studies indicate that the anterior cingulate cortex and the lateral prefrontal cortex are the core brain systems that underlie the executive and attentional processes influencing math performance (Beringer & Richards, 2002; Geary, 2007). According to the Swanson and Jarman (2006) math meta-analysis, deficits in controlled attention (focus) to verbal information differentiated children with MLD when compared to average achievers. Since the brain regions that support the attentional control and inhibitory control components of the executive system appear to contribute to math learning, the implications of this research for the population with ADHD will require further investigation (Geary, 2007; Kane & Engle, 2002). Several researchers suggest that individual differences in working memory capacity and retrieval efficiency are significantly related to the ability to inhibit irrelevant associations (Conway, Cowan, Bunting, Therriault, & Minkoff, 2002; Geary, 2007; Geary, Hoard, Nugent, & Byrd-Craven, 2007).

Children with MLD also often demonstrate procedural impairments in counting; arithmetic strategy use; and the executive functions of organizing, monitoring, and sequencing the steps required in more complex problem solving (Bull, 2007; Geary, 2004, 2007). Although evidence that a deficient number sense (primary ability) may also contribute to procedural deficits (secondary abilities) was provided by Barth, Kanwisher, and Spelke (2002), ample evidence supports the significant role that executive, attention, and working memory processes play in different aspects of mathematical learning. For instance, Lee, Ng, Ng, and Pee (2006) studied the neurological systems required to solve algebraic tasks and found that at different stages of the problem-solving process, different cognitive and language processes were utilized. Not only does the complexity of the task require unique cognitive contributions, but Cowan, Elliott, and Saults (2002) provide evidence that age-related changes in working memory, processing speed, strategy use, and decay of information can contribute to differential performance on academic tasks.

Speed of processing is also a core cognitive mechanism in the working memory system (Deary, 2000; Geary, 2007; Jensen, 1998). The fast and automatic use of primary and secondary abilities, particularly overlearned abilities, obviously results in less of a drain on verbal working memory resources (Gigerenzer & Selten, 2001; Kanwisher, McDermott, & Chun, 1997). According to Geary (2007), the benefit of processing speed is that it "enables larger amounts of information to be simultaneously represented in working memory, and thus more information . . . can be considered when explicit problem solving becomes necessary, that is, when conditions are variant or novel" (p. 483). Therefore, cognitive processing speed and efficiency certainly have the potential to influence both rote and novel math problem solving.

Long-Term Memory System

A characteristic of many individuals with MLD is the inability to store and retrieve number combinations in long-term memory. Several sources for this problem have been suggested, including general impairments in semantic associations, phonological coding, inhibitory processes, and processing speed (Bull, 2007; Dehaene, Spelke, Pinel, Stanescu, & Tsivkin, 1999; Geary, 2004; Jordan, Hanich, & Kaplan, 2003). Other researchers suggest that the difficulty children with MLD experience with retrieval of number facts may be the result of language deficits (Dehaene, 1997; Jordan et al., 2003). Geary (1993, 2004) has categorized individuals with MLD who experience difficulty with their long-term memory system as demonstrating a semantic memory disorder (see Table 7.1). However, other researchers have challenged the validity of this classification (Landerl, Bevan, & Butterworth, 2004; Swanson & Jerman, 2006).

Investigating the interaction of task and cognitive processing demands, Fuchs and colleagues (2006) found that the long-term memory system plays a mediating role in several different task demands, such as single-digit arithmetic, algorithmic computation, and word problems. With an adult population referred for learning problems, Cirino and colleagues (2002) found that semantic retrieval and executive processes played a significant predictive role in computational performance. However, in a more recent study with a similar adult population (Cirino et al., 2007), they found that semantic retrieval and visual–spatial processes predicted about 30% of the variance for calculation performance, whereas executive processes made no unique contribution. The differences between Cirino and colleagues' first and second studies may have been due in part to the neuropsychological tasks used in the studies. Nevertheless, it appears from this and other research that an individual who demonstrates deficits with such processes as orthographic coding, naming, or semantic memory may be at risk for underachievement in certain areas of mathematics, particularly calculation.

Visual–Spatial System

Some researchers propose that impairments in visual–spatial working memory and/or reasoning are defining features for some individuals with MLD (Geary, 2007). However, other researchers challenge the idea that visual–spatial skills may play a role in mathematical learning (Barnes, Fletcher, & Ewing-Cobbs, 2007; Cirino et al., 2002). According to Bull (2007), the differences researchers are finding related to the role of visual–spatial skills in mathematical learning may be more a function of the task demands than of the validity of the construct. In the Barnes and colleagues (2007) study, children were required to perform simple arithmetic tasks. When children were asked to perform more complex tasks (e.g., estimation, word problems, geometry), visual–spatial working memory and reasoning were stronger performance predictors (Barnes et al., 2007; Geary, 2007). Interestingly, Bull suggests that the visual–spatial system may play a different role when an individual chooses to use different cognitive and language processes to solve a problem:

> Poor visuospatial skills may only predict MLD when an alternative representational basis (verbal) for numbers cannot be easily utilized, for example, when there are corresponding language problems or when poor number sense limits the association of nonverbal representations to the verbal number system. (p. 267)

The significance of this statement for the adolescent and adult populations with LD or ADHD should not be overlooked by professionals involved in diagnostic decision making and accommodation selection.

Fluid Reasoning

The important role of fluid or nonverbal reasoning in mathematical learning is supported by empirical evidence (Fuchs et al., 2006; Geary,

2007; Procter, Floyd, & Shaver, 2005). According to Cattell (1963, p. 3), "fluid general ability shows more in tests requiring adaptation to new solutions," whereas crystallized abilities are primarily the results of schooling and acculturation. Fluid reasoning involves strategic problem solving and abstract reasoning (Geary, 2007). Although working memory is a primary cognitive system underlying fluid reasoning, it does not explain all of the individual variance (Geary, 2007; Stanovich, 1999; Stanovich & West, 2000). According to Embretson (1995), working memory capacity and the ability to make inferences explain almost all of the variance in fluid reasoning tasks; however, when she separated out their contributions to fluid reasoning, the ability to draw and apply inferences during problem solving explained about two-thirds of the variance, whereas working memory contributed only one-third. Interestingly, the same brain regions that support attentional control and the inhibitory control components of executive functioning also direct explicit reasoning and problem-solving abilities (Fugelsang & Dunbar, 2005; Geary, 2007; Kane & Engle, 2002; Stavy, Goel, Critchley, & Dolan, 2006). As clearly stated by Geary (2007), "Once attention is focused, intelligent people are able to represent more information in working memory than are other people and more easily manipulate this information. The manipulation in turn is guided and constrained by reasoning and inference making mechanisms" (p. 487). This multiplicity of cognitive systems is important for professionals to keep in mind as they make diagnostic decisions about the causes of an adolescent's or adult's math underachievement.

Ellie's profile (Figure 7.1) demonstrates that deficits in fluid reasoning, processing speed, spatial working memory, and visual–spatial reasoning have significantly influenced her ability to learn quantitative concepts. However, we note that her strong verbal abilities allow her to succeed in the areas of reading and writing. Ellie is an individual whose MLD functionally limits her ability to learn mathematical concepts. A programmatic math course substitution will probably be appropriate in Ellie's case.

Verbal Ability System

The relationship between verbal ability in general quantitative literacy is important to a better understanding of individuals with LD or ADHD who are experiencing difficulties with various math skills. Researchers are providing evidence that children with specific language disorders demonstrate difficulty in the production of number–word sequences, basic calculation, fact retrieval, and procedural strategies (Donlan, 2007). However, many students with specific language disorders also

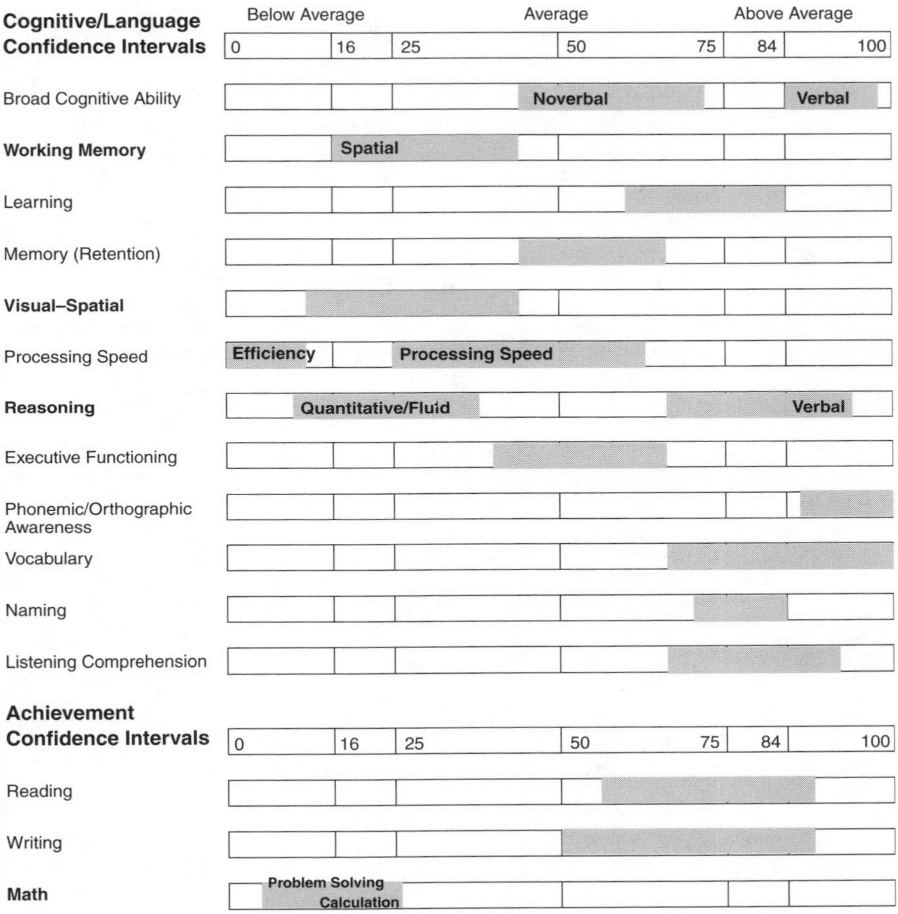

Cognitive/Language Confidence Intervals

	Below Average			Average			Above Average
	0	16	25	50	75	84	100

Broad Cognitive Ability — **Noverbal** ... **Verbal**

Working Memory — **Spatial**

Learning

Memory (Retention)

Visual–Spatial

Processing Speed — **Efficiency** ... **Processing Speed**

Reasoning — **Quantitative/Fluid** ... **Verbal**

Executive Functioning

Phonemic/Orthographic Awareness

Vocabulary

Naming

Listening Comprehension

Achievement Confidence Intervals

	0	16	25	50	75	84	100

Reading

Writing

Math — **Problem Solving** / **Calculation**

FIGURE 7.1. Assessment profile for Ellie, an individual with math LD (MLD).

appear to demonstrate average conceptual understanding (Donlan, 2007; Koponen, Mononen, Rasanen, & Ahonen, 2006). An adolescent or adult with LD or ADHD who exhibits verbal ability deficits may demonstrate difficulty with some aspects of math learning (e.g., calculation), but may perform within the average or above-average range on nonverbal or fluid problem-solving tasks.

David (see Figure 7.2) is a young man with LD (oral language) and ADHD who demonstrates underachievement in certain math skills but excels at others, particularly if accommodations are provided. When we review his profile, his verbal deficits are apparent (e.g., verbal working memory, orthographic coding, naming, and listening comprehension). In addition, we note that specific executive functioning deficits co-occur with his verbal ability deficits, influencing his ability to perform on math fluency and/or calculation problems. However, his strong visual working memory, visual–spatial reasoning, and fluid reasoning contribute to his stronger performance on quantitative problem solving.

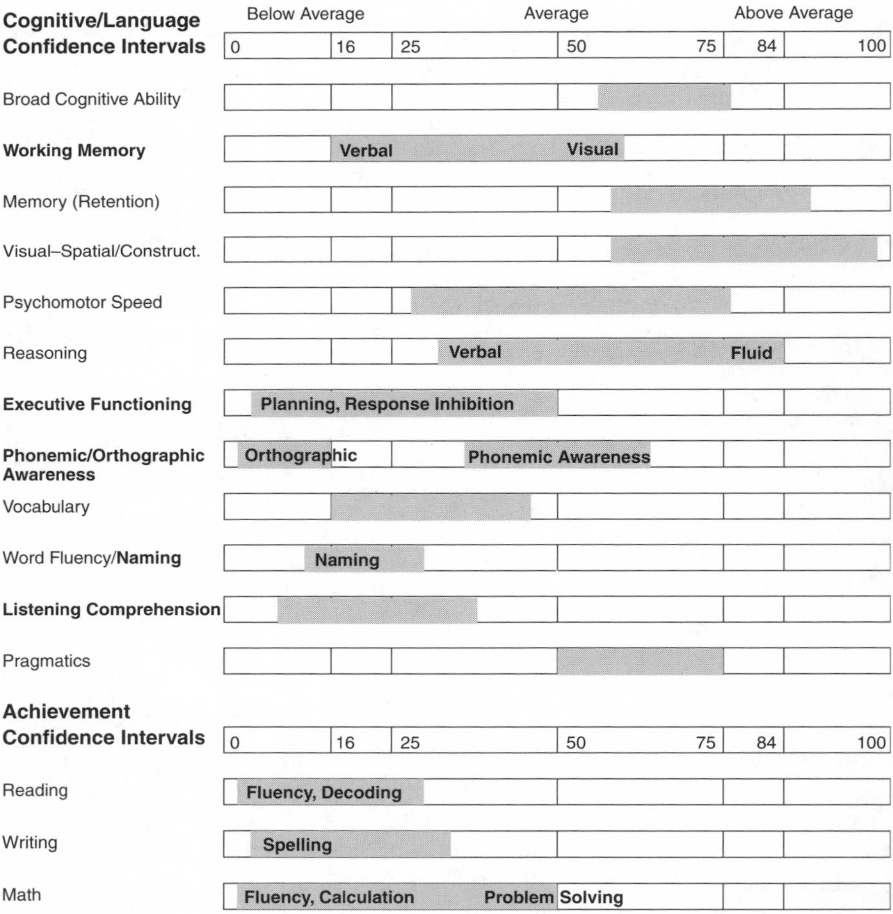

Cognitive/Language Confidence Intervals	Below Average			Average		Above Average	
	0	16	25	50	75	84	100
Broad Cognitive Ability							
Working Memory		Verbal		Visual			
Memory (Retention)							
Visual–Spatial/Construct.							
Psychomotor Speed							
Reasoning				Verbal		Fluid	
Executive Functioning		Planning, Response Inhibition					
Phonemic/Orthographic Awareness	Orthographic			Phonemic Awareness			
Vocabulary							
Word Fluency/Naming		Naming					
Listening Comprehension							
Pragmatics							
Achievement Confidence Intervals	0	16	25	50	75	84	100
Reading	Fluency, Decoding						
Writing	Spelling						
Math	Fluency, Calculation		Problem Solving				

FIGURE 7.2. Assessment profile for David, an individual with MLD and ADHD.

Graphomotor System

Berninger and Richards (2002) remind us that the graphomotor system is essential for completing math items when students are asked to compute on paper. Therefore, the graphomotor problems experienced by many individuals with LD or ADHD, as discussed in Chapter Six, can also have an impact on math production tasks. In fact, in a longitudinal study investigating the math performance of young children, Fayol, Barrouillet, and Marinthe (1998) found that neuropsychological tasks measuring fine motor ability significantly predicted arithmetic skills. The relationship of the graphomotor system to math performance has not received substantial attention from researchers. However, for adolescents and adults with LD or ADHD, graphomotor competence has clinical significance for the interpretation of test performance and/or for accommodation selection.

Mathematical Task Demands and Mediating Cognitive Processes

The assessment tools used to evaluate an individual's math competency often requires the individual to manipulate written numerals and symbols to solve problems. Such tasks are *abstract* and require a meaningful understanding of the mathematical concepts involved. If an examinee is experiencing difficulty with abstract tasks, professionals are encouraged to evaluate math knowledge by providing *concrete* experiences. At the concrete level, the examinee actually manipulates objects to illustrate relationships and solve problems. An examiner may also decide to evaluate an adolescent or adult at the *semiconcrete* level of learning. At this level, an individual is asked to solve problems by using aids that are slightly more abstract than a three-dimensional manipulative—for example, by drawing a diagram, drawing a picture, or making tallies to represent numbers. Bringing the level of learning down from abstract to concrete provides the examiner information about the type of accommodations that may be most effective. Each level of representation (i.e., abstract, concrete, and semiconcrete) draws upon different cognitive and linguistic processes. Further research is needed in which the direct and indirect influences of representational levels on math performance is investigated with both adolescents and adults.

Different task requirements also appear to draw upon a variety of cognitive and linguistic processes. For instance, Fuchs and colleagues (2006) explored the cognitive correlates that third graders drew upon across arithmetic, algorithmic computation, and arithmetic word problems. First, their data support a partially hierarchical model of mathematical development, which has been proposed by other researchers (Aunola, Leskinen, Lerkkanen, & Nurmi, 2004). Therefore, arithmetic calculation is a significant path to algorithmic computation and to arithmetic word problems. However, Fuchs and colleagues also note that algorithmic computation was not a strong predictor of ability to do word problems in their study. Therefore, the procedural competencies required for algorithmic computation did not appear to be essential to conceptualizing relations among numbers. Arithmetic calculation was a strong predictor of success with algorithmic computation and problem solving. The cognitive correlates most closely associated with arithmetic calculation appeared to be attention, processing speed, and phonological coding. For algorithmic computation, attention and arithmetic computation were the strongest predictors—not working memory, long-term memory, or phonological coding. For word problems, nonverbal problem solving, sight word efficiency, and language were the strongest predictors. In the Fuchs and colleagues research, the attentional processes of working memory capacity appeared to influence math performance significantly across task demands.

Professionals working with adolescents and adults must be cautious in interpreting the Fuchs and colleagues (2006) research, as a child population was studied. As noted earlier, Cowan and colleagues (2002) provide evidence of age-related changes in working memory, processing speed, strategy use, and decay of information. In addition, Floyd, Evans, and McGrew (2003), using cognitive clusters from the WJ III Tests of Cognitive Abilities (WJ III COG; Woodcock et al., 2001b) that measure specific Cattell–Horn–Carroll (CHC) abilities, investigated which of these measures best predicted performance on the WJ III ACH (Woodcock et al., 2001a) Math Calculation and Math Reasoning Clusters across ages ranging from 6 to 19 years in the WJ III normative data. Comprehension–Knowledge demonstrated a moderate relationship with Math Calculation after the early school-age years, and a moderate relationship with Math Reasoning. Fluid Reasoning, Short-Term Memory, and Working Memory generally demonstrated moderate relationships with the mathematics clusters. Processing Speed demonstrated a moderate relationship with Math Reasoning during the elementary school years, and a moderate to strong relationship with Math Calculation skills. For younger children, Long-Term Retrieval demonstrated a moderate relationship with the math clusters, and Auditory Processing demonstrated a moderate relationship with Math Calculation. The Visual–Spatial Cluster did not demonstrate a significant relationship with either of the math clusters across the age span. This research supports the hypothesis that different cognitive and linguistic processes appear to be utilized in solving specific types of math tasks, depending on an individual's age and ability.

Assessment of Mathematics Achievement

Diagnostic math achievement tests include various tasks for professionals to use in measuring different aspects of mathematics (e.g., calculation, quantitative knowledge, problem solving). Depending on the particular test, quantitative knowledge may be assessed on one subtest, as on the WRAT4 (Wilkinson with Robertson, 2004), or across several subtests, such as the WJ III ACH (Woodcock et al., 2001a) Calculation, Quantitative Reasoning, and Applied Problems subtests. Sometimes similar types of test items are scattered throughout a measure rather than clustered together.

The cause(s) for an individual's underachievement on math tests should be investigated through a comprehensive evaluation in which possible reasons for the underachievement are considered, such as instructional history, task format, cognitive and linguistic factors, reading abilities, motivation, and apprehension about math learning (i.e., "math anxiety"). Identifying the reason(s) for underachievement provides a framework for selecting effective accommodations for testing, instructional, or work situations. Professionals are encouraged to answer the seven questions posed in Figure 7.3 to guide their decision making during assessment and selection of accommodations related to mathematics.

Assessment of Calculation

Calculation skills are measured in a variety of ways across psychometric measures. A test of computation may be timed (the WRAT4 Math Computation subtest) or untimed (the Numerical Operations subtest of the Wechsler Individual Achievement Test—Second Edition; Wechsler, 2001). Adolescents or adults with retrieval problems may appear to have poorly developed calculation skills if they are assessed only on a timed subtest. The WJ III ACH Math Fluency subtest is designed and normed specifically to measure math calculation fluency. This timed task can then be compared to the WJ III ACH Calculation subtest (untimed) to help sort out accuracy from fluency issues.

Items on a calculation test are also often organized in various ways that can influence examinee performance. Sometimes single-operation items are grouped together (e.g., addition, subtraction). Other tests mix items involving different types of operations, requiring that the exam-

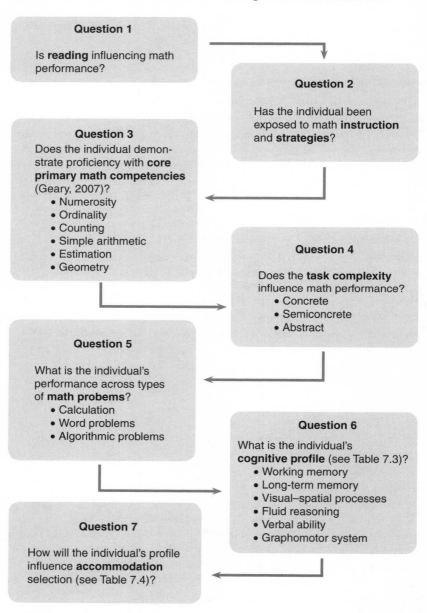

Question 1

Is **reading** influencing math performance?

Question 2

Has the individual been exposed to math **instruction** and **strategies**?

Question 3

Does the individual demonstrate proficiency with **core primary math competencies** (Geary, 2007)?
- Numerosity
- Ordinality
- Counting
- Simple arithmetic
- Estimation
- Geometry

Question 4

Does the **task complexity** influence math performance?
- Concrete
- Semiconcrete
- Abstract

Question 5

What is the individual's performance across types of **math probems**?
- Calculation
- Word problems
- Algorithmic problems

Question 6

What is the individual's **cognitive profile** (see Table 7.3)?
- Working memory
- Long-term memory
- Visual–spatial processes
- Fluid reasoning
- Verbal ability
- Graphomotor system

Question 7

How will the individual's profile influence **accommodation** selection (see Table 7.4)?

FIGURE 7.3. Questions to support decision making for the accommodation of mathematics difficulties.

inee attend closely to the operational signs. The format of a calculation test can also influence an examinee's performance. Some tests (e.g., WRAT4 Math Computation) place many problems on a page, which can cause anxiety or confusion that is ancillary to math knowledge. Other tests (e.g., WJ III ACH Calculation) place each problem in a separate box, whereas still others place no barriers between problems.

In addition, the response mode often differs among calculation measures. Some tests provide multiple-choice responses, while others require the examinee to generate oral or written answers. Most calculation tests require the student to write or mark the answers. A few tests do not use a paper-and-pencil format, but require oral answers to problems presented on an easel. A professional trying to understand why an individual performs poorly on a calculation task should consider the influence of the task format and the requirements for accessing and responding to items. In addition, the clinician should examine the direct and indirect relationships of an examinee's primary math knowledge, working memory system (attention, executive, and processing speed), long-term memory system, verbal ability system, and graphomotor abilities to his or her calculation performance.

Assessment of Math Knowledge Application

Application of math knowledge is also assessed via several different types of tasks. Some subtests measure an examinee's knowledge of quantitative facts learned in school (e.g., WJ III ACH Quantitative Knowledge). Application of math knowledge through problem solving is another type of task. On many problem-solving tasks, an examinee must read the problems; when an individual is required to read problems on his or her own before solving them, reading difficulties can interfere. Some test directions suggest that examinees read the problems themselves, but encourage them to ask for help with unknown words. Despite this encouragement, some individuals will not ask for help, and their scores may be depressed because of their reading abilities. A professional trying to understand why an individual performs poorly on applied math problems is encouraged to look at the relationship of this performance to the individual's primary math knowledge, fluid reasoning system, working memory system (attention, executive, and processing speed), long-term memory system, verbal ability system, and graphomotor abilities.

Accommodations for Mathematics Difficulties

The selection of accommodations for an individual demonstrating functional limitations in learning math requires a professional to examine several factors, including (but not limited to) (1) the individual's cognitive, language, and affective profile; (2) the type of math learning (e.g., calculation, applied problem solving); and (3) the specific instruction, test, or work requirements in which quantitative literacy is required. Table 7.4 provides a list of options for accommodating difficulties with mathematics and science content. The four most commonly suggested accommodations for math disorders are extra time, calculators, read-alouds, and graphic organizers. However, very little research about the effectiveness of such accommodations is available, particularly for adolescents and/or adults with LD or ADHD, who are required to master higher-level math problems.

Extended time during test taking—an accommodation that is commonly provided to individuals with MLD and ADHD—has not been well researched, and results have been somewhat unclear (Alster, 1997; Johnson, 2000; Munger & Loyd, 1991; Tindal & Ketterlin-Geller, 2004). As noted by Fuchs, Fuchs, Eaton, Hamlett, and Karns (2000), the majority of studies examining the effectiveness of extra time on math tests for students both with and without LD or ADHD lack population specificity and usually have confounding treatment variables. However, two recent studies provide professionals with a better understanding of the role of extended time for adolescents with LD. We (Cohen et al., 2005) conducted two studies to investigate the influence of extended time and content knowledge on the performance of ninth-grade students who took a statewide mathematics test with ($n = 1,250$) and without ($n = 1,250$) extended time. Both studies suggested that students were not accurately characterized by their accommodation status, but rather by their content knowledge. That is, knowing students' accommodation status contributed little to understanding the differences in students' test performance. Rather, the data suggested as a more likely explanation that mathematics competency differentiated the groups of student learners, regardless of their accommodation and/or reading levels. The findings do not suggest that extra time was not beneficial, but rather that both math knowledge and extended time significantly influenced the scores for students receiving the accommodation. The accommodation cannot compensate for deficits in math knowledge and/or learning. However, there is plenty of research evidence to support providing extended time to many individuals with MLD, because their deficits in working memory, processing speed, lexical access, and/or language affect their ability to process mathematical information quickly.

The use of calculators as accommodations for students with disabilities during mathematics testing is discussed thoroughly in Chapter Eight. As noted in that chapter, the effectiveness of calculators in the testing context differs primarily by the type of item content. However,

TABLE 7.4. Math and Science Accommodation Options

Working memory deficit	Long-term memory deficit	Visual–spatial deficit	Verbal ability deficit	Reasoning deficit	Graphomotor deficit
Extended time	Extended time	Extended time	Extended time	Extended time	Extended time
Read-alouds[a]	Read-alouds[a]	Verbal cues	Read-alouds[a]	Graphic organizers	Touch screen
Graphic organizers	Embedded e-text supports[b]	Think-alouds	Graphic organizers	Think-alouds	Mouse options
Embedded e-text supports[b]	Presentational	Embedded e-text supports[b]	Modified language	Cognitive strategies[c]	Calculators
Formula calendar	Translational	Navigational	Think-alouds		
Color-coding symbols	Enrichment	Translational	Embedded e-text supports[b]		
Cognitive strategies[c]	Notational	Explanatory	Navigational		
	Color-coding symbols	Illustrative	Translational		
	Calculators	Summarizing	Explanatory		
		Instructional	Illustrative		
		Enrichment	Summarizing		
		Cognitive strategies[c]	Instructional		
			Enrichment		
			Cognitive strategies[c]		
			Color-coding symbols		

[a]When reading deficits are also documented.
[b]Embedded e-text supports are discussed in Chapter Five (see especially Table 5.3).
[c]See Miller (1996) for cognitive strategies.

research evidence pertaining to cognitive deficits influencing calculation competencies as discussed throughout this chapter certainly justi-
fies allowing many individuals with MLD and ADHD to use calculators
as accommodations for instruction, in testing, and in work environments.

The use of read-alouds during math assessments is beginning to
receive greater attention from professionals as a result of the increase
in high-stakes tests in the world of school and work (Tindal & Ketterlin-
Geller, 2004). Again, the majority of this research is flawed by methodology errors, such as nonspecific selection of participants (e.g., students
with disabilities in general rather than those with LD or ADHD), provision of only one accommodation to the research participants, little participant training or history with the type of read-aloud investigated, and
few item-level data. However, if a professional is concerned that poor
reading skills will limit an individual's ability to access math knowledge
or will influence the construct validity of a measure, a read-aloud is an
appropriate accommodation.

Graphic organizers are often suggested by professionals as appropriate accommodations for individuals with MLD. However, little research
evidence is available to support their use as accommodations for adolescents and/or adults with MLD. As graphic organizers rely on visual–
spatial reasoning skills and lend themselves to higher-level mathematics, their importance to the adolescent and adult populations requires
greater research attention. Recently, Ives (2007) provided evidence that
the use of graphic organizers in secondary algebra instruction for students with LD and ADHD was very effective. However, in this study no
differentiation was made between types of LD (e.g., dyslexia, MLD).
Therefore, the effectiveness of graphic organizers with certain LD and
ADHD profiles will require further investigation.

Let's consider the effectiveness of math accommodations for Ellie
(Figure 7.1), who demonstrates MLD. Cognitively, Ellie demonstrates
superior verbal abilities, but much weaker visual–spatial abilities and
abstract reasoning involving numbers, proportions, and so forth. This
suggests that she will benefit from detailed verbal explanations of visual,
conceptual, and procedural math information. Also, she may require
individual assistance with the interpretation of graphs, charts, and
other complex visual data. Some of the embedded e-text supports listed
in Table 7.4 may be effective in providing the prompts and scaffolding
necessary for her to understand math concepts.

Academically, Ellie demonstrates facility with only basic operations
(addition, subtraction, multiplication) and knowledge of relatively few
math-related facts (e.g., the length of a standard ruler and the units in

our monetary system). She does not generally attempt math problems involving long division, fractions, decimals, percentages, geometry, or algebra; her efforts to solve practical problems are often hindered by her weak knowledge of operations, formulas, and math-related facts. Thus, in addition to being permitted to use a formula sheet and a calculator, Ellie may benefit from one-on-one guidance about procedural steps and the reasons behind them. Her investment and understanding may be enhanced by a Socratic approach (e.g., "What is this problem asking? What are the pertinent numbers? If you had to guess without doing any calculations, what estimate would you make? Why?").

Science

Adolescents with LD or ADHD often do not participate in rigorous secondary curricula that would prepare them for pursuing careers in science or mathematics (Gregg, 2007; Mastropieri & Scruggs, 1992). Alston, Bell, and Hampton (2002) surveyed 140 parents and 323 teachers regarding entry into science and engineering careers for secondary students with LD. These two groups were assessed on their perceptions of eight variables: (1) faculty access, (2) expense of accommodations, (3) role models, (4) teachers' understanding of students' academic needs, (5) amount of learning time, (6) students' aptitude and educational preparation, (7) career guidance, and (8) employers' attitudes. The results of both surveys revealed that parents, more than teachers, felt that secondary schools were not making the necessary efforts to accommodate students with LD in science curricula. In addition, both teachers and parents felt that employers in the science and engineering fields would be reluctant to hire individuals with LD.

The data on individuals with LD or ADHD in postsecondary education science and engineering programs are nonexistent. Although several national surveys track the number of students with disabilities in higher education (e.g., the National Center for Education Statistics Survey, the National Postsecondary Student Aid Survey, and the Postsecondary Students Longitudinal Study), a 2006 review by the National Science Foundation of the results from these assessments provides no record of the number of science and engineering bachelor's and master's degrees awarded to persons with LD or ADHD. The reason for this paucity of data is that a diagnosis of LD or ADHD does not tend to be part of comprehensive postsecondary academic institutional records. In addition, no data are available on trends in graduate enrollment for students with LD or ADHD, since the National Science Foundation's

(2006) Survey of Graduate Students and Postdoctorates in Science and Engineering did not collect information specific to the populations of students with LD or ADHD. What we do know from the Foundation's survey is that as of 2006, only 1% of all science and engineering doctoral degrees were awarded to individuals with disabilities.

Research to date has provided very little empirical evidence about difficulties that individuals with LD or ADHD may face in learning scientific concepts. An adolescent with either disorder may encounter difficulty in learning specific science content because of an inefficient verbal working memory system, long-term memory system, fluid reasoning system, verbal ability system, and/or graphomotor processes. Therefore, the accommodations listed in Table 7.4 are possible options for adolescents or adults who are dealing with science content. However, there is no specific research evidence on the effectiveness of these options with science tasks for the adolescent population with LD or ADHD.

On the other hand, a great deal of interesting research related to the use of cognitive and metacognitive strategy instruction for enhancing science performance among adolescents in general is providing professionals with possibilities for accommodating the learning and testing environments for the populations with LD and ADHD. Researchers have provided evidence that when students with and without disabilities are introduced to specific cognitive and metacognitive strategies, instructional and test performance improves (Conley, 2004; Olson & Land, 2007; Schumaker & Deshler, 2006). The strategies with the most empirical evidence for enhancing academic performance are those that focus on planning and goal setting; activating prior knowledge; forming interpretations; and reflecting, relating, and evaluating (Conley, 2008). The goal of cognitive strategy instruction is to help adolescents and adults learn to be strategic learners, so that their use of cognitive and technology tools or accommodations to be effective in school will generalize to the world of work. As noted by Conley (2008),

> To successfully operate in college and in the workplace, now and in the future, adolescents will need to master cognitive strategies for reading, writing, and thinking in complex situations where texts, skills, or requisite knowledge are fluid and not always clearly understood. (p. 85)

Science Writer II, developed by the Center for Applied Special Technology (*www.cast.org/research/projects/tws.html*), is an innovative, evidence-based tool that employs "universal design for learning" (see Chapter One) to teach middle school children science. Although it was not designed for secondary or postsecondary students, it does demonstrate the effectiveness of providing a supportive, technology-rich learning environment. Science Writer II is a technology-based writing approach that provides learning tools (embedded e-text supports; see Chapter Five) to aid students in the process of writing science reports. Prompts related to both writing and the scientific process tailored for individual student profiles are built into the program. In addition, several forms of assistive technology (AT), such as text-to-speech (TTS) software and vocabulary help, are integrated throughout the program.

As noted in Chapter Five, a great many adolescents or adults with LD or ADHD demonstrate serious reading difficulties. Therefore, it is very likely that such students will need alternative media (alt media— e.g., e-text or books on tape) and AT (e.g., TTS software) to succeed in science courses. David is an excellent example of an individual who can learn science or math concepts if he is provided with appropriate accommodations in gaining access to information and demonstrating his learning. David has been struggling with his math and science courses in high school. Since his current math instructor is quite verbal and uses manipulatives and graphics during his teaching, David is able to keep up in class. However, when doing his outside coursework and when taking tests, he has usually had the problems read to him. Although David and the math instructor have developed acceptable shorthand for certain vocabulary words, he does still need to write numbers and variables.

The professionals at David's high school have decided that his science and math coursework should be placed in an electronic format on a Web/CT Vista profile accessed through an alt media repository (e.g., *www.amac.uga.edu*). This allows David constant access to his material; it also provides him with AT software such as a math/word processor and scientific graphing calculator software. He is now quite successful in using the keyboard and toolbar icons to record his answers in his math course; he only solicits help from the teacher when he needs to record answers in complete sentences. By utilizing online support through Web/CT Vista and helpful AT software, the instructor is now able to record all chapter reviews, test questions, and the attached figures, using specialized authoring tools. All review and test questions are voiced in the background (which David can access and repeat at the push of a button); each figure is described; and all of the figure measurements have been keyed to individual points, which he can touch to activate. Thus David can independently access the review/test to get the information he needs, enter Alt-Tab to go to his notes, record his answers, and then use Alt-Tab to return to the text for the next question. David is very excited about his ability to complete his work independently. Since he uses earphones, the rest of the class is not disturbed by the teacher reading the problems; nor do they hear David's answers.

Foreign Languages

The ability to learn a second language requires specific cognitive and linguistic abilities as well as general aptitude. Evidence-based research has documented that several linguistic processing deficits demonstrated by adolescents and young adults with dyslexia have a negative impact on their learning a foreign language (Downey, Snyder, & Hill, 2000; Ganschow & Sparks, 1995; Ganschow, Sparks, Javorsky, Pohlman, & Bishop-Marbury, 1991, Sparks, 1995; Smythe, Everatt, & Salter, 2004).

For many individuals with certain types of LD (i.e., dyslexia, oral language disorders), learning a second language to the level of proficiency required at the secondary or postsecondary level may be all but impossible. Such individuals may demonstrate sufficient difficulty on phonemic, orthographic, morphemic, or syntactic awareness tasks in their first language to provide evidence that learning a second language will present significant barriers. These abilities and the types of measures used to assess them are discussed in Chapter Five. In addition to measuring these abilities, an evaluator should take an adolescent's or adult's other cognitive, language, achievement, and emotional functioning into consideration when investigating his or her potential for learning a second language. Finally, an individual's actual exposure to learning a second language should be considered, along with all of the other diagnostic information. Professionals are encouraged to use the questions presented in Figure 7.4 to guide their decision making for determining appropriate accommodations for a student attempting to learn a second language.

The transparency of the language must also be considered when determining the appropriateness of accommodations. "Transparency" refers to the relationship between the written symbols of a language and their associated sounds in speech. For instance, Spanish and Italian are considered to have more transparent/shallow orthographies, since they have a high correspondence between written symbols and speech sounds. Other languages, such as English and French, are considered to have more inconsistent orthographies, since they have a much more inconsistent (irregular) correspondence between symbols and sounds. Therefore, a student's evaluation profile should be considered in relation to the orthography he or she is attempting to learn. A student may be more successful in learning a more transparent language (e.g., Spanish) with accommodations, but may not be able to learn a more opaque language (e.g., French).

There is no one "second-language" test a clinician can use to determine whether an individual's LD would make learning a second language difficult or impossible. Rather, standardized, descriptive, and informal data collected during a comprehensive evaluation provide the evidence necessary for such a decision. Central to a professional's deci-

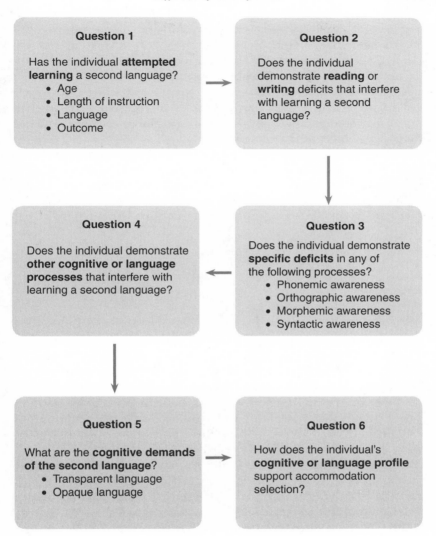

FIGURE 7.4. Questions to support decision making for the accommodation of difficulties with learning a second language.

sion making about whether to support a foreign language substitution is his or her understanding of the difference between language aptitude and LD. According to Carroll (1981), foreign language aptitude should "be defined in terms of prediction of rate of learning" (p. 91). Different types of LD are defined by significant cognitive and linguistic deficits that impair or functionally limit a person's ability to learn certain content (e.g., a second language). However, the rate of learning is not the same as the ability or inability to learn.

The Modern Language Aptitude Test (MLAT; Carroll & Sapon, 2002) is a standardized instrument that assesses an individual's rate of learning a foreign language. Again, rate of learning is not equal to inability to learn. In fact, the MLAT manual can be used as support *not* to use the test as "the" diagnostic evidence of LD:

> The MLAT does not claim to say whether an individual has a "language block" or some inherited disposition or rate which will prevent him or her from learning a foreign language. As far as is known, any individual who is able to use his mother tongue in the ordinary affairs of everyday life can also acquire similar competence in a second language, given time and opportunity. (Carroll & Sapon, 2002, p. 23)

Moreover, as discussed above, the determination of whether an individual's LD will functionally limit the learning of a second language should not be based on a single measure, but rather on a comprehensive evaluation.

Joyce (see Figure 7.5) is an excellent example of a high-functioning college student with dyslexia for whom the learning of a second language is significantly hindered by her cognitive and language-processing deficits (e.g., verbal working memory capacity, phonemic and orthographic awareness, orthographic fluency, and naming). She reports that she is currently experiencing great difficulty learning Spanish at college. In high school she attempted to learn German, but failed it in two consecutive semesters and was then allowed to substitute a course on German culture for the language course. Joyce was advised at her college to at least attempt Spanish in college before requesting a course substitution. Therefore, she enrolled in an introductory Spanish course, but failed it despite working closely with her teacher and a tutor throughout the semester. Her Spanish teacher has suggested that she seek current documentation to support her appeal for a foreign language substitution.

Course Substitutions

Both secondary and postsecondary programs of study require students to take certain core courses in order to graduate. Mathematics and for-

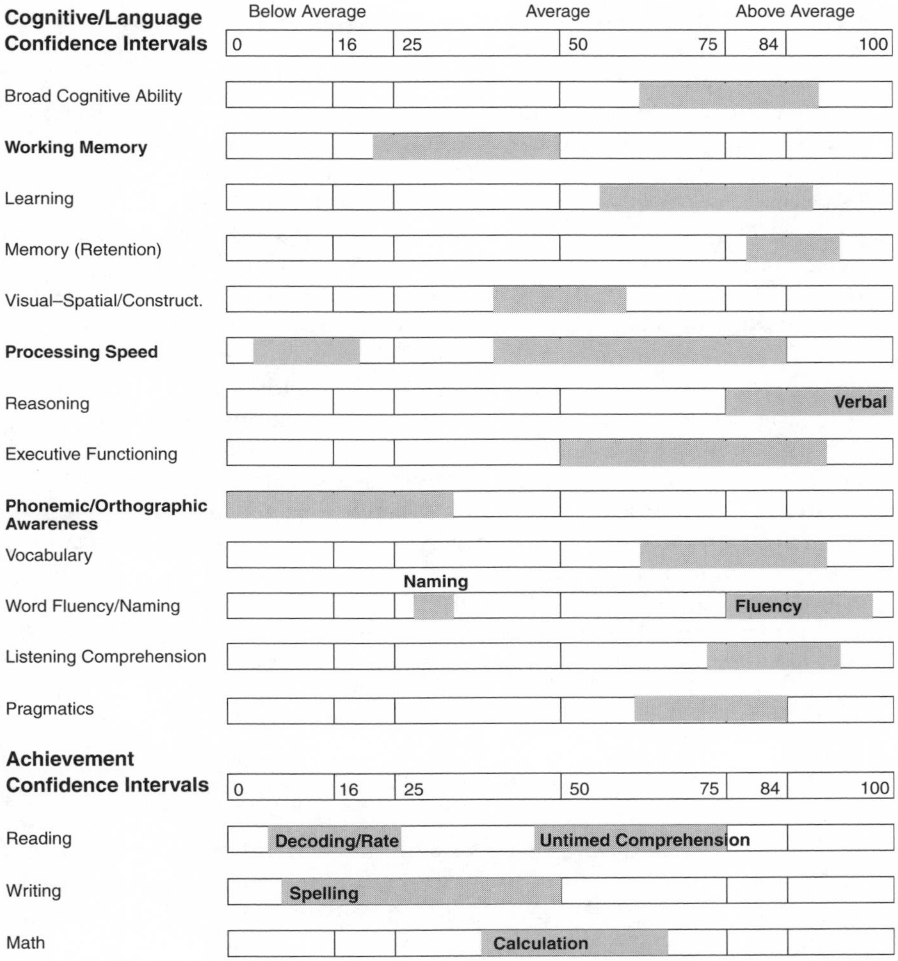

FIGURE 7.5. Assessment profile for Joyce, an individual with dyslexia.

eign language requirements are central to many academic programs of study. As discussed throughout this chapter, meeting these requirements may present a difficult obstacle for some students with LD or ADHD, even with accommodations. Section 504 of the Rehabilitation Act of 1973 (see Chapter Two) lists several alternative accommodations, such as "substitution of specific courses," as appropriate in particular situations (34 C.F.R. §104.44(a) and (d)(1)). However, there has been much debate both in the courts and at academic institutions about the relative necessity of specific mathematics and foreign language courses to a particular student's program of study (e.g., *Guckenburger v. Boston University*, 1997, 1998). There is wide but not universal agreement on the options available to students for accommodations in and/or substitutions for mathematics and foreign language courses (Wolinsky & Whelan, 1999). Students are often allowed to substitute a "programmatic" requirement for foreign language if their documentation provides evidence of significant phonemic and orthographic awareness deficits impacting on the learning of a second language. Depending on the severity of the disability, a student may be allowed accommodations to the course "requirements" rather than a full substitution of the course. For instance, if the student's documents provide support, the following accommodations to the course requirements may be allowed: borrowing lab tapes; dictating sections on tape; dictations repeated by instructors; word processing with language spell checks; writing dictation questions before composing responses; extending time to formulate replies on an oral examination; and the oral component counted less toward the final grade, or not graded. As noted by Scott (2002), "Institutions need to carefully and proactively assess how they will provide equal access to such programmatic requirements" (p. 320). What is apparent is that a comprehensive evaluation of an individual's cognitive, language, achievement, affective abilities is essential to the process of determining whether a substitution for a mathematics or foreign language course is appropriate for a specific student.

Implications for Assessment and Accommodation

✓ The term "quantitative literacy" is often used, rather than the term "mathematics," to refer to the quantitative knowledge and skills necessary for an adult to function adequately in the workplace, home, and community.

✓ Individuals with LD in mathematics (math LD or MLD) appear to be a heterogeneous group exhibiting several different learning profiles.

✓ Two significant limitations of research on math disorders involve (1) the different eligibility criteria used to identify populations of individuals with MLD, and (2) the restricted tools employed to measure performance.

✓ The capacity to learn mathematical concepts, according to Geary (2007), requires an individual to utilize both primary and secondary cognitive abilities.

✓ Numerous studies provide evidence that individuals with MLD do not perform as well as their peers on tests of verbal working memory capacity.

✓ A characteristic of many individuals with MLD is the inability to store and retrieve number combinations from long-term memory.

✓ The important role of fluid or nonverbal reasoning in mathematical learning is supported by empirical evidence.

✓ The relationship between verbal ability in general and quantitative knowledge is important to a better understanding of the difficulties experienced by individuals with LD or ADHD as they attempt math problems.

✓ The graphomotor system is essential for completing math items when students are asked to compute on paper.

✓ Different mathematical task requirements draw upon a variety of cognitive and linguistic processes.

✓ Diagnostic math achievement tests include various tasks for professionals to use in measuring different aspects of mathematics (e.g., calculation, quantitative knowledge, problem solving).

✓ The cause(s) for an individual's underachievement on math tests should be investigated through a comprehensive evaluation in which possible reasons for this underachievement are considered, such as instructional history, task format, cognitive and linguistic factors, reading abilities, motivation, and apprehension about math learning (i.e., "math anxiety").

✓ The four most commonly suggested accommodations for math disorders are extra time, read-alouds, calculators, and graphic organizers (concept or knowledge maps).

✓ Research to date has provided very little empirical evidence related to difficulties that individuals with LD or ADHD may face in learning scientific concepts.

✓ The ability to learn a second language requires specific cognitive and linguistic abilities as well as general aptitude.

✓ Certain individuals with LD (i.e., dyslexia, oral language) cannot learn a second language to the level of proficiency required at the secondary or postsecondary level.

✓ Substitutions of specific courses may be appropriate in particular situations for particular individuals whose LD affects their learning of mathematics, science, or foreign languages.

CHAPTER EIGHT

Accommodations on Large-Scale Assessments

Kathy, first mentioned in the text of Chapter Two, is a European American political science major interested in a law career. She is currently preparing to take the Law School Admission Test (LSAT). Although Kathy received accommodations during her undergraduate years for substantial limitations (reading and writing) resulting from her LD and ADHD, her documentation is over 3 years old. She has sought an evaluation to update her accommodation documentation, in order to receive extra time when she takes the LSAT.

Josiah, an African American student, was diagnosed with LD (dyslexia) in first grade and received special education services through his sophomore year in high school. His parents recognized his talents in art and nurtured these abilities throughout his school years. Unfortunately, Josiah is seriously considering dropping out of school, because of his concern that he will not pass his 10th-grade statewide assessment of reading and writing. He has just completed a comprehensive evaluation to help identify effective accommodations to be used both in the classroom and on high-stakes tests.

Standards-based reforms and changes in professional licensing requirements have led to an increase in large-scale assessments as the gateways to promotion, graduation, and career attainment. These high-stakes tests are increasingly central to accountability across the lifespan. In addition, as a result of the No Child Left Behind (NCLB) Act's mandates, elementary and secondary outcomes measured by large-scale assessments are now tied to school funding. As a result of the focus on high-stakes testing, research pertaining to accommodations in testing rather than to those in instructional or work environments now dominates the literature (Gregg, 2008).

This chapter focuses on the evidence-based literature pertaining to the accommodation of adolescents and adults with LD and ADHD on large-scale assessments. The reader is referred back to Chapters Five, Six, and Seven for instructional accommodations. The accommodations discussed here adjust the manner in which testing situations are presented and/or evaluated, so that individuals with disabilities can access and/or demonstrate knowledge in a fair and equitable manner. As a guide for professionals, definitions of terms used in the adaptation of testing are provided in Table 8.1.

Unfortunately, research examining the effectiveness of accommodations on large-scale assessments specifically for adolescents or adults

TABLE 8.1. Accommodation Terminology

Term	Meaning
Accommodations	Changes to instructional, testing, or work situations that allow an individual access to or demonstration of knowledge without altering standards or expectations.
Differential-boost hypothesis	Hypothesis that an accommodation should improve the performance of students with disabilities to a significantly greater extent than it improves the performance of students without disabilities.
Interaction hypothesis	Hypothesis that (1) when test accommodations are given to individuals with disabilities, their test scores will improve; and (2) students without disabilities will not exhibit higher scores when taking the test with those accommodations.
Modifications	Changes to instruction, testing, or work situations that alter standards or expectations.
Read-alouds	Accommodations in which printed text is read aloud, either by a person or by technological means (e.g., a screen reader).
Universal design for learning (UDL)	Multiple means of providing opportunities to acquire and demonstrate learning more flexibly, so that accommodations become unnecessary.
Universal design for testing (UDT)	Multiple means of constructing and administering tests more flexibly, so that accommodations become unnecessary.

with LD or ADHD is lacking not only in quantity, but in sophisticated design methods. For instance, when Sireci, Li, and Scarpati (2003) reviewed the accommodation literature, they found that only 41% of the studies investigated were published in peer-reviewed journals, and that quasi- or nonexperimental designs were the most frequently used methodologies. More alarming was the fact that they found no experimental designs at the secondary level and only one involving postsecondary students. More recently, a colleague and I (Gregg & Nelson, 2008) conducted a meta-analysis of the extended-time test accommodation literature specific to adolescents and adults with LD. Of the nine empirical-based studies identified in this literature search, five involved the performance of participants with and without LD on postsecondary college entrance examinations. The generalizability of this body of research to the broad range of abilities represented by the adolescent and adult population with LD is highly questionable.

The literature focusing on test accommodations provides some insight into the frequency with which accommodations are used, but more often than not the researchers do not isolate subgroups of students with specific disabilities (e.g., LD, ADHD); rather, they investigate "students with disabilities" as a general group. Another limitation of many such studies is that the participants were often given several accommodations at one time, making the effectiveness of any one accommodation difficult to determine. Both of these factors suggest that any generalizations about the construct validity and/or effectiveness of specific accommodations for individuals with LD or ADHD should be cautiously explored. Several published reviews of the accommodation literature highlight the need for better research methodologies and more specifically defined populations (Calahan-Laitusis, 2003; Chi & Pearson, 1999; Gregg, 2008; Johnstone, Altman, Thurlow, & Thompson, 2006; MacArthur, 2006; Sireci, 2004; Sireci, Li, & Scarpati, 2003; Thompson, Blount, & Thurlow, 2002; Tindal & Fuchs, 1999; Tindal & Ketterlin-Geller, 2004).

Rationales for Providing Test Accommodations

A test accommodation should not change the content being evaluated; nor should it provide unfair advantage to the individual using it. Clinical data, legal mandates, and professional standards all provide important information to guide professionals in selecting appropriate and effective test accommodations. In addition, current evidence-based research should support professional decision making.

Clinical Rationale

Kathy's profile (Figure 8.1) provides the clinical rationale to support a request for extended time on a high-stakes test. Kathy's performance on different reading comprehension measures also demonstrates the importance of considering the type of task format in relation to the severity of a person's functional limitation. Kathy's strong verbal reasoning and oral language abilities appear to have helped her compensate for her problems with reading decoding on certain reading comprehension measures. Her difficulties with decoding, resulting from deficits with phonemic and orthographic awareness, prevent her from reading fluently. However, when she was administered the Comprehension portion of the Nelson–Denny Reading Test (Brown et al., 1993), she reported afterwards to the clinician that she did not read the passages, but guessed at the answers by using her strong verbal reasoning and language skills. As discussed in Chapter Five, this is not an uncommon strategy for poor decoders. On the Woodcock–Johnson III Tests of Achievement (WJ III ACH) Passage Comprehension subtest (Woodcock et al., 2001a), an untimed cloze task, Kathy was able to linguistically predict correct answers without reading the short passages. However, on the Gray Oral Reading Tests—Fourth Edition (GORT-4; Wiederholt & Bryant, 2001), she was required to read aloud and answer questions. Her comprehension on the GORT-4 was adequate, but her rate and accuracy of reading were significantly low. On the LSAT, the passage length and complexity will prohibit Kathy from relying simply on guessing. Therefore, she should receive extra time or a read-aloud as an accommodation on the test administration, because of her significant functional limitations in reading decoding and fluency. However, the testing agency has decided to deny her access to either of these accommodations (see Chapter Two).

Legal Rationale

Legal protection of the right for adolescents and adults with LD or ADHD to receive testing accommodations is provided by several pieces of legislation, some of which I have discussed in Chapter Two: the 14th Amendment to the U.S. Constitution; Title VI of the Civil Rights Act of 1964; the Equal Educational Opportunities Act of 1974; Section 504 of the 1973 Rehabilitation Act; the Americans with Disabilities Act (ADA) of 1990; the Individuals with Disabilities Education Improvement Act of 2004 (IDEA 2004); and the NCLB Act of 2001. As also discussed in Chapter Two, secondary students are protected by entitlement laws, whereas postsecondary institutions operate under eligibility laws. The

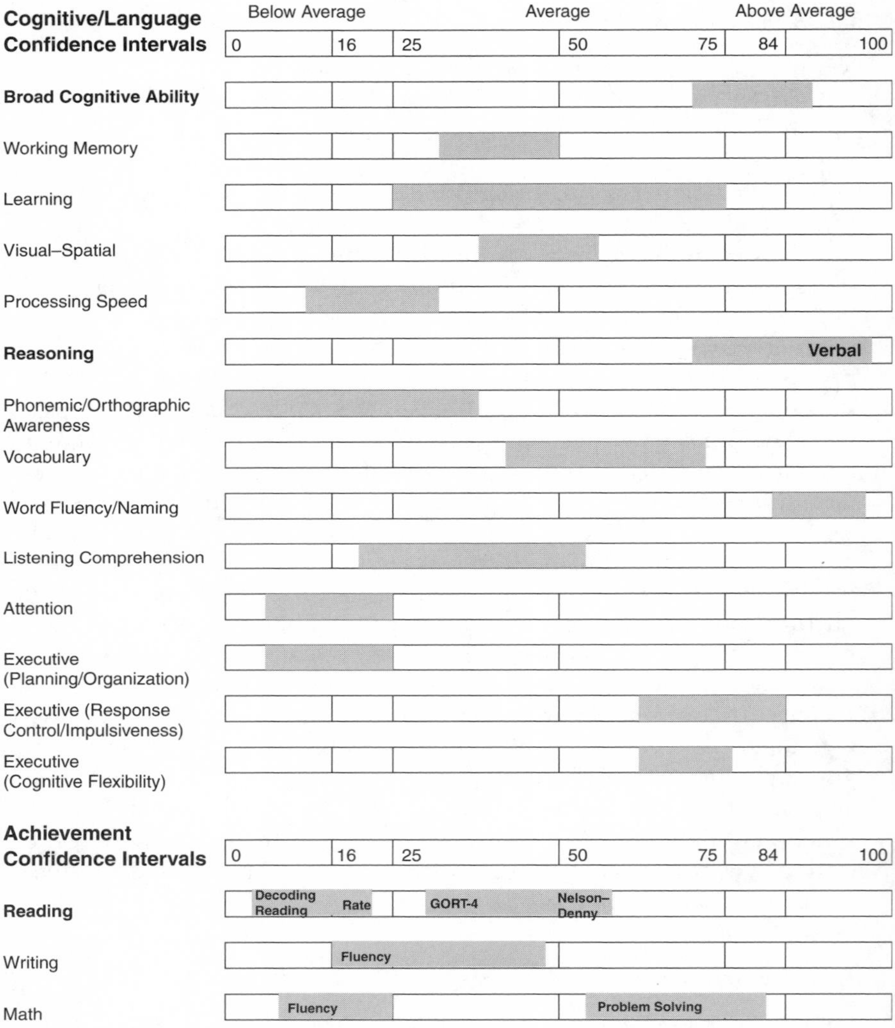

Cognitive/Language Confidence Intervals	Below Average			Average		Above Average	
	0	16	25	50	75	84	100
Broad Cognitive Ability							
Working Memory							
Learning							
Visual–Spatial							
Processing Speed							
Reasoning						Verbal	
Phonemic/Orthographic Awareness							
Vocabulary							
Word Fluency/Naming							
Listening Comprehension							
Attention							
Executive (Planning/Organization)							
Executive (Response Control/Impulsiveness)							
Executive (Cognitive Flexibility)							

Achievement Confidence Intervals							
	0	16	25	50	75	84	100
Reading	Decoding Reading	Rate	GORT-4	Nelson–Denny			
Writing		Fluency					
Math		Fluency		Problem Solving			

FIGURE 8.1. Assessment profile for Kathy, an individual with LD and ADHD.

accommodation documentation requirements are not identical across sets of legislation. Therefore, there is no guarantee that students who received accommodations in high school will be eligible for them in a postsecondary learning or work environment.

At the secondary level, adolescents are provided rights under IDEA 2004, which requires that students with disabilities be provided appropriate accommodations in both instructional and testing situations. Students must have their accommodation needs specified in their individualized education programs (IEPs). The IEP team determines whether specific accommodations are consistent with federal and state guidelines. It is important to understand that the right for an adolescent to receive an accommodation in one situation does not generalize to all settings. Secondary schools must have accountability systems that provide ongoing evaluation of individual students' needs for specific accommodations, as well as of these accommodations' effectiveness (Almond, Lehr, Thurlow, & Quenemoen, 2002; Gregg & Lindstrom, 2007).

As a result of the mandatory, standards-driven reform of the NCLB Act of 2001, students with disabilities must be included in the assessments of mathematics and of reading or language arts that states administer to monitor "adequate yearly progress" toward academic proficiency for all students. The accommodation of students with disabilities on mandatory high-stakes tests has heightened concerns over test construct validity, as well as the effectiveness of specific types of accommodations for learning proficiency. Federal legislation protecting adolescents with LD or ADHD (IDEA 2004 and the NCLB Act) does caution that only "appropriate" and "reasonable" accommodations should be provided to a student. Therefore, states are left with the responsibility of determining how the rules for ensuring valid and reliable decision making remain consistent with professional and technical standards. Josiah's assessment profile (Figure 8.2) provides strong evidence to support his need for effective accommodations on his state's high-stakes tests.

The ADA and Section 504 of the Rehabilitation Act provide the legal support necessary for adults to access accommodations at postsecondary learning or work environments. Legally, to access an accommodation, an adult must demonstrate a "physical or mental impairment that substantially limits one or more . . . major life activities" as compared to the average person in the general population (see Chapter Two for an in-depth discussion). According to court rulings in the cases of *Bartlett v. New York State Board of Law Examiners* (1997, 1998, 1999, 2000, 2001]) and *Turner et al. v. American Association of Medical Colleges* (2006), accommodation decision making under ADA and Section 504 must be based on a comprehensive evaluation, and single test scores should not be used to support or reject access to specific accommodations. The

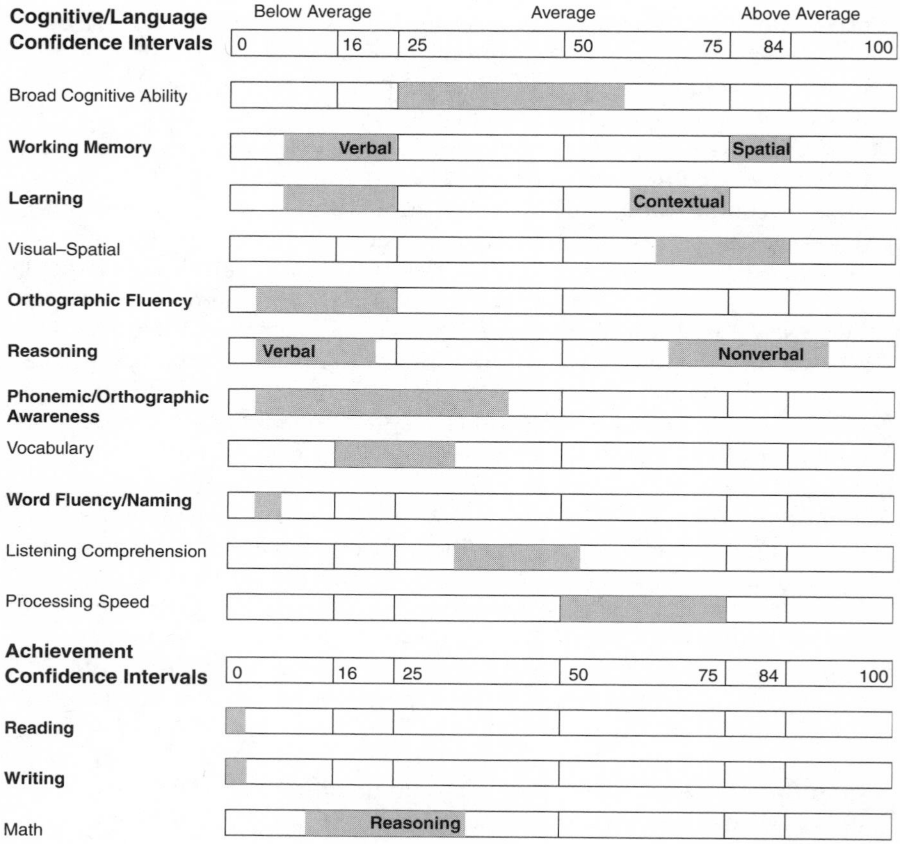

FIGURE 8.2. Assessment profile for Josiah, an individual with dyslexia.

courts thus appear to look unfavorably at relying on single cutoff scores, and favorably on the use of clinical judgment for accommodation decision making.

Professional Standards Rationale

In addition to legal guidelines, professionals developing accommodation policy, procedures, and decision-making practices usually depend upon the *Standards for Educational and Psychological Testing* (American Educational Research Association [AERA] et al., 1999). These standards, though not legally binding, are a widely respected guide to the best practices that have evolved over several decades (Koenig & Bachman, 2004). The *Standards* volume recommends selecting accommodations on the basis of existing research (Standards 10.2 and 10.8) and consistently following clearly delineated policies describing the rationale and procedures for accommodation decision making, as well as possible limits on the validity of inferences that can be made (Standards 10.4 and 10.5). Linn (2002) provides an excellent review of all the standards that apply specifically to high-stakes testing.

Types of Test Accommodations

The four categories of testing accommodations most frequently utilized by professionals in both secondary and postsecondary settings are accommodations in the presentation, response, scheduling/timing, and setting of assessments. An excellent resource for professionals seeking the most recent research related to accommodations is the National Center on Educational Outcomes (NCEO), a federally funded project that since 1990 has maintained a systematic database on the participation of students with disabilities in large-scale testing programs. The NCEO provides professionals with a wealth of state-level data and other resources pertaining to state compliance and the accommodation of high-stakes testing (see *www.education.umn.edu/nceo*).

Test Presentation Accommodations

The purpose of a test presentation accommodation is to provide an individual with *access* to content, most often print material, by an alternative means. Such accommodations include the use of a human reader or a screen reader; alternative media (alt media—e.g., electronic text [e-text], audiotaped text); alternative language structures (simplified syntax); and alternative formats (e.g., large print). Read-alouds, or oral presentations of print, are among the most frequently investigated and used testing accommodations across disabilities (Sireci, Li, & Scarpati, 2003; Thompson, Bount, & Thurlow, 2002). Chapter Five discusses many of these types of accommodations in detail. For Josiah (Figure 8.2), a read-aloud will be an essential accommodation in testing his knowledge on any large-scale assessment.

Test Response Accommodations

Test response accommodations give an individual equal opportunity to *demonstrate* knowledge by an alternative means. These accommodations include writing directly on a test booklet; giving oral responses; using a human assistant (e.g., a scribe); and employing speech-to-text (STT) software or other tools (e.g., a calculator). Commonly used technology response accommodations other than those just mentioned include word processing with spell checkers; abbreviation expanders (programs that allow students to type abbreviations for frequently used words or phrases and press the space bar/mouse to select the complete word or phrase); and outlining software programs (Gregg, Morgan, Lindstrom, & Coleman, 2008).

Test Scheduling/Timing Accommodations

Test scheduling/timing accommodations are adjustments to the time provided to complete a test (e.g., extended time, unlimited time, frequent breaks, testing over multiple days). Receiving extra time on a test has been studied more than any other accommodation for students with disabilities (Chi & Pearson, 1999; Gregg, 2008; Sireci, Li, & Scarpati, 2003; Thompson, Blount, & Thurlow, 2002). The profiles of both Kathy (Figure 8.1) and Josiah (Figure 8.2) support a need for extra time on a high-stakes test.

Test Setting Accommodations

Test setting accommodations alter the testing environment (e.g., a private room, a quiet room, a small-group setting). Although test setting accommodations are often recommended by professionals for the adolescent and adult populations with LD and ADHD, only anecdotal evidence is available to support the effectiveness of such accommodations in practice.

Accommodations on Different Types of Large-Scale Assessments

Reading Test Accommodations

Read-aloud technology, such as text-to-speech (TTS) software or some other oral presentation of print (e.g., a human reader), is an accommodation often recommended by professionals for individuals with LD. However, it is important to be aware that using a read-aloud to accommodate an examinee who is taking a test designed to measure "reading competency" is very controversial. First, the use of read-alouds on reading tests challenges traditional definitions of "reading" as an individual reading print. Second, since the majority of reading tests were designed to measure reading as thus traditionally defined, the construct validity of a standardized reading measure is affected. In a review of the validity issues surrounding accommodations on the National Assessment of Educational Progress (NAEP), Sireci (2004) suggests that the use of read-alouds on reading tests is likely to change the construct measured. If the construct validity of a measure is changed as a result of an accommodation, test scores cannot be compared across populations (i.e., examinees with and without accommodations), and inferences pertaining to score interpretation are jeopardized. Sireci provides some suggestions on how to compare scores obtained with and without read-aloud accommodations; he suggests treating them as two different test forms and then equating them. He also strongly encourages the continuing development of universal design for testing (UDT), which will make accommodation unnecessary.

Some researchers suggest that using a read-aloud accommodation with other accommodations may lead to better test performance than using a read-aloud as the only modification to the testing situation. For instance, Calhoon, Fuchs, and Hamlett (2000) found that individuals with disabilities often did better on constructed-response items than on multiple-choice items across different read-aloud formats; the read-aloud formats appeared to have an indirect effect on performance. As read-aloud assistive technology (AT) and various alt media continue to be refined, and as their use becomes more standard practice for individuals with reading disorders, the need for more empirically based research on the effectiveness of these technologies will only continue to grow.

For many adolescents and adults with LD, extra time during test taking has proven to be an extremely effective accommodation on reading tests (Gregg & Nelson, 2008). According to Sireci (2004), flexible time limits reduce unintended "speededness" effects and do not alter the construct validity of a reading test. In addition, several studies provide evidence that extra time is not going to improve performance if an individual does not know the content (Cohen et al., 2005; Mandinach, Bridgeman, Cahalan-Laitusis, & Trapani, 2005). These studies highlight the fact that accommodations do not replace instruction, but rather facilitate access to or production of knowledge.

Recently, we (Lindstrom & Gregg, 2007) investigated the factor structure of the SAT Reasoning Test across two groups of students (students without disabilities tested under standard time conditions, and students with LD and ADHD tested with extended time) to determine whether the test appeared to be measuring the same constructs for both groups. Invariance across the two groups was supported for all parameters of interest, suggesting that the scores on the Critical Reading, Mathematics, and Writing sections of the SAT Reasoning Test can be interpreted in the same way when students are granted extended time. More measurement invariance research is needed across other high-stakes tests (e.g., the GRE, graduation/exit examinations, etc.) to determine whether or not the factor structure changes if extended time is provided to examinees with LD. If it does not, it will be hard to support the argument that when examinees are granted extended time, the construct validity of a test is compromised.

Writing Test Accommodations

Written language disorders are exhibited by a significantly large percentage of adolescents and adults with LD and ADHD (see Chapter Six for an in-depth discussion). Commonly requested accommodations on writing assessments for individuals with these disorders include extra time, word processors, spell checkers, word prediction software, and TTS technology.

The effectiveness of word processing as an accommodation on large-scale assessments of writing for adolescents and/or adults with LD or ADHD has been virtually unexamined (Cahalan-Laitusis, 2003; Gregg, 2008). Unfortunately, researchers reporting small differences in scores between word-processed and handwritten versions of timed essay writing tests reviewed studies conducted a decade or more ago (Hollenbeck, Tindal, Harniss, & Almond, 1999; MacArthur & Graham, 1987). Since that time, word processing and other technologies have been more fully integrated into school curricula. As discussed in Chapter Six, we (Gregg, Coleman, Davis, & Chalk, 2007) recently studied college writers with and without dyslexia who were required to write a timed impromptu essay similar to tasks found on high-stakes writing tests (e.g., high school graduation tests, postsecondary entrance examinations). We investigated the influence of handwritten, typed, and typed/edited formats on these students' writing quality scores. Our results suggest that legibility problems can easily influence raters' perceptions of competence, because a writer who is slow and laborious in forming letters and words may sacrifice verbosity and thinking and planning time. In addition, we did not find that handwritten scores were superior to word-processed scores for either group, as past research suggests. Providing the response accommodation of word processing for many adolescents and adults with LD or ADHD thus appears to have strong empirical evidence. The effects of word processing on the overall writing quality scores of examinees with and without LD have yet to be explored.

As also discussed in Chapter Six, ample research supports the effectiveness of spell checkers and word prediction programs for enhancing the spelling performance of adolescent writers with LD. Speech recognition software and TTS software have likewise gained support as ways to enhance the writing performance of adolescents and adults with LD who demonstrate spelling, handwriting, and fluency problems. However, no empirically based evidence is currently available to support the effectiveness of these technologies as accommodations on large-scale assessments of writing for the adolescent and adult populations with LD and ADHD (Gregg & Nelson, 2008).

Mathematics Test Accommodations

Three commonly suggested accommodations on large-scale assessments of mathematics are read-alouds, extra time, and calculators. However, very little research has examined the effectiveness of such testing accommodations, particularly for adolescents and/or adults with LD and ADHD (Gregg & Nelson, 2008). The use of read-alouds during math assessments is beginning to receive greater attention, as noted in Chapter Seven. Tindal and Ketterlin-Geller (2004), reviewing the research on mathematics test accommodations relevant to the NAEP, conclude that read-aloud accommodations benefit younger "students with disabilities" and "students with low reading skills." In addition, they suggest that the construct validity of mathematics tests is not altered when a read-aloud is used.

Plenty of research evidence indicates that many individuals with LD and ADHD should be provided extended time as a result of deficits in working memory, processing speed, lexical access, and/or language, which have an impact on their ability to process mathematical information quickly (Swanson & Jerman, 2006). Unfortunately, as noted by Fuchs and colleagues (2000b), many studies investigating the effectiveness of extra time on math tests for students with and without disabilities lack population specificity and usually have confounding treatment variables. In the Gregg and Nelson (2008) meta-analysis, extended time on large-scale assessments did have a significantly positive effect on the scores of adolescents and adults with LD.

In addition, recent research provides professionals with a better understanding of the role of extended time for the population with LD. As described in Chapter Seven, we (Cohen et al., 2005) conducted two studies to investigate the influence of extended time and content knowledge on the performance of ninth-grade students who took a statewide mathematics tests with ($n = 1,250$) and without ($n = 1,250$) the accommodation of only extended time. The results of both studies indicated that adolescents for whom items were functioning differently were not accurately characterized by their accommodation status, but rather by their content knowledge. That is, the data suggested that mathematics competency differentiated the groups of learners, regardless of their accommodation and/or reading levels. The findings do not suggest that extra time was not beneficial, but rather that math knowledge and extended time significantly influenced the scores for individuals with the accommodation. The accommodation cannot make up for deficits in math knowledge.

In another study, we (Lindstrom & Gregg, 2007) found that the use of extended time did not change the construct validity of the Mathematics section of the SAT for examinees with LD taking the test with this accommodation. However, the total mean scores differed significantly between these two groups, with the examinees with LD scoring lower than their peers with no disabilities. As in the Cohen and colleagues (2005) studies, individual differences appeared to be more the results of math competency than of the use of extended time as an accommodation.

Research on the use of calculators during high-stakes math testing suggests that "the effect of calculator use differs by the item types included in the tests" rather than by the characteristics of the populations studied (Cohen & Kim, 1992, p. 305). For instance, Scheuneman, Camara, Cascallar, and Lawrence (2002) found that calculator use favored fraction items but not reasoning items. Most interesting was their finding that calculator use was inversely related to test completion, and that more capable students used them more often than less capable students. In a thorough review of the literature investigating the research on mathematics tests accommodations relevant to NAEP testing, Tindal and Ketterlin-Geller (2004) conclude: "Research in mathematics testing accommodations highlights specific accommodations that function interactively by the characteristics of individual items and in reference to specific skills of individuals (not their disabilities)" (p. 10). However, my review of the literature specific to adolescents and adults with LD (Gregg, 2008) identified no studies in which the effectiveness of calculators on math tests was investigated.

Accommodations on Postsecondary Entrance and Licensure Examinations

An adolescent or adult with LD or ADHD must submit documentation to testing agencies as proof of a disability when requesting accommodations for postsecondary entrance or licensure examinations. In Chapter Two, I have discussed the types of information generally required by postsecondary testing agencies for approving accommodations on a high-stakes test. However, it is important for a consumer to remember that the documentation guidelines, eligibility criteria, and review processes are not identical across testing agencies. What appears most elusive are eligibility criteria that are reliably followed by reviewers to operationalize functional limitations. In other words, do the review policies or instructions provided to reviewers (often unpublished) at a particular agency specify that an individual's achievement scores must fall below the 16th percentile in order for a functional limitation to be identified? Brinckerhoff and Banerjee (2007) suggest otherwise: "The assumption that testing agencies are guided solely by psychometric evidence is simplistic because it minimizes the purpose of the disability documentation and the different perspectives towards disability documentation held by different stakeholders in high-stakes assessment" (p. 249). However, when one reviews the documentation guidelines across the majority of high-stakes testing agencies, no statements are provided about how reviewers are supposed to define substantial limitations. If individuals with disabilities are going to be given or denied accommodations, it behooves testing agencies to be specific in their guidelines as to how substantial limitations are defined and operationalized. If testing agencies are not using psychometric data alone to drive decision making, Kathy (Figure 8.1) should have had no difficulty obtaining the accommodation of extended time on the LSAT.

Brinckerhoff and Banerjee (2007) suggest that most testing agencies anchor decision making in their notion of "independent verifiability" of information. They define this construct to mean that an examinee's documentation (clinical report) must be written by a clinician to provide a clear case for external reviewers to follow. However, "independent verifiability" is also not clearly defined in the policies and procedures published by many testing agencies for consumers to use in preparing their documentation for accommodation review. The documentation guidelines provided by a testing agency are usually not where a consumer finds ambiguity. Rather, the specific eligibility criteria used by the accommodation reviewers employed by a testing agency to include or exclude an accommodation request are often very unclear. Both clinical evaluators and testing agencies should be required to provide clear criteria for how a behavior is or is not determined to be functionally limiting.

Brinckerhoff and Banerjee (2007) note: "By necessity, testing agencies make determinations about accommodations based on a 'moment-in-time' approach. In other words, accommodation decisions are based on information that is provided to the testing agency at the time of application by the test taker" (p. 256). Therefore, professionals must ensure that all information, historical or psychometric, provides clear and concise support for the requested accommodation(s). Banerjee and Shaw

(2007) also suggest that evaluators build a strong case for accommodations by providing (1) multiple sources of diagnostic information; (2) a consistent pattern (history) of a functional limitation; (3) evidence of the effectiveness of an accommodation; and (4) evidence of tests taken with and without an accommodation as proof of the accommodation's effectiveness (context relevance). Although these suggestions appear theoretically sound, the problem is that Banerjee and Shaw are asking evaluators to follow poor measurement practice. The effectiveness of an accommodation on one standardized high-stakes tests does not validate or invalidate its effectiveness on another measure. The two measures are more often normed on very different populations, measure different content, use different items, use different measurement models, and were administered at different points of time. Having no history of standardized accommodations does not validate or invalidate the need for accommodations on a postsecondary entrance or licensure exam.

As an example, we (Gregg, Coleman, Lindstrom, & Lee, 2007; see also Chapter Two of this book) discuss a 35-year-old African American woman named Jovita who scored at the 96th percentile on a verbal index of an intelligence measure. Jovita was raised in an abusive home in a poor Southern town, never received special education, and had no history of being tested for a disability. At the time of her postsecondary evaluation, her reading scores were markedly low: the 6th percentile on the WJ III ACH Word Attack subtest (Woodcock et al., 2001a); the 15th percentile on the WJ III ACH Letter–Word Identification subtest; the 20th percentile on the Comprehension portion of the Nelson–Denny Reading Test (Brown et al., 1993); and the 25th percentile on the WJ III ACH Reading Fluency subtest. Jovita was denied the accommodation of extended time on a high-stakes postsecondary graduate-level entrance examination, for two reasons. First, the testing agency's representatives stated in her rejection letter that because her scores on the last two reading measures mentioned above were "average" (>16th percentile), they felt that her functional limitations in reading were not sufficient to constitute a "disability." Second, since Jovita had not received accommodations before and had no history of special services, it did not appear that her underachievement was the result of a disability. As we (Gregg, Coleman, Lindstrom, & Lee, 2007) have stated, "It is difficult to view such a judgment as being equitable, justifiable, or within the spirit of the ADA" (p. 267). LD or ADHD is not defined, clinically or legally, by any one single behavior (e.g., discrepancy, underachievement, history of accommodations). Rather, substantial limitations are defined by the *condition*, *manner*, and *duration* of an individual's learning in our current on- and offline technical world of school and work.

Accommodations Allowed in Standardized Testing

Test accommodations are not universally approved across secondary/postsecondary institutions, states, or testing agencies. On standardized high-stakes tests, the decision to allow or prohibit the use of an accommodation relates to whether it changes the construct validity of the measure. Accommodations that significantly influence the interpretation of a test's construct validity are often referred to as "nonstandard," "invalid," or "not okay." The NCEO provides updated lists of what accommodations are considered "valid" in individual states' high-stakes tests. In addition, most testing agencies provide consumers with a list of "valid" accommodations provided on a specific test. However, there is a great deal of controversy in the literature and among professionals as to what constitutes a "valid" or "invalid" accommodation.

Computer-Based Testing

Brinckerhoff and Banerjee (2007) have noted an increase in the use of computer-based (CB) high-stakes testing by many of the major testing agencies. At first glance, one might consider CB testing a better alternative than traditional paper-and-pencil measures for students with specific print disabilities. Unfortunately, many of these CB tests are not accessible to screen readers and other forms of AT. In addition, Thompson, Thurlow, Quenemoen, and Lehr (2002), in a thorough review of the positives and negatives of CB instruction, also note that the practice has often been to "simply take the paper-and-pencil test and put it on to the computer" (p. 1).

However, the future of CB testing holds great potential for individuals with print disabilities. As noted by Haladyna (2002), "online web testing is coming of age" (p. 357). Unfortunately, at this time little evidence-based research has examined the equivalence of CB to paper-and-pencil testing. One promising use of CB testing that may prove to be effective for individuals with print disabilities involves high-fidelity simulations. The Dental Interactive Simulation Corporation, several dental agencies, and the Educational Testing Service (ETS) have partnered to produce a series of simulations and scoring methods for patient problems (Haladyna, 2002). Some licensure agencies, such as some states' medical licensing boards and the National Council of Architectural Registration Boards, have also developed simulations to be used as part of their examinations. According to Haladyna, "As we improve our understanding of the theories driving these developments and as technologies improve for designing simulations and the scoring engine, this innovation in the testing of cognitive abilities will be more widespread" (p. 362). Researchers developing new types of AT will need to work closely with the instructional designers and measurement experts developing CB testing, to ensure that individuals with LD and ADHD will have easy access to these new means of assessment.

CB essay scoring is also increasing across testing agencies assessing writing proficiency. Researchers at ETS have developed e-Rater, which is a computer program used in conjunction with human scorers to evaluate writing samples (see *www.ets.org*). The implications of CB scoring of writing produced by individuals with written language disorders remain unexplored at this time.

Questions to Guide Decision Making in Test Accommodation Selection

The selection of effective test accommodations depends upon a professional's sensitivity to individual differences (cognitive and language processes), task format (e.g., structured vs. free responses auditory vs. visual modalities), and response choices (e.g., written, oral, electronic). As I have stressed throughout this book, information from an adolescent's or adult's psychological evaluation should always guide professional decision making. Matching an individual's profile to specific types of accommodations enhances the probability that the accommodations will be effective. In addition to informed professional judgment, reliable procedures/policies for selecting accommodations are essential to valid accommodation decision making (Fuchs et al., 2000a; Hollenbeck et al., 1999). Several researchers are attempting to develop theory-driven guidelines for matching individual student profiles with test accommodations (Elliott, 2006; Helwig & Tindal, 2003; Kopriva, 2002; Siskind, 2004); currently, however, there is no available research evidence on the application of these models for the adolescent and/or adult populations with LD and ADHD. To guide professionals in the selection of testing accommodations, Figure 8.3 provides seven steps to inform decision making. The steps are discussed below.

• *Step 1 (examinee's profile)*. The first step in choosing testing accommodations is to review an examinee's profile (i.e., behavioral/affective, cognitive, language, academic achievement, other life experiences). Underachievement should not be the sole basis for selecting testing accommodations. For instance, an adolescent with ADHD may dem-

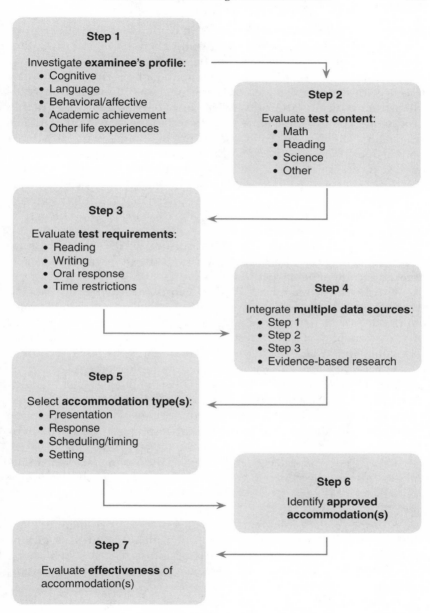

FIGURE 8.3. Seven steps in selecting accommodations for large-scale assessments.

onstrate significant underachievement in reading because of executive processing deficits (e.g., inferencing, comprehension monitoring). Presentation accommodations may not be as effective for this individual as scheduling/timing and setting accommodations. However, an adolescent with dyslexia may demonstrate functional limitations in reading as the result of significant deficits in phonemic and orthographic processing. For this individual, accommodations in test presentation (e.g., e-text, screen reader) and test scheduling/timing (e.g., extra time) would appear to be appropriate. In addition to psychological assessment data, a professional should give consideration to a student's history, including academic achievement and social/work experiences.

• *Step 2 (test content)*. In step 2, the professional carefully examines the content being tested. For instance, if math skills (e.g., problem solving) are what a test is measuring, the ancillary reading demands of the task should not penalize a student with print disabilities. In this situation, a student should be provided with e-text and a screen reader to access the content being measured.

• *Step 3 (task requirements)*. Step 3 consists of examining the task requirements during testing. For instance, a professional should evaluate the degree of structure required to complete test items (e.g., print presentation, oral vs. written responses, modality, time). An examinee's functional limitations should then be compared to the task demands.

• *Step 4 (multiple data sources)*. In step 4 a professional incorporates multiple data sources (the information collected during steps 1–3, plus other data). In particular, professionals should consider any available evidence-based research on the use of specific accommodations by examinees with similar profiles during the testing of the same types of items.

• *Step 5 (accommodation type)*. In step 5, a professional uses the information reviewed in step 4 to select the type(s) of accommodation(s) appropriate for the test (presentation, response, scheduling/timing, setting).

• *Step 6 (approved accommodation[s])*. Prior to providing an examinee access to an accommodation, a professional will need to ensure that it is approved for the type of test administered. Test publishers, test agencies, and state and federal agencies will make this information available to professionals.

• *Step 7 (effectiveness)*. Step 7 consists of following a standardized and systematic method to record the effectiveness of specific testing accommodations for an examinee. As we (Gregg & Lindstrom, 2007) have noted elsewhere, "At any given time, an outside reviewer should be able to evaluate the progress a student is making when specific accommodations are provided" (p. 309).

Strategic Use of Accommodations

Unfortunately, many individuals are provided with test accommodations but are given very little training in how to make strategic use of them, particularly in a high-stakes testing situation. Teaching an adolescent or adult specific strategies for how and when to use an accommodation is essential to any kind of positive outcome. For instance, Brincker-hoff and Banerjee (2007) encourage training in active listening for any student being introduced to e-text. Accommodations such as alt media (e.g., e-text, audiotaped text) and AT (e.g., TTS software) are often recommended for students with print disabilities to use on high-stakes tests. Although physical space (i.e., for the use of an alt media format) is a necessary first step, such examinees also need cognitive access in the form of explicit strategies for active engagement with the format. Similarly, individuals with LD or ADHD who are provided extended time should also gain proficiency with learning strategies that will help them to structure time management and organization if the extra time is going to be effective.

Test Accommodation Measurement Considerations

Providing test accommodations to qualified individuals is designed to promote fairness in testing and lead to accurate interpretation of the examinees' test scores (Sireci & Pitoniak, 2006). Accommodations are intended to provide equal access by removing unnecessary barriers (e.g., construct-irrelevant variance). Controversy over providing a specific accommodation arises when there is reason to believe that the accommodation may change the test's construct, thus altering the comparability of scores derived from the accommodated test. The three major concerns about tests taken with an accommodation are whether the accommodation (1) alters the skill being measured, (2) precludes the comparison of scores between examinees, or (3) would allow examinees without disabilities to benefit if they were granted the same accommodation.

Alteration of Measured Skills

Many accommodations do not appear to alter the constructs being measured. For instance, a reading test written in large print should not change the underlying construct the test was intended to measure, because the skill of reading can still be assessed unless reading the large print requires the examinee to take more time. Test accommodations are provided to remove construct-irrelevant barriers to test performance, while maintaining the integrity of the construct being measured (Sireci, Li, & Scarpati, 2003). For instance, Josiah (Figure 8.2) demonstrates significant functional limitations in the area of reading. If he takes a test designed to measure mathematics, his inability to read the problems may be considered extraneous to the math construct targeted by the test, but will certainly affect his test performance if he is not allowed to have a read-aloud accommodation.

Two situations have the potential to influence construct validity when a test accommodation is provided. The first one is that if the construct intended to be measured by a test changes because of the accommodation, and the new characteristic measured represents a different and unintended construct, then construct-relevant variance is present (Sireci & Parker, 2005). The second situation, construct underrepresentation, occurs if the accommodation itself removes or replaces portions of the test content. Thus, although an accommodation is designed to promote fairness in testing, the degree to which the accommodation strengthens validity is inversely related to the degree to which the accommodation alters the construct or lessens the content being measured (Sireci, Scarpati, & Li, 2005).

The accommodation of extra time has received a great deal of attention, particularly from testing agencies. This is quite understandable when one considers the number of accommodation requests such agencies receive each year. For instance, Brinckerhoff and Banerjee (2007) report that in 2005 ETS received over 10,000 requests for accommodations, and that the majority of these requests were for extended time. When one is considering whether extra time changes the construct validity of a test, the first question to be addressed pertains to whether the construct being measured by the assessment measure is speed. On tests of pure speed, individual differences depend entirely upon the speed of performance, and items are relatively easy. On tests of power, the differences are not contingent on speed, and the items increase in difficulty (Ofiesh et al., 2005). According to the *Standards* volume, "Speededness is a test characteristic dictated by the test's time limits, that results in a test taker's score being dependent on the rate at which work is performed as well as the correctness of the response. . . . speededness is often an undesirable characteristic" (AERA et al., 1999, p. 182). Tests such as the SAT and the Graduate Record Examination (GRE) are generally designed to minimize the importance of speed (Bridgeman, Curley, & Trapani, 2001).

Investigations of the effect of extra time on high-stakes test performance have not usually found reliability to be an issue (Bennett, Rock,

Kaplan, & Jirele, 1988; Lindstrom & Gregg, 2007; Morgan & Huff, 2002). Again, the challenge that is usually raised relates to construct validity. However, as noted by Gersten and Baker (2002), "the traditional validity and reliability indexes provided by test developers, although essential, serve only as a point of departure—a necessary but not sufficient condition for understanding the ultimate validity of an assessment" (p. 49). Unfortunately, many of our current high-stakes tests are asked to serve a variety of purposes, some of which are not always what the test was originally designed to measure. Current best practice is to view validity as a "unitary concept that incorporates the use of a variety of types of evidence and logical analyses to make an evaluation of the degree to which the specific use or interpretation of assessment results is justified" (Linn, 2002, p. 32).

Score Comparability

Some researchers approach the issue of score comparability (e.g., the question of whether the scores of examinees taking a test with extended time are genuinely comparable to those of examinees taking the test without this accommodation) by investigating only one type of validity— the predictive validity of a measure. For instance, do the scores for students who receive the accommodation of extra time on the SAT have the same predictive power as the scores for students who do not take the test with extended time? First, predictive validity is a statistical methodology that provides a means of inferring the extent to which a measure (e.g., the SAT) relates to an external standard (e.g., first-year college grade point average [GPA]). This type of validity is referred to as "criterion-related validity," and several potential problems can influence the results of studies using it. These include (but are not limited to) (1) identification of a suitable criterion, (2) insufficient sample size, (3) criterion contamination, (4) restriction of criterion range, and (5) unreliability of the predictor score (see Crocker & Algina, 1986, for an in-depth discussion of these problems). According to Crocker and Algina (1986),

> For most clinical, educational, or personnel uses, a single test score provides insufficient data for making important decisions about individual examinees. In the event that one or more useful predictor variables have already been identified, the validation question is whether the new predictor can make a significant improvement in the predictor criterion performance when added to these other predictors. (p. 230)

In addition, professionals are strongly encouraged to read the entire published report or journal article for a study comparing the scores of students taking a test with and without extended time, in order to evaluate the results in the context of the entire study. Far too often, one sentence is extracted from a detailed technical report and used out of context. For instance, several studies have been used to argue that the scores of students who took entrance examinations with extended time overpredicted their first-year GPA. Such observations have been made about the SAT (Cahalan, Mandinach, & Camara, 2002), the LSAT (Wightman, 1993), the GRE (Willingham et al., 1988), and the Miller Analogies Test (Zurcher & Bryant, 2001).

Let's use one of these studies as an example to reinforce the need to review the entire technical report or published research study. If we read further into the technical report of the Cahalan and colleagues (2002) study, we find that when the predicted GPA was analyzed by using both the SAT and high school GPA (combined), as suggested by the College Board, predictive accuracy for the accommodated group was similar to that for the nonaccommodated examinees (Sireci, Zanetti, & Berger, 2003). In addition, when Cahalan and colleagues broke the scores in their study down by gender, the females taking the test with extended time demonstrated underprediction, and the males using this accommodation showed a trivial overprediction. Very interestingly, Cahalan and colleagues found that the differences in predictive validity between administrations of the SAT with standard and extended time were smaller than those found across different ethnic groups (Bridgeman et al., 2001). Informed consumers must take the responsibility of reviewing, in depth and with critical eyes, the technical reports and/or journal articles providing evidence of specific accommodations' effects on individual performance.

Determining score comparability also requires the investigation of measurement equivalence/invariance. A test fulfills the requirement of measurement invariance when it is shown to measure the same attribute under different conditions (Meade & Lautenschlager, 2004). These conditions may include the stability of measurement across different populations and/or different methods of test administration. Tests of measurement equivalence/invariance are typically conducted with methodologies such as confirmatory factor analysis (CFA). Unfortunately, many companies publishing high-stakes tests do not have research available to demonstrate whether the test scores of individuals with LD or ADHD using an accommodation (e.g., extended time) are comparable to those of individuals not provided with this accommodation.

One exception to this observation is the College Board. As described earlier in this chapter, we (Lindstrom & Gregg, 2007) recently compared the scores of 2,475 students with LD or ADHD taking the SAT

Reasoning Test with only the accommodation of extended time to those of 2,475 nondisabled peers taking the test without accommodations. As noted earlier, we found no evidence to suggest that the scores on the Critical Reading, Mathematics, and Writing sections of this test should have different interpretations for these two groups. Therefore, extended time did not change the construct validity of the measure.

Researchers using differential item functioning (DIF) as a methodology to investigate item bias are also providing invaluable studies. The presence of DIF (biased items) on a test poses a serious threat to the validity of the test used. According to Standard 7.3 (AERA et al., 1999),

> When credible research reports that differential item functioning exists across age, gender, racial/ethnic, cultural, disability, and/or linguistic groups in the population of test takers in the content domain measured by the test, test developers should conduct appropriate studies when feasible. Such research should seek to detect and eliminate aspects of test design, content, and format that might bias test scores for particular groups. (p. 81)

For instance, we (Cohen et al., 2005) used a mixed DIF model to investigate the performance of examinees with and without LD who were administered a statewide mathematics test. As noted in earlier mentions of this study, all individuals with LD were given only extended time as an accommodation. We found that DIF on the mathematics test was not related to the use of extended time, but rather to item content.

Multivariate generalizability theory (G-theory; Brennan, 1992, 2001), another methodology used to explore accommodation effectiveness, goes beyond estimation of variance due to disability or accommodation type and provides a means of investigating more detailed information about measurement conditions. Unfortunately, the use of G-theory is significantly lacking to date in studies of the adolescent and adult populations with LD or ADHD. In education or work settings, adolescents and adults are nested within programs or businesses, and then further nested within institutions or states. The result is that individuals within each setting are linked by common experiences and exposure to information (Guion, 1995). Few studies related to the adolescent or adult populations with LD or ADHD account for the reality that these individuals are incorporated within institutions, or that test items may be representative of different subcategories within the larger construct being measured. Therefore, the variance attributable to factors extraneous to the individuals' abilities–disabilities or to the items themselves may confound the results. G-theory allows researchers to more accurately gauge the contribution of many factors that may influence scores on tests taken with and without accommodations.

Specificity of Test Accommodation Benefits

Accommodations are assumed to have a beneficial influence on the test scores of examinees receiving them, but not to provide accommodated individuals with an advantage over nonaccommodated examinees (Shepard, Taylor, & Betebenner, 1998; Zuriff, 2000). For instance, as noted previously, some professionals are concerned that the scores of students taking a test with extended time overpredict their first-year GPA. Therefore, they conclude that examinees taking a test with extended time may have an unfair advantage over those individuals who do not receive this accommodation. In response to this inference, some researchers propose using the "interaction hypothesis" or "maximum-potential hypothesis" to interpret score comparability. This hypothesis suggests that an accommodation should benefit test scores *only* for students who need the accommodation, not for students who do not need the accommodation (Shepard et al., 1998; Zuriff, 2000). According to Sireci, Lee, and Scarpati (2003), the interaction hypothesis purports "that there is an interaction between accommodation condition (accommodated versus standard test administration) and type of student (e.g., students with disabilities versus students without disabilities) with respect to test performance" (p. 5). Another construct proposed to address the interpretation of test accommodations is the "differential-boost hypothesis," in which researchers argue that an accommodation should improve the performance of students with disabilities to a significantly greater extent than it improves the performance of students without disabilities (Fuchs & Fuchs, 1999; Pitoniak & Royer, 2001).

In a thorough investigation of the accommodation literature, Sireci and colleagues (2005) provide evidence of the problems associated with the interaction hypothesis and suggest that the construct be reexamined. They note that although extra time on a test can benefit all examinees, individuals with disabilities demonstrate significantly greater gains than those of their nondisabled peers. Therefore, for individuals with disabilities, the gain is significantly great to warrant the accommodation. As mentioned previously, we (Gregg & Nelson, 2008) conducted a meta-analysis on the effects of extended time on the standardized administration of tests for adolescents and adults with LD. The results of this analysis suggest that such individuals benefit significantly more from receiving the accommodation of extended time than do their peers who demonstrate no disabilities. This finding supports the differential-boost hypothesis and provides evidence for the effectiveness of extended time as an accommodation on standardized tests of reading, mathematics, and writing for the adolescent and adult populations with LD (Fuchs & Fuchs, 1999). In addition, our meta-analysis indicates that despite receiving extended time on standardized test administrations, the academic performance of the population with LD is still significantly below that of their peers. As we (Cohen et al., 2005) have noted, accommodations are only one aspect of providing access to learning for this population.

Implications for Assessment and Accommodation

✓ Standards-based reforms and changes in professional licensing requirements have led to an increase in high-stakes tests as the gateways to promotion, graduation, and career attainment.

✓ Test accommodations should not change the content being evaluated; nor should they provide unfair advantage to the individual using it.

✓ Clinical data, legal mandates, and professional standards all provide important information to guide professionals in selecting appropriate and effective test accommodations.

✓ The four categories of testing accommodations most frequently utilized by professionals in both secondary and postsecondary settings are accommodations in the presentation, response, scheduling/timing, and setting of assessments.

✓ For many adolescents and adults with LD or ADHD, extra time during test taking has proven to be an extremely effective accommodation.

✓ Test accommodations are not universally approved across secondary/postsecondary institutions, states, or testing agencies.

✓ The selection of effective test accommodations depends on a professional's sensitivity to individual differences (cognitive and language processes), task format (e.g., structured vs. free responses, auditory vs. visual modalities), and response choices (e.g., written, oral, electronic).

✓ The three major concerns related to tests taken with an accommodation are whether the accommodation (1) alters the skill being measured, (2) precludes the comparison of scores between examinees, or (3) would allow examinees without disabilities to benefit if they were granted the same accommodation.

References

Abbott, R., & Berninger, V. (1993). Structural equation modeling of relationships among developmental skills and writing skills in primary and intermediate grade students. *Journal of Educational Psychology, 85*, 478–508.

Abidin, R. R., & Robinson, L. L. (2002). Stress biases or professionalism: What drives teachers' referral judgments of students with challenging behaviors? *Journal of Emotional and Behavioral Disorders, 10*(4), 202–212.

Achenbach, T. M., & Rescorla, L. A. (2001). *Manual for the ASEBA school-age forms and profiles.* Burlington: University of Vermont, Research Center for Children, Youth, and Families.

Adams, M. J. (1990). *Beginning to read: Thinking and learning about print.* Cambridge, MA: MIT Press.

Albertsons, Inc., v. Kirkingburg, 119 S. Ct. 2162 (1999).

Allen, L. M., Conder, R. L., Green, P., & Cox, D. R. (1997). *CARB 97 manual for the Computerized Assessment of Response Bias.* Durham, NC: CogniSyst.

Alliance for Excellent Education. (2006). *Who's counted? Who's counting?: Understanding high school graduation rates.* Washington, DC: Author.

Allport, G. W. (1954). *The nature of prejudice.* Reading, MA: Addison-Wesley.

Allyn, F. A., & Burt, J. S. (1998). Pinch my wig or winch my pig: Spelling, spoonerisms and other language skills. *Reading and Writing: An Interdisciplinary Journal, 10*, 51–74.

Almond, P. J., Lehr, C., Thurlow, M. L., & Quenemoen, R. (2002). Participation in large-scale state assessment and accountability systems. In G. Tindal & T. M. Haladyna (Eds.), *Large-scale assessment programs for all students: Validity, technical adequacy, and implementation* (pp. 341–370). Mahwah, NJ: Erlbaum.

Alster, E. H. (1997). The effects of extended time on algebra test scores for college students with and without learning disabilities. *Journal of Learning Disabilities, 30*, 222–227.

Alston, R. J., Bell, T. J., & Hampton, J. L. (2002). Learning disability and career entry into the sciences: A critical analysis of attitudinal factors. *Journal of Career Development, 28*, 263–275.

Alvarez, V., & Adelman, H. S. (1986). Over-statements of self-evaluations by students with psychoeducational problems. *Journal of Learning Disabilities, 19*, 567–571.

Alverman, D., & Rush, L. S. (2004). Literacy intervention programs at the middle and high school levels. In T. L. Jetton & J. A. Dole (Eds.), *Adolescent literacy research and practice* (pp. 210–227). New York: Guilford Press.

American Educational Research Association, American Psychological Association, & National Council on Measurement in Education. (1999). *Standards for educational and psychological testing* (2nd ed.). Washington, DC: American Educational Research Association.

American Psychiatric Association. (1980). *Diagnostic and statistical manual of mental disorders* (3rd ed.). Washington, DC: Author.

American Psychiatric Association. (1994). *Diagnostic and statistical manual of mental disorders* (4th ed.). Washington, DC: Author.

American Psychiatric Association. (2000). *Diagnostic and statistical manual of mental disorders* (4th ed., text rev.). Washington, DC: Author.

American Psychological Association. (2001). *Publication manual of the American Psychological Association* (5th ed.). Washington, DC: Author.

Americans with Disabilities Act (ADA) of 1990, Public Law No. 101-336, 104 Stat. 327.

Andersen, S. L., & Teicher, M. H. (2000). Sex differences in dopamine receptors and their relevance to AD/HD. *Neuroscience and Biobehavioral Reviews, 24*(1), 137–141.

Anderson, K. G. (1997). Gender bias in special education referrals. *Annals of Dyslexia, 47*, 151–162.

Anderson-Inman, L. (2004). Reading on the Web: Making the most of digital text. *Wisconsin State Reading Association Journal, 4*, 8–14.

Anderson-Inman, L., & Horney, M. A. (2007). Supported eText: Assistive technology through text transformations. *Reading Research and Practice, 14*, 153–160.

Anderson-Inman, L., & Horney, M. A. (2008). *Supported e-text.* Eugene, OR: National Center for Supported e-Text. Retrieved July 24, 2008, from *ncset. uoregon.edu/index.php?option=com_content&task=blogsection&id=8&Itemi d=88*

Anderson-Inman, L., Horney, M. A., Chen, D., & Lewin, L. (1994, April). Hypertext literacy: Observations from the Electro Text project. *Language Arts, 71*, 37–45.

Angold, A., Costello, E. J., & Erkanli, A. (1999). Comorbidity. *Journal of Child Psychiatry, 40*(1), 57–87.

Arnau, R. C., & Thompson, B. (2001). Second order confirmatory factor analysis of the WAIS-III. *Assessment, 7*(30), 237–246.

Arnsten, A. F. T., Steere, J. C., & Hunt, R. D. (1996). The contribution of alpha2 noradrenergic mechanism to prefrontal cortical cognitive function. *Archives of General Psychiatry, 53*, 448–455.

Asperger, H. (1944). Die "Autistischen Psychopathen" im Kindesalter. *Archiv für Psychiatrie und Nervenkrankheiten, 117*, 76–136.

Assistive Technology Act of 1998, Public Law No. 105-394, 112 Stat. 3627 (1998).

Assistive Technology Act of 2004, Public Law No. 108-364, 118 Stat. 1707 (2004).

Association on Higher Education and Disability (AHEAD). (2007). *AHEAD best practices: Disability documentation in higher education.* Retrieved June 2007, from *www.ahead.org/resources/bestpracticesdoc.htm*

Au, K. (1998). Social constructivism and the school literacy learning of students of diverse backgrounds. *Journal of Literacy Research, 30,* 297–319.

August, G. J., Stewart, M. A., & Holmes, C. S. (1983). A four-year follow-up of hyperactive boys with and without conduct disorder. *British Journal of Psychiatry, 143,* 192–198.

Aunola, K., Leskinen, E., Lerkanen, M., & Nurmi, J. (2004). Developmental dynamics of math performance from preschool to grade 2. *Journal of Educational Psychology, 96,* 699–713.

Awh, E., Vogel, E. K., & Oh, S. H. (2006). Interactions between attention and working memory. *Neuroscience, 139,* 201–208.

Baddeley, A. (2000). The episodic buffer: A new component of working memory? *Trends in Cognitive Sciences, 4,* 417–423.

Baddeley, A. (2007). *Working memory, thought, and action.* New York: Oxford University Press.

Baddeley, A., & Hitch, G. (1974). Working memory. In G. H. Bower (Ed.), *The psychology of learning and motivation: Advances in research and theory* (Vol. 8, pp. 47–89). New York: Academic Press.

Baddeley, A., Logie, R., & Nimmo-Smith, I. (1985). Components of fluent reading. *Journal of Memory and Language, 24,* 119–135.

Badian, N. A. (1983). Dyscalculia and nonverbal disorders of learning. In H. R. Myklebust (Ed.), *Progress in learning disabilities* (Vol. 5, pp. 235–264). New York: Grune & Stratton.

Ball, A. F. (1992). Cultural preferences and the expository writing of African American adolescents. *Written Communication, 9,* 510–532.

Ball, A. F. (1996). Expository writing patterns of African American students. *English Journal, 85,* 27–36.

Ball, A. F. (1999). Evaluating the writing of culturally and linguistically diverse students: The case of the African American vernacular English speaker. In C. R. Cooper & L. Odell (Eds.), *Evaluating writing* (pp. 225–248). Urbana, IL: National Council of Teachers of English.

Ball, A. F. (2006). Teaching writing in culturally diverse classrooms. In C. A. MacArthur, S. Graham, & J. Fitzgerald (Eds.), *Handbook of writing research* (pp. 293–310). New York: Guilford Press.

Bandalos, D., & Gregg, N. (2008). *Latent means and covariance differences with measurement equivalence in adults with LD versus the WJ III normative sample.* Unpublished manuscript.

Bandura, A. (1995). Experience of personal and collective efficacy in changing societies. In A. Bandura (Ed.), *Self-efficacy in changing societies* (pp. 1–45). New York: Cambridge University Press.

Bandura, A., Barbaranelli, C., Capara, G. V., & Pastorelli, C. (2001). Self-efficacy beliefs as shapers of children's aspirations and career trajectories. *Child Development, 72*, 187–206.

Banerjee, M., & Brinckerhoff, L. C. (2007). *Technological preparedness for college: Implications for high school transition planning and postsecondary disability service providers.* Workshop presented at the 19th Annual Postsecondary Training Institute, Center on Postsecondary Education and Disability, University of Connecticut, Saratoga Springs, NY.

Banerjee, M., & Gregg, N. (in press). Redefining accessibility on high-stakes tests for postsecondary college students with LD in an era of technology. *Learning Disabilities: A Multidisciplinary Journal.*

Banerjee, M., & Shaw, S. (2007). High stakes test accommodations: Documentation review by testing agencies in an era of change. *Assessment for Effective Instruction, 32*(3), 171–180.

Bangert-Drowns, R. L. (1993). The word processor as an instructional tool: A meta-analysis of word processing in writing instruction. *Review of Educational Research, 63*, 69–93.

Bannan-Ritland, B. (2002). Computer-mediated communication, eLearning and interactivity: A review of the research. *Quarterly Review of Distance Education, 3*(2), 161–179.

Barkley, R. A. (2004). Driving impairments in teens and young adults with attention-deficit/hyperactivity disorder. *Psychiatric Clinics of North America, 27*(2), 233–260.

Barkley, R. A. (2006). *Attention-deficit hyperactivity disorder: A handbook for diagnosis and treatment* (3rd ed.). New York: Guilford Press.

Barkley, R. A., & Edwards, G. (2006). Diagnostic interviews, behavior rating scales, and the medical examination. In R. A. Barkley, *Attention-deficit hyperactivity disorder: A handbook for diagnosis and treatment* (3rd ed., pp. 337–368). New York: Guilford Press.

Barkley, R. A., Fischer, M., Edelbrock, C. S., & Smallish, L. (1990). The adolescent outcome of hyperactive children diagnosed by research criteria: An 8-year prospective follow-up study. *Journal of the American Academy of Child and Adolescent Psychiatry, 29*, 546–557.

Barkley, R. A., Fischer, M., Smallish, L., & Fletcher, K. (2006). Young adult outcome of hyperactive children: Adaptive functioning in major life activities. *Journal of the American Academy of Child and Adolescent Psychiatry, 45*(2), 192–202.

Barkley, R. A., Murphy, K. R., & Kwasnik, D. (1996). Psychological adjustment and adaptive impairments in young adults with ADHD. *Journal of Attention Disorders, 1*, 41–54.

Barnes, M. A., Fletcher, J. M., & Ewing-Cobbs, L. (2007). Mathematical disabilities in congenital and acquired neurodevelopment al disorders. In D. B. Berch & M. M. M. Mazzocco (Eds.), *Why is math so hard for some children?: The nature and origins of mathematical learning difficulties and disabilities* (pp. 195–218). Baltimore: Brookes.

Barnett, D. W., & Zucker, K. B. (1990). *The personal and social assessment of chil-*

dren: An analysis of current status and professional practice issues. Boston: Allyn & Bacon.

Barr, C. L. (2002). Genetics of childhood disorders: XXII. ADHD, Part 6: The dopamine D4 receptor gene. *Journal of the American Academy of Child and Adolescent Psychiatry, 40,* 118–121.

Barry, T. D., Lyman, R. D., & Klinger, L. G. (2002). Academic underachievement and attention-deficit/hyperactivity disorder: The negative impact of symptom severity on school performance. *Journal of School Psychology, 40,* 259–283.

Barth, H., Kanwisher, N., & Spelke, E. (2002). The construction of large number representation in adults. *Cognition, 86,* 201–221.

Bartlett v. New York State Board of Law Examiners, 970 F. Supp. 1094 (S.D.N.Y. 1997) [Bartlett I]; aff'd 2 F. Supp. 2d 3888 (S.D.N.Y., 1997) (Bartlett II); aff'd in part, rev'd & remanded in part, 156 F.3d 321 (2nd Cir. 1998) (Bartlett III); vacated and remanded, 119 S. Ct. 3288 (1999) (Bartlett IV); aff'd in part & remanded, 226 F. 3d 69 (2d Cir. 2000) (Bartlett V); 2001 WL 930792 (S.D.N.Y. Aug. 15, 2000) (Bartlett VI).

Barton, R. S., & Fuhrman, B. S. (1994). Counseling and psychotherapy for adults with learning disabilities. In P. J. Gerber & H. B. Reiff (Eds.), *Learning disabilities in adulthood: Persisting problems and evolving issues* (pp. 82–92). Austin, TX: Pro-ED.

Bear, G. G., Minke, K. M., Griffin, S. M., & Deemer, S. A. (1998). Achievement related perceptions of children with learning disabilities and normal achievement: Group and developmental differences. *Journal of Learning Disabilities, 31,* 91–104.

Becker, H. J. (1999). *Internet use by teachers: Conditions of professional use and teacher-directed student use.* Irvine, CA: Center for Research on Information Technology and Organizations.

Bennett, R. E., Rock, D. A., Kaplan, B. A., & Jirele, T. (1988). Psychometric characteristics. In W. W. Willingham (Ed.), *Testing handicapped people* (pp. 83–97). Boston: Allyn & Bacon.

Benson, J. (1998). Developing a strong program of construct validation: A test anxiety example. *Educational Measurement: Issues and Practice, 17,* 10–22.

Berch, D. B., & Mazzocco, M. M. M. (Eds.). (2007). *Why is math so hard for some children?: The nature and origins of mathematical learning difficulties and disabilities.* Baltimore: Brookes.

Bereiter, C., & Scardamalia, M. (1985). Cognitive copying strategies and the problem of "inert knowledge." In S. F. Chipmon, J. W. Segal, & R. Glaser (Eds.), *Thinking and learning skills: Research and open questions* (pp. 65–80). Hillsdale, NJ: Erlbaum.

Berndt, T. J., & Burgy, L. (1996). Social self-concept. In B. A. Bracken (Ed.), *Handbook of self concept* (pp. 171–209). New York: Wiley.

Berninger, V. W. (Ed.). (1994). *The varieties of orthographic knowledge* (2 vols.). Dordrecht, The Netherlands: Kluwer Academic.

Berninger, V. W. (1996). *Reading and writing acquisition: A developmental neuropsychological perspective.* Boulder, CO: Westview Press.

Berninger, V. W. (2001). Understanding the "lexia" in dyslexia: A multidisciplinary team approach to learning disabilities. *Annals of Dyslexia, 51,* 1–16.

Berninger, V. W., Abbott, R. D., Thomson, J., Wagner, R., Swanson, H. L., Wijsman, E. M., et al. (2006). Modeling phonological core deficits within a working memory architecture in children and adults with developmental dyslexia. *Scientific Studies of Reading, 10*(2), 165–198.

Berninger, V. W., & Richards, T. L. (2002). *Brain literacy for educators and psychologists.* San Diego, CA: Academic Press.

Berninger, V. W., & Winn, W. D. (2006). Implications of advancements in brain research and technology for writing development, writing instruction, and educational evaluation. In C. A. MacArthur, S. Graham, & J. Fitzgerald (Eds.), *Handbook of writing research* (pp. 96–114). New York: Guilford Press.

Berthiaume, K. S. (2006). Story comprehension and academic deficits in children with ADHD: What is the connection? *School Psychology Review, 35,* 309–323.

Biancarosa, G., & Snow, C. E. (2004). *Reading Next: A vision for action and research in middle and high school literacy. A report to the Carnegie Corporation of New York.* Washington, DC: Alliance for Education.

Biber, D. (1988). *Variation across speech and writing.* Cambridge, UK: Cambridge University Press.

Biber, D., Conrad, S., & Reppen, R. (1998). *Corpus linguistics: Investigating language structure and uses.* Cambridge, UK: Cambridge University Press.

Bibler, V. S. (1984). Thinking as creation: Introduction to the logic of mental dialogue. *Soviet Psychology, 22,* 29–54.

Biederman, J., Faraone, S. V., Milberger, S., Curtis, S., Chen, L., Marrs, A., et al. (1996). Predictors of persistence and remission of ADHD into adolescence: Results from a four-year prospective follow-up study. *Journal of the American Academy of Child and Adolescent Psychiatry, 35,* 343–351.

Biederman, J., Faraone, S., Spencer, T., Wilens, T., Norman, D., Lapey, K. A., et al. (1993). Patterns of psychiatric comorbidity, cognition, and psychosocial functioning in adults with attention deficit hyperactivity disorder. *American Journal of Psychiatry, 150,* 1792–1798.

Biederman, J., Newcorn, J., & Sprich, S. (1991). Comorbidity of attention deficit hyperactivity disorder with conduct, depressive, anxiety, and other disorders. *American Journal of Psychiatry, 148,* 564–577.

Black, A., & Watts, D. (1993). Proof-reading monospaced and proportionally-spaced typefaces: Should we check typewritten or typeset text? *Visible Language, 27,* 362–377.

Blackwell, L. S., Trzesniewski, K. H., & Dweck, C. S. (2007). Implicit theories of intelligence predict achievement across an adolescent transition: A longitudinal study and an intervention. *Child Development, 78*(1), 246–263.

Boekaerts, M., & Niemivirta, M. (2000). Self-regulated learning: Finding a balance between learning and ego-protective goals. In M. Boekaerts, P. R. Pintrick, & M. Zeidner (Eds.), *Handbook of self-regulation* (pp. 417–450). San Diego, CA: Academic Press.

Bong, M., & Skaalvik, E. M. (2003). Academic self-concept and self-efficacy: How different are they really? *Educational Psychology Review, 15,* 1–40.

Bonk, C. J., & Reynolds, T. H. (1992). Early adolescent composing within a generative–evaluative computerized prompting framework. *Computers in Human Behavior, 8,* 39–62.

Bookshare.Org (2007). *Individual subscriptions.* Retrieved March 5, 2007, from *www.bookshare.org/web/AboutIndividualSubscriptions.html*

Boone, K. B. (2007). *Assessment of feigned cognitive impairment: A neuropsychological perspective.* New York: Guilford Press.

Bowden, S., Gregg, N., Bandalos, D., Davis, M., Coleman, C., Holdnack, J., et al. (2008). Latent means and covariance differences with measurement equivalence in college students with developmental difficulties versus the WAIS-III/WMS-III normative sample. *Journal of Educational and Psychological Measurement, 68*(4), 621–642.

Bowden, S. C., Cook, M. J., Bardenhagen, F. J., Shores, E. A., & Carstairs, J. R. (2004). Measurement invariance of core cognitive abilities in heterogeneous neurological and community samples. *Intelligence, 33,* 363–389.

Bowden, S. C., Shores, A., & Mathias, J. L. (2006). Does effort suppress cognition after traumatic brain injury?: A re-examination of the evidence for the Word Memory Test. *The Clinical Neuropsychologist, 20,* 858–872.

Bracken, B. A. (2005). Reynolds Intellectual Assessment Scales and the Reynolds Intellectual Screening Test. In R. A. Spies & B. S. Plake (Eds.), *The sixteenth mental measurements yearbook* (pp. 892–894). Lincoln, NE: Buros Institute of Mental Measurements.

Brackett, J., & McPherson, A. (1996). Learning disabilities diagnosis in postsecondary students: A comparison of discrepancy-based diagnostic models. In N. Gregg, C. Hoy, & A. Gay (Eds.), *Adults with learning disabilities: Theoretical and practical perspectives* (pp. 68–84). New York: Guilford Press.

Bragg, D. D., Kim, E., & Barnett, E. A. (2006). Creating access and success: Academic pathways reaching underserved students. In D. D. Bragg & E. A. Barnett (Eds.), *Academic pathways to and from the community college* (pp. 5–20). San Francisco: Jossey-Bass.

Brennan, R. L. (1992). Generalizability theory. *Educational Measurement: Issues and Practice, 11,* 27–34.

Brennan, R. L. (2001). *Generalizability theory.* New York: Springer-Verlag.

Bridgeland, J. M., Dilulio, J. J., & Morison, K. B. (2006, March). *The silent epidemic: Perspectives of high school dropouts.* Washington, DC: Civic Enterprises.

Bridgeman, B., Curley, W. E., & Trapani, C. (2001). *To what extent is the SAT I speeded? Is the SAT I speeded?: Is the SAT I differentially speeded for ethnic/gender groups?* Princeton, NJ: Educational Testing Service.

Bridgeman, B., Harvey, A., & Braswell, J. (1995). Effects of calculator use on scores on a test of mathematic reasoning. *Journal of Educational Measurement, 32*(4), 323–340.

Bridgeman, B., Trapani, C., & Curley, E. (2003). *Impact of fewer questions per section on SAT I scores* (College Board Research Report No. 2003-2). New York: College Board.

Brigham, N., Morocco, C. C., Clay, K., & Zigmond, N. (2006). What makes a high school a good high school for students with disabilities. *Learning Disabilities Research and Practice, 21*(30), 184–190.

Brinckerhoff, L., McGuire, J., & Shaw, S. (2002). *Postsecondary education and transition for students with learning disabilities*. Austin, TX: Pro-ED.

Brinckerhoff, L. C., & Banerjee, M. (2007). Misconceptions regarding accommodations on high-stakes tests: Recommendations for preparing disability documentation for test takers with learning disabilities. *Learning Disabilities Research and Practice, 22*, 246–256.

Brown, J. I., Fishco, V. V., & Hanna, G. (1993). *Nelson–Denny Reading Test*. Itasca, IL: Riverside.

Brown, T. E. (1996). *Brown Attention-Deficit Disorder (ADD) Scales*. San Antonio, TX: Psychological Corporation.

Brown, T. E. (2000). Attention-deficit disorders with obsessive–compulsive disorder. In T. E. Brown (Ed.), *Attention-deficit disorders and comorbidities in children, adolescents, and adults* (pp. 209–230). Washington, DC: American Psychiatric Press.

Brown, W. E., Eliez, S., Menon, V., Rumsey, J. M., White, C. D., & Reiss, A. L. (2001). Preliminary evidence of widespread morphological variations of the brain in dyslexia. *Neurology, 56*, 781–783.

Brownell, H. H., Carroll, J. J., Rehak, A., & Wingfield, A. (1992). The use of pronoun anaphora and speaker mood in the interpretation of conversational utterances by right hemisphere brain-damaged patients. *Brain and Language, 42*, 121–147.

Bruce, B., & Levin, J. (1997). Educational technology: Media for inquiry, communication, construction, and expression. *Journal of Educational Computing Research, 17*(1), 79–102.

Bruck, M. (1992). Persistence of dyslexics' phonological awareness deficits. *Developmental Psychology, 28*, 874–886.

Bruck, M. (1993). Component spelling skills of college students with childhood diagnoses of dyslexia. *Learning Disability Quarterly, 16*, 171–184.

Bruck, M., & Waters, G. (1990). Effects of reading skill on component spelling skills. *Applied Psycholinguistics, 9*, 77–92.

Buehl, M. M., Alexander, P. A., & Murphy, P. K. (2002). Beliefs about schooled knowledge: Domain specific or domain general? *Contemporary Educational Psychology, 27*, 415–449.

Buhusi, C. V., & Meck, W. H. (2005). What makes us tick?: Functional and neural mechanisms of interval timing. *Nature Review Neuroscience, 6*, 755–765.

Bull, R. (2007). Neuropsychological factors. In D. B. Berch & M. M. M. Mazzocco (Eds.), *Why is math so hard for some children?: The nature and origins of mathematical learning difficulties and disabilities* (pp. 265–278). Baltimore: Brookes.

Burgstahler, S. (2003). *DO-IT: Helping students with disabilities transition to college and careers*. Minneapolis, MN: National Center on Secondary Education and Transition. Retrieved March 28, 2007, from *www.ncset.org/publications/viewdesc.asp?id=1168*

Burrell, S., & Warboys, L. (2000, July). *Special education and the juvenile justice system*. Washington, DC: Office of Juvenile Justice and Delinquency Prevention. Retrieved January 7, 2007, from *www.ncjrs.org/html/ojjdp/2000_6_5/ contents.html*

Burt, J. S., & Fury, M. B. (2000). Spelling in adults: The role of reading skills and experience. *Reading and Writing, 13,* 1–30.

Burt, J. S., & Shrubsole, C. S. (2000). Processing of phonological representations and adult spelling proficiency. *Australian Journal of Psychology, 52*(2), 100–109.

Busse, J., Berninger, V., Smith, D., & Hildebrant, D. (2001). Assesment for math talent and disability: A developmental model. In J. Andrews, D. Saklofske, & H. Jansen (Eds.), *Handbook of psychoeducational assessment: Ability, achievement, and behavior in children* (pp. 225–253). New York: Academic Press.

Butler, D. (1998). Metacognition and learning disabilities. In B. Y. L. Wong (Ed.), *Learning about learning disabilities* (2nd ed., pp. 277–307). San Diego, CA: Academic Press.

Bynner, J. (1998). Education and family components of identity in the transition from school to work. *International Journal of Behavioral Development, 22,* 29–53.

Bynner, J., & Parson, S. (1997). *Does numeracy matter?: Evidence from the National Child Development Study on the impact of poor numeracy on adult life.* London: Basic Skills Agency.

Byrne, B., Olson, R. K., Samuelsson, S., Wadsworth, S., Corley, R., DeFries, J. C., et al. (2006). Genetic and environmental influences on early literacy. *Journal of Research in Reading, 29,* 33–49.

Cahalan, C., Mandinach, E., & Camara, W. (2002). *Predictive validity of SAT I: Reasoning tests for test takers with learning disabilities and extended time accommodations* (College Board Research Report No. 2002-05). New York: College Board.

Cahalan-Laitusis, C. (2003). *Accommodations on high stakes writing tests for students with disabilities.* Princeton, NJ: Educational Testing Service. Retrieved August 2007, from *www.ets.org/research.html*

Cain, K., & Oakhill, J. (Eds.). (2007). *Children's comprehension problems in oral and written language: A cognitive perspective.* New York: Guilford Press.

Cain, K., Oakhill, J., & Elbro, C. (2002). The ability to learn new word meanings from context by school-age children with and without language comprehension difficulties. *Journal of Child Language, 30,* 681–694.

Cain, K., Oakhill, J. V., & Lemmon, K. (2004). Individual differences in the inference of word meanings from context: The influence of reading comprehension, vocabulary knowledge, and memory capacity. *Journal of Educational Psychology, 96,* 671–681.

Calhoon, M. B., Fuchs, L. S., & Hamlett, C. L. (2000). Effects of computer-based test accommodations on mathematics performance assessments for secondary students with learning disabilities. *Learning Disability Quarterly, 23,* 271–282.

Cannito, M., Jarecki, J., & Pierce, R. S. (1986). Effects of thematic structure on syntactic comprehension in aphasia. *Brain and Language, 27,* 310–321.

Cantwell, D. P., & Baker, L. (1989). Stability and natural history of DSM-III childhood diagnoses. *Journal of the American Academy of Child and Adolescent Psychiatry, 28,* 691–700.

Carl D. Perkins Vocational and Applied Technology Education Act of 1998, Public Law No. 105-332, 20 U.S.C. 2301 (1998).

Carlisle, J. (1995). Morphological awareness and early reading achievement. In L. B. Feldman (Ed.), *Morphological aspects of language processing* (pp. 189–209). Hillsdale, NJ: Erlbaum.

Carlisle, J. (2000). Awareness of the structure and meaning of morphologically complex words: Impact on reading. *Reading and Writing: An Interdisciplinary Journal, 12,* 169–190.

Carlisle, J. (2004). Morphological processes that influence learning to read. In C. A. Stone, E. R. Silliman, B. J. Ehren, & E. Apel (Eds.), *Handbook of language and literacy: Development and disorders* (pp. 318–339). New York: Guilford Press.

Carlisle, J., & Rice, M. S. (2002). *Improving reading comprehension: Research-based principles and practices.* Baltimore: York Press.

Carlisle, J., & Stone, A. (2003). The effects of morphological structure on children's reading of derived words. In E. Assink & D. Santa (Eds.), *Reading complex words: Cross-language studies* (pp. 27–52). New York: Kluwer Academic.

Carlson, G. A. (1998). Mania and ADHD: Comorbidity or confusion? *Journal of Affective Disorders, 51,* 177–187.

Carnevale, A. P., & Fry, R. A. (2000). *Crossing the great divide: Can we achieve equity when Generation Y goes to college?* Princeton, NJ: Educational Testing Service.

Carr, T. H., & Posner, M. I. (1994). The impact of learning to read on the functional anatomy of language processing. In B. de Gelder & J. Morais (Eds.), *Language and literacy: Comparative approaches* (pp. 32–42). Cambridge, MA: MIT Press.

Carroll, J. B. (1981). Twenty-five years of research on foreign language aptitude. In K. C. Diller (Ed.), *Individual differences and universals in language learning aptitude* (pp. 83–118). Rowley, MA: Newbury House.

Carroll, J. B. (1993). *Human cognitive abilities: A survey of factor analytic studies.* New York: Cambridge University Press.

Carroll, J. B. (2005). The three-stratum theory of cognitive abilities. In D. P. Flanagan & P. L. Harrison (Eds.), *Contemporary intellectual assessment: Theories, tests, and issues* (2nd ed., pp. 69–76). New York: Guilford Press.

Carroll, J. B., & Sapon, S. M. (2002). *Modern Language Aptitude Test manual.* Bethesda: Second Language Testing.

Carrow-Woolfolk, E. (1996). *Oral and Written Language Scales (OWLS).* Circle Pines, MN: American Guidance Service.

Caruso, J. C., & Cliff, N. (1999). The properties of equally and differentially weighted WAIS-III factor scores. *Psychological Assessment, 11,* 198–206.

Case, R., Kurland, M. D., & Goldberg, J. (1982). Operational efficiency and the growth of short-term memory span. *Journal of Experimental Child Psychology, 33,* 386–404.

Castellanos, F. X., Marvasti, F. F., Ducharme, J. L., Walter, J. M., Israel, M. E.,

Krain, A., et al. (2000). Executive function oculomotor tasks in girls with ADHD. *Journal of the American Academy of Child and Adolescent Psychiatry, 39,* 644–650.

Cattell, R. B. (1943). The measurement of intelligences. *Psychological Bulletin, 40,* 153–193.

Cattell, R. B. (1963). Theory of fluid and crystallized intelligence: A critical experiment. *Journal of Educational Psychology, 54,* 1–22.

Catts, H. W., Adlof, S. M., & Ellis, W. S. (2006). Language deficits in poor comprehenders: A case for the simple view of reading. *Journal of Speech, Language, and Hearing Research, 49,* 278–293.

Chadwick, O., Taylor, E., Taylor, A., Hepinstall, E., & Danckaerts, M. (1999). Hyperactivity and reading disability: A longitudinal study of the nature of the association. *Journal of Child Psychology and Psychiatry, 40,* 1039–1050.

Chaffee Amendment to the Copyright Act, Public Law No. 104-197.17 (1996).

Chapman, J. W. (1988). Learning disabled children's self-concepts. *Review of Educational Research, 58*(3), 347–371.

Chapman, S. B., Culhane, K. A., Levin, H. S., Harwood, H., Mendelsohn, D., Ewing-Cobbs, et al., (1992). Narrative discourse after closed head injury in children and adolescents. *Brain and Language, 43,* 42–65.

Charness, N. (1991). Expertise in chess: The balance between knowledge and search. In K. A. Ericsson & J. Smith (Eds.), *Toward a general theory of expertise: Prospects and limits* (pp. 30–62). Cambridge, UK: Cambridge University Press.

Chen, X. (2005). *First generation students in postsecondary education: A look at their college transcripts.* Washington, DC: U.S. Department of Education, National Center for Education Statistics. Retrieved December 11, 2005, from *nces. ed.gov/pubsearch/pubsinfo.asp?pubid=2005171*

Chi, C. W. T., & Pearson, P. D. (1999, June). *Synthesizing the effects of test accommodations for special education and limited English proficient students.* Paper presented at the National Conference on Large Scale Assessment, Snowbird, UT.

Chickering, A. W., & Erhman, S. C. (2004). *Implementing the seven principles: Technology as lever.* Retrieved December 4, 2004, from *www.tltgroup.org/programs.seven.html*

Christle, C. A., Jolivette, K., & Nelson, C. M. (2000). *Youth aggression and violence: Risk, resilience, and prevention.* Arlington, VA: ERIC Clearinghouse on Disabilities and Gifted Education. Retrieved January 16, 2006, from *ericec. org/digests/e602.html*

Chronicle of Higher Education. (2007). Almanac. Retrieved January 15, 2007, from *chronicle.com/free/almanac/2006*

Cirino, P. T., Morris, M. K., & Morris, R. D. (2002). Neuropsycholgical concomitants of calculation skills in college students referred for learning difficulties. *Developmental Neuropsychology, 21,* 201–218.

Cirino, P. T., Morris, M. K., & Morris, R. D. (2007). Semantic, executive, and visuospatial abilities in mathematical reasoning of referred college students. *Assessment, 14,* 94–104.

Civil Rights Restoration Act of 1987, Public Law 100-259, 102 Stat. 28 (1988).

Claude, D., & Firestone, P. (1995). The development of ADHD boys: A 12-year follow-up. *Canadian Journal of Behavioural Science, 27,* 226–249.

Clever, A., Bear, G. G., & Juvonen, J. (1992). Discrepancies between competence and importance in self-perceptions of children in integrated classrooms. *Journal of Special Education, 26,* 125–138.

Cobin, D. (2003). *Adult numeracy: Review of research and related literature.* London: National Research and Development Centre for Adult Literacy and Numeracy.

Cohen, A., Gregg, N., & Deng, M. (2005). The role of extended time and item content on a high-stakes mathematics test. *Learning Disabilities Research and Practice, 20,* 225–233.

Cohen, A. S., & Kim, A. (1992). Detecting calculator effects on item performance. *Applied Measurement in Education, 5,* 303–320.

Cohen, D. J., & Snowden, J. L. (2008). The relationship between document familiarity, frequency, and prevalence, and document literacy performance among adult readers. *Reading Research Quarterly, 43*(1), 9–26.

Coiro, J. (2003). Reading comprehension on the Internet: Expanding our understanding of reading comprehension to encompass new literacies. *The Reading Teacher, 56,* 458–464. (Also available at *www.readingonline.org/ electronic/elec_index.asp?HREF=/electronic/rt/2-03_Column*)

Coiro, J. (2006). *Exploring changes to reading comprehension on the Internet: Paradoxes and possibilities for diverse adolescent readers.* Unpublished doctoral dissertation, University of Connecticut.

Coiro, J., & Dobler, E. (in press). Exploring the online reading comprehension strategies used by sixth-grade skilled readers to search for and locate information on the Internet. *Reading Research Quarterly.*

Coleman, C., & Gregg, N. (2004, June). *The role of dyslexia and ADHD screeners in identifying college students with and without reading disorders and ADHD.* Paper presented at the meeting of the Society for the Scientific Study of Reading, Amsterdam.

Coleman, C., & Gregg, N. (2005, July). *Assessing adult writing disorders: Beyond standardized test scores.* Paper presented at the 9th European Congress of Psychology, Granada, Spain.

Coleman, C., Gregg, N., McLain, L., & Belair, L. (in press). Spelling and writing fluency: A comparison of performance errors and verbosity across young adults with and without dyslexia. *Assessment for Effective Intervention.*

Coleman, C., Lindstrom, J., & Gregg, N. (2007). *Comprehending the Nelson–Denny Reading Comprehension Test without reading it.* Unpublished manuscript, University of Georgia.

Coles, G. (1987). *The learning mystique: A critical look at "learning disabilities."* New York: Pantheon.

Compton, J. I., Cox, E., & Laanan, F. S. (2006). Adult learners in transition. In F. S. Laanan (Ed.), *Understanding students in transition: Trends and issues* (pp. 73–80). San Francisco: Jossey-Bass.

Conley, M. W. (2004). *Connecting standards and assessment through literacy.* Boston: Allyn & Bacon.

Conley, M. W. (2008). Cognitive instruction for adolescents: What we know about the promise, what we don't know about the potential. *Harvard Educational Review*, 84–106.

Conners, C. K., & Multi-Health Systems Staff. (2000). *Conners' Continuous Performance Test II: Computer program for Windows, technical guide, and software manual.* Toronto: Multi-Health Systems.

Connor, D. F. (2006). Stimulants. In R. A. Barkley, *Attention-deficit hyperactivity disorder: A handbook for diagnosis and treatment* (3rd ed., pp. 608–648). New York: Guilford Press.

Conway, A. R., Cowan, N., Bunting, M. F., Therriault, D. J., & Minkoff, S. R. B. (2002). A latent variable analysis of working memory capacity, short-term memory capacity, processing speed, and general fluid intelligence. *Intelligence, 30*, 163–183.

Conway, A. R., Kane, M. J., Bunting, M. F., Hambrick, D. Z., Wilhelm, O., & Engle, R. (2005). Working memory span tasks: A methodological review and user's guide. *Psychonomic Bulletin and Review, 12*, 769–786.

Conway, A. R., Kane, M. J., & Engle, R. (2003). Working memory capacity and its relation to general intelligence. *Trends in Cognitive Sciences, 7*, 547–552.

Cooper, C. R., & Odell, L. (Eds.). (1977). *Evaluating writing: Describing, measuring, judging.* Urbana, IL: National Council of Teachers of English.

Cooper, C. R., & Odell, L. (Eds.). (1999). *Evaluating writing: The role of teachers' knowledge about text, learning, and culture.* Urbana, IL: National Council of Teachers of English.

Corley, M. A., & Taymans, J. (2002). Adults with learning disabilities: A review of the literature. *Review of Adult Learning and Literacy, 3*. Retrieved June 2007, from *www.ncsall.net/?id=771 &pid=575*

Cornelissen, P., Munro, N., Fowler, S., & Stein, J. (1993). The stability of binocular fixation during reading in adults and children. *Developmental Medicine and Child Neurology, 35*, 777–787.

Cosden, M., Brown, C., & Elliott, K. (2002). Development of self-understanding and self-esteem in children and adults with learning disabilities. In B. Y. L. Wong & M. Donahue (Eds.), *Social dimensions of learning disabilities* (pp. 33–51). Mahwah, NJ: Erlbaum.

Council of State Administrators of Vocational Rehabilitation (CSAVR). (2005). *CSAVR response to the Government Accountability Office (GAO) audit of the vocational rehabilitation program.* Bethseda, MD: Author.

Cowan, N. (1997). *Attention and memory: An integrated framework.* New York: Oxford University Press.

Cowan, N. (2005). *Working memory capacity.* New York: Psychology Press.

Cowan, N., Elliott, E. M., & Saults, J. S. (2002). The search for what is fundamental in the development of working memory. *Advances in Child Development and Behavior, 29*, 1–49.

Crocker, J., & Major, B. (1989). Social stigma and self-esteem: The self-protective properties of stigma. *Psychological Review, 96*, 608–630.

Crocker, L., & Algina, J. (1986). *Introduction to classical and modern test theory.* New York: Harcourt Brace Jovanovich.

Cumming, G., & Finch, S. (2005). Inference by eye: Confidence intervals and how to read pictures of data. *American Psychologist, 60*, 170–180.

Cunningham, A. E., Perry, K. E., & Stanovich, K. E. (2001). Converging evidence for the concept of orthographic processing. *Reading and Writing, 14,* 549–568.

Cunningham, A. E., & Stanovich, K. D. (1990). Assessing print exposure and orthographic processing skill in children: A quick measure of reading experience. *Journal of Educational Psychology, 82*(4), 733–740.

Curie, M. (1923). *Pierre Curie* (C. Kellog & V. Kellog, Trans.). New York: Macmillan.

Curry, D., Schmitt, M. J., & Waldron, S. (1996). *A framework for adult numeracy standards: The mathematical skills and abilities adults need to be equipped for the future.* Retrieved February 25, 2007, from *www.literacynet.org/ann/framework.html*

DAISY Consortium. (2007). *FAQ.* Retrieved March 5, 2007, from *www.daisy.org/about_us/g_faq.asp#a_24*

Damasio, A. R. (1994). *Descartes' error: Emotion, reason, and the human brain.* New York: Putnam.

Daneman, M., & Carpenter, P. A. (1980). Individual differences in working memory and reading. *Journal of Verbal Learning and Verbal Behavior, 19,* 450–466.

Daneman, M., & Merikle, P. M. (1996). Working memory and language comprehension: A meta-analysis. *Psychonomic Bulletin and Review, 3*(4), 422–433.

Daniel, S. S., Walsh, A. K., Goldstone, D. B., Arnold, E. M., Reboussin, B. A., & Wood, F. B. (2006). Suicidality, school dropout, and reading problems among adolescents. *Journal of Learning Disabilities, 39*(6), 507–516.

Darwin, C. (1958). *Autobiography.* London: Collins. (Original work published 1887)

Day, J., & Newburger, E. (2002). *The big payoff: Educational attainment and synthetic estimates of work-life earnings* (Current Population Reports No. P23-210). Washington, DC: U.S. Bureau of the Census.

Deacon, H., Parrila, R., & Kirby, J. (2006). Processing of derived forms in high-functioning dyslexics. *Annals of Dyslexia, 56*(1), 103–128.

Deary, I. J. (2000). *Looking down on human intelligence: From psychophysics to the brain.* Oxford, UK: Oxford University Press.

DeFries, J. C., & Baker, L. A. (1983). Parental contributions to longitudinal stability of cognitive measures in the Colorado Family Reading Study. *Child Development, 54*(2), 388–395.

Dehaene, S. (1997). *The number sense: How the mind creates mathematics.* New York: Oxford University Press.

Dehaene, S., Spelke, E., Pinel, P., Stanescu, R., & Tsivkin, S. (1999). Sources of mathematical thinking: Behavioral and brain-imaging evidence. *Science, 284,* 970–974.

Delis, D. C., Kaplan, E., & Kramer, J. H. (2001). *Delis–Kaplan Executive Function System (D-KEFS).* San Antonio, TX: Psychological Corporation.

Dendy, C. A. Z. (2006). *Teenagers with ADD and ADHD: A guide for parents and professionals* (2nd ed.). Bethesda, MD: Woodbine House.

Dennis, J. L., & Swinthe, Y. (2001). Pencil grasp and children's handwriting legibility during different length writing tasks. *American Journal of Occupational Therapy, 55,* 171–183.

Deshler, D. D., Ellis, E. S., & Lenz, B. K. (1996). *Teaching adolescents with learning disabilities: Strategies and methods* (2nd ed.). Denver, CO: Love.

Deshler, D. D., & Lenz, B. K. (1989). The strategies instructional approach. *International Journal of Disability, Development and Education, 3*(2), 15–23.

Deshler, D. D., & Schumaker, J. B. (1993). Strategy mastery by at-risk students: Not a simple matter. *Elementary School Journal, 94*(2), 153–167.

Deul, R. K. (1992). Motor skill disorder. In S. R. Hooper, G. W. Hynd, & R. E. Mattison (Eds.), *Developmental disorders: Diagnostic criteria and clinical assessment* (pp. 239–282). Hillsdale, NJ: Erlbaum.

DiMaio, S., Grizenko, N., & Joober, R. (2003). Dopamine genes in attention-deficit hyperactivity disorder: A review. *Journal of Psychiatric Neuroscience, 28,* 27–38.

Disability Rights Advocates. (2005, Fall). High stakes testing and students with learning disabilities. *The Briefcase,* pp. 12–13.

Dombrowski, S. C., Kamphaus, R. W., & Reynolds, C. R. (2004). After the demise of the discrepancy: Proposed learning disabilities diagnostic criteria. *Professional Psychology: Research and Practice, 35,* 364–372.

Donlan, C. (2007). Mathematical development in children with specific language impairments. In D. B. Berch & M. M. M. Mazzocco (Eds.), *Why is math so hard for some children?: The nature and origins of mathematical learning difficulties and disabilities* (pp. 151–172). Baltimore: Brookes.

Downey, D., Snyder, L., & Hill, B. (2000). College students with dyslexia: Persistent linguistic deficits and foreign language learning. *British Journal of Dyslexia, 6,* 101–111.

Duke, N., Pressley, M., & Hildren, K. (2004). Difficulties with reading comprehension. In C. A. Stone, E. R. Silliman, B. J. Ehren, & K. Apel (Eds.), *Handbook of language and literacy: Development and disorders* (pp. 501–520). New York: Guilford Press.

Dukes, L. L., Shaw, S., & Madaus, J. (2007). How to complete a summary of performance for students exiting to postsecondary education. *Assessment for Effective Intervention, 32,* 143–159.

Durant, J. E., Cunningham, C. E., & Voelker, S. (1990). Academic, social and general self-concept of behavioral subgroups of learning disabled children. *Journal of Educational Psychology, 82,* 657–663.

Durston, S., Hulshoff, H. F., Schanck, H. G., Buitelaar, J. K., Steenhuis, M. P., Minderaa, R. B., et al. (2004). Magnetic resonance imaging of boys with attention-deficit/hyperactivity disorder and their unaffected siblings. *Journal of the American Academy of Child and Adolescent Psychiatry, 43,* 332–240.

Dweck, C. S. (2002). The development of ability conceptions. In A. Wigfield & J. Eccles (Eds.), *The development of achievement motivation* (pp. 34–54). San Diego, CA: Academic Press.

Eccles, J. (1983). Expectancies, values, and academic behaviors. In J. T. Spence (Ed.), *Achievement and achievement motives: Psychological and sociological approaches* (pp. 75–146). San Francisco: Freeman.

Eccles, J., & Wigfield, A. (1995). In the mind of the actor: The structure of adolescents' achievement task values and expectancy-related beliefs. *Personality and Social Psychology Bulletin, 21*(3), 215–225.

Eden, G. F., Van Meter, J. W., Rumsey, J. M., Maisog, J. M., Woods, R. P., & Zeffro, T. A. (1996). Abnormal processing of visual motion in dyslexia revealed by functional brain imaging. *Nature, 382,* 66–69.

Education for All Handicapped Children Act of 1975, Public Law 94-142, 89 Stat. 773 (1975).

Educational Testing Service. (2005). *One-third of a nation: Rising dropout rates and declining opportunities.* Princeton, NJ: Author.

Educational Testing Service. (2006a). *New policy regarding LD and LD/ADHD documentation shelf-life.* Office of Disability Policy, Princeton, NJ. Available at *www.ets.org/portal/site/ets/menuitem*

Educational Testing Service. (2006b). *Resources for test takers with disabilities: Tips for evaluators.* Office of Disability Policy, Princeton, NJ. Available at *www.ets.org/portal/site/ets/menuitem*

Educational Testing Service. (2007). *Policy statement for documentation of a learning disability in adolescents and adults.* Retrieved January 24, 2008, from *www.ets.org/portal/site/ets/menuitem*

Einstein, A. (1970). Autobiographical notes. In P. A. Schilpp (Ed.), *Albert Einstein: Philosopher-scientist* (p. 9). LaSalle, IL: Open Court.

Elbaum, B., & Vaughn, S. (2003). Self-concept and students with learning disabilities. In H. L. Swanson, K. R. Harris, S. Graham (Eds.), *Handbook of learning disabilities* (pp. 229–241). New York: Guilford Press.

Elementary and Secondary Education Act of 1965, Public Law No. 89-10, 79 Stat. 27 (1965).

Elliott, C. D. (1990). *Differential Ability Scales (DAS).* San Antonio, TX: Psychological Corporation,

Elliott, C. D. (2007). *Differential Ability Scales–II (DAS-II).* San Antonio, TX: Harcourt Assessment.

Elliott, S. (2006). *Selecting accommodations wisely: Facilitating test access and enhancing implementation integrity.* Paper presented at the 2006 Educational Testing Service Symposium on Accommodating Students with Disabilities on State Assessments, Princeton, NJ.

Embretson, S. E. (1995). The role of working memory capacity and general control processes in intelligence. *Intelligence, 20,* 169–189.

Emerson, C. (1983). The outer word and inner speech: Bakhtin, Vygotsky, and the internationalization of language. *Critical Inquiry, 10,* 245–264.

Engel-Ortlieb, D. (1981). Discourse processing in aphasics. *Text, 1,* 361–383.

Engle, R. W., Cantor, J., & Carullo, J. J. (1992). Individual differences in working memory and comprehension: A test of four hypotheses. *Journal of Experimental Psychology: Learning, Memory, and Cognition, 18,* 972–992.

Engle, R. W., Tuholski, S. W., Laughlin, J. E., & Conway, A. R. A. (1999). Working memory, short-term memory, and general fluid intelligence: A latent variable approach. *Journal of Experimental Psychology: General, 128,* 309–331.

Englert, C. S. (1990). Unraveling the mysteries of writing through strategy instruction. In T. E. Scruggs & B. Y. L. Wong (Eds.), *Intervention research in learning disabilities* (pp. 186–223). New York: Springer-Verlag.

Englert, C., & Mariage, T. (1991). Shared understandings: Structuring the writing experience through dialogue. *Journal of Learning Disabilities, 24,* 330–342.

Englert, C. S., Mariage, T. V., & Dunsmore, K. (2006). Tenets of sociocultural theory in writing instruction research. In C. A. MacArthur, S. Graham, & J. Fitzgerald (Eds.), *Handbook of writing research* (pp. 208–221). New York: Guilford Press.

Ericsson, K. A. (1996). The acquisition of expert performance. In K. A. Ericsson (Ed.), *The road to excellence* (pp. 1–50). Mahwah, NJ: Erlbaum.

Ericsson, K. A. (1997). Deliberate practice and the acquisition of expert performance: An overview. In H. Jorgensen & A. C. Lehmann (Eds.), *Does practice make perfect?: Current theory and research on instrumental music practice* (pp. 9–51). Oslo: NMH-Publikasjoner.

Ericsson, K. A., & Kintsch, W. (1995). Long-term working memory. *Psychological Review, 105,* 211–245.

Evans, J. J., Floyd, R. G., McGrew, K. S., & Leforgee, M. H. (2002). The relations between measures of Cattell–Horn–Carroll (CHC) cognitive abilities and reading achievement during childhood and adolescence. *School Psychology Review, 31,* 246–262.

Eviatar, Z., Ganayim, D., & Ibrahim, R. (2004). Orthography and the hemispheres: Visual and linguistic aspects of letter processing. *Neuropsychology, 18,* 174–184.

Eyestone, L. L., & Howell, R. J. (1994). An epidemiological study of attention-deficit hyperactivity disorder and major depression in a male prison population. *Bulletin of the American Academy of Psychiatry and Law, 22,* 181–193.

Faraone, S. V., Biederman, J., Wozniak, J., Mundy, E., Mennin, D., & O'Donnell, D. (1997). Is comorbidity with ADHD a marker for juvenile-onset mania? *Journal of the American Academy of Child and Adolescent Psychiatry, 36,* 1046–1055.

Faraone, S. V., Doyle, A., Mick, E., & Biederman, J. (2001). Meta-analysis of the association between the 7-repeat allele of the dopamine D4 receptor gene and attention deficit hyperactivity disorder. *American Journal of Psychiatry, 158,* 1052–1057.

Faraone, S. V., & Doyle, A. E. (2001). The nature and heritability of attention-deficit/hyperactivity disorder. *Child and Adolescent Psychiatric Clinics of North America, 10,* 299–316.

Fayol, M., Barrouillet, P., & Marinthe, C. (1998). Predicting arithmetical achievement from neuropsychological performance: A longitudinal study. *Cognition, 68,* 63–70.

Fecho, B. (2000). Critical inquiries into language in an urban classroom. *Research in the Teaching of English, 34,* 368–395.

Fein, D., Stevens, M., Dunn, M., Waterhouse, L., Allen, D., Rapin, I., et al. (1999). Subtypes of pervasive developmental disorder: Clinical characteristics. *Child Neuropsychology, 5,* 1–23.

Fergusson, D. M., & Lynskey, M. T. (1996). Adolescent resiliency to family adversity. *Journal of Child Psychology and Psychiatry, 37,* 281–292.

Ferri, B. A. (1997). *The construction of identity among women with learning disabilities: The many faces of the self.* Unpublished doctoral dissertation, University of Georgia.

Fink, R. (1998). Literacy development in successful men and women with dyslexia. *Annals of Dyslexia, 48,* 311–347.

Finucci, J. M., Isaacs, S. D., Whitehouse, C. C., & Childs, B. (1982). Empirical validation of reading and spelling quotients. *Developmental Medicine and Child Neurology, 24,* 733–744.

Fischer, F. W., Shankweiler, D., & Liberman, I. Y. (1985). Spelling proficiency and sensitivity to word structure. *Journal of Memory and Language, 24,* 423–441.

Fischer, M., Barkley, R. A., Smallish, L., & Fletcher, K. (2002). Young adult follow-up of hyperactive children: Self-reported psychiatric disorders, comorbidity, and the role of childhood conduct problems. *Journal of Abnormal Child Psychology, 30,* 463–475.

Fisher, S. E., Francks, C., McCracken, J. T., McGough, J. J., Marlow, A. J., MacPhie, L., et al. (2002). A genomewide scan for loci involved in attention-deficit/hyperactivity disorder. *American Journal of Human Genetics, 70,* 1183–1196.

Fitzgerald, J. (2006). Multilingual writing in preschool through 12th grade: The last 15 years. In C. A. MacArthur, S. Graham, & J. Fitzgerald (Eds.), *Handbook of writing research* (pp. 337–356). New York: Guilford Press.

Flanagan, D. P., & Harrison, P. L. (Eds.). (2005). *Contemporary intellectual assessment: Theories, tests, and issues* New York: Guilford Press.

Flanagan, D. P., & Kaufman, A. S. (2004). *Essentials of WISC-IV assessment.* New York: Wiley.

Flanagan, D. P., Keiser, S., Bernier, J. E., & Ortiz, S. O. (2003). *Diagnosis of learning disability in adulthood.* Boston: Allyn & Bacon.

Flanagan, D. P., & Mascolo, J. T. (2005). Psychoeducational assessment and learning disability diagnosis. In D. P. Flanagan & P. L. Harrison (Eds.), *Contemporary intellectual assessment: Theories, tests, and issues* (pp. 521–556). New York: Guilford Press.

Flanagan, D. P., McGrew, K., & Ortiz, S. (2000). *The Wechsler Intelligence Scales and Gf-Gc theory: A contemporary approach to interpretation.* Needham Heights, MA: Allyn & Bacon.

Flanagan, D. P., & Ortiz, S. (2001). *Essentials of cross-battery assessment.* New York: Wiley.

Fletcher, J. M., Lyon, G. R., Barnes, M., Stuebing, K. K., Francis, D. J., Olson, R. K., et al. (2001, August). *Classification of learning disabilities: An evidence-based evaluation.* Paper presented at the U.S. Department of Education LD Summit, Washington, DC.

Fletcher, J. M., & Reschly, D. J. (2005). Changing procedures for identifying learning disabilities: The danger of perpetuating old ideas. *The School Psychologist, 59,* 10–15.

Floyd, R. G., Clark, M. H., & Shadish, W. R. (2008). The exchangeability of intelligent quotients: Implications for professional psychology. *Professional Psychology: Research and Practice, 39,* 414–423.

Floyd, R. G., Evans, J. J., & McGrew, K. S. (2003). Relations between measures of Cattell–Horn–Carroll (CHC) cognitive abilities and mathematics achievement across the school-age years. *Psychology in the Schools, 40,* 155–171.

Floyd, R. G., Gregg, N., Keith, T. Z., & Meisinger, E. C. (2008). *Explanation of reading comprehension from early childhood using models from CHC theory: Support for integrative models of reading comprehension.* Manuscript submitted for publication.

Flynn, J. R. (1984). The mean IQ of Americans: Massive gains 1932 to 1978. *Psychological Bulletin, 95*(1), 29–51.

Flynn, J. R. (1987). Massive IQ gains in 14 nations: What IQ tests really measure. *Psychological Bulletin, 101*(2), 171–191.

Flynn, J. M., & Rahbar, M. H. (1994). Prevalence of reading failure in boys compared with girls. *Psychology in the Schools, 31,* 66–71.

Foorman, B. R. (1994). Phonological and orthographic processing: Separate but equal? In V.W. Berninger (Ed.), *The varieties of orthographic knowledge: Vol. 1. Theoretical and developmental issues* (pp. 321–357). Dordrecht, The Netherlands: Kluwer Academic.

Fourqurean, J. M., Meisgeier, C., Swank, P. R., & Williams, R. E. (1991). Correlates of postsecondary employment outcomes for young adults with learning disabilities. *Journal of Learning Disabilities, 24*(7), 400–405.

Frank, A. R., Sitlington, P. L., & Carson, R. R. (1995). Young adults with behavioral disorders: A comparison with peers with mild disabilities. *Journal of Emotional and Behavioral Disorders, 3,* 156–164.

Frazier, T., Youngstrom, E., Glutting, J., & Watkins, M. (2007). ADHD and achievement: A meta-analysis of the child, adolescent, and adult literature with a concomitant study using college students. *Journal of Learning Disabilities, 40,* 49–65.

Frederick, R. I., & Bowden, S. C. (in press). The test validation summary: Part I. Essential test classification characteristics.

Frith, U. (1980). Unexpected spelling problems. In U. Frith (Ed.), *Cognitive processes in spelling* (pp. 495–515). London: Academic Press.

Frith, U. (1999). Paradoxes in the definition of dyslexia. *Dyslexia: An International Journal of Research and Practice, 5,* 192–214.

Fuchs, D., Mock, D., Morgan, P. L., & Young, C. L. (2003). Responsiveness-to-intervention: Definitions, evidence, and implications for the learning disabilities construct. *Learning Disabilities Research and Practice, 18,* 157–171.

Fuchs, L. S., Compton, D. L., Fuchs, D., Paulsen, K., Bryant, J. D., & Hamlett, C. L. (2005). The prevention, identification, and cognitive determinants of math difficulty. *Journal of Educational Psychology, 97,* 493–513.

Fuchs, L. S., & Fuchs, D. (1999). Fair and unfair testing accommodations. *School Administrator, 56,* 24–29.

Fuchs, L. S., Fuchs, D., Compton, D. L., Powell, S. R., Seethalter, P. M., Capizzi, A. M., et al. (2006). The cognitive correlates of third-grade skill in arithmetic, algorithmic computation, and arithmetic word problems. *Journal of Educational Psychology, 98,* 29–43.

Fuchs, L. S., Fuchs, D., Eaton, S., Hamlett, C. L., & Karns, K. (2000b). Supplementing teachers' judgments of mathematics test accommodations with objective data sources. *School Psychology Review, 29,* 65–85.

Fuchs, L. S., Fuchs, D., Eaton, S. B., Hamlett, C. B., Binkley, E., & Crouch, R. (2000a). Using objective data sources to enhance teacher judgments about test accommodations. *Exceptional Children, 67*(1), 67–81.

Fuchs, L. S., Fuchs, D., & Maxwell, L. (1988). The validity of informal reading comprehension measures. *Remedial and Social Education, 9,* 20–28.

Fugelsang, J. A., & Dunbar, K. N. (2005). Brain-based mechanisms underlying complex causal thinking. *Neuropsychologia, 43,* 1204–1213.

Gal, I., van Groenestijn, M., Manly, M., Schmitt, M. J., & Trout, D. (2005). Adult numeracy and its assessment in the ALL survey: A conceptual framework and pilot results. In T. S. Murray, Y. Clermont, & M. Binkley (Eds.), *Measuring adult literacy and life skills: New frameworks for assessment* (pp. 137–191). Ottawa: Statistics Canada.

Galda, L., & Beach, R. (2001). Response to literature as a cultural activity. *Reading Research Quarterly, 36,* 64–73.

Gallagher, R., & Appenzeller, T. (1999). Beyond reductionism: Introduction to a special issue on complex systems. *Science, 284,* 79–92.

Ganschow, L., & Sparks, R. (1995). Effects of direct instruction in Spanish phonology on the native-language skills and foreign-language aptitude of at-risk foreign language learners. *Journal of Learning Disabilities, 28,* 107–110.

Ganschow, L., Sparks, R., Javorsky, J., Pohlman, J., & Bishop-Marbury, A. (1991). Identifying native language difficulties among foreign language learners in college: A "foreign" language learning disability? *Journal of Learning Disabilities, 24,* 530–541.

Gardner, H. (1983). *Frames of mind: The theory of multiple intelligences.* New York: Basic Books.

Garrett, A., Mazzocco, M., & Baker, L. (2006). Development of the metacognitive skills of prediction and evaluation in children with and without math disabilities. *Learning Disabilities Research and Practice, 21,* 77–88.

Geary, D. C. (1993). Mathematical disabilities: Cognitive, neuropsychological, and genetic components. *Psychological Bulletin, 114,* 345–362.

Geary, D. C. (2001). From infancy to adulthood: The development of numerical abilities. *European Child and Adolescent Psychiatry, 9,* 11–16.

Geary, D. C. (2004). Mathematics and learning disabilities. *Journal of Learning Disabilities, 37,* 4–15.

Geary, D. C. (2007). An evolutionary perspective on learning disability in mathematics. *Developmental Neuropsychology, 32,* 471–519.

Geary, D. C., Hoard, M. K., Byrd-Craven, J., & Desota, M. (2004). Strategy choices in simple and complex addition: Contributions of working memory and counting knowledge for children with mathematical disability. *Journal of Experimental Child Psychology, 88,* 121–151.

Geary, D. C., Hoard, M. K., Byrd-Craven, J., Nugent, L., & Numtee, C. (2007). Cognitive mechanisms underlying achievement deficits in children with mathematical learning disability. *Child Development, 78,* 1343–1359.

Geary, D. C., Hoard, M. K., Nugent, L., & Byrd-Craven, J. (2007). Strategy use, long-term memory, and working memory capacity. In D. B. Berch & M. M. M. Mazzocco (Eds.), *Why is math so hard for some children?: The nature and origins of mathematical learning difficulties and disabilities* (pp. 83–106). Baltimore: Brookes.

Geary, D. C., & Widaman, K. F. (1992). Numerical cognition: On the convergence of componential and psychometric models. *Intelligence, 16*, 47–80.

Gerber, P. J., Ginsberg, R., & Reiff, H. B. (1992). Identifying alterable patterns in employment success for highly successful adults with learning disabilities. *Journal of Learning Disabilities, 25*, 475–487.

Gerber, P. J., & Reiff, H. B. (1991). *Speaking for themselves: Ethnographic interviews with adults with learning disabilities*. Anne Arbor: University of Michigan Press.

Gersten, R., & Baker, S. (2002). The relevance of Messick's four faces for understanding the validity of high-stakes assessments. In G. Tindal & T. M. Haladyna (Eds.), *Large-scale assessment programs for all students: Validity, technical adequacy, and implementation* (pp. 49–66). Mahwah, NJ: Erlbaum.

Gervais, R. O., Rohling, M. L., Green, P., & Ford, W. (2004). A comparison of WMT, CARB, and TOMM failure rates in non-head injury disability claimants. *Archives of Clinical Neuropsychology, 19*, 475–487.

Gigerenzer, G., & Selten, R. (Eds.). (2001). *Bounded rationality: The adaptive toolbox*. Cambridge, MA: MIT Press.

Gillberg, C. (1992). The Emmanuel Miller Memorial Lecture 1991: Autism and autistic-like conditions: Subclasses among disorders of empathy. *Journal of Child Psychology and Psychiatry, 33*, 813–842.

Gillberg, C. (1998). Asperger syndrome and high-functioning autism. *British Journal of Psychiatry, 172*, 200–209.

Gillberg, C., & Ehlers, S. (1998). High-functioning people with autism and Asperger syndrome: A literature review. In E. Schopler, G. B. Mesibov, & L. J. Kunce (Eds.), *Asperger syndrome or high-functioning autism?* (pp. 79–106). New York: Plenum Press.

Gilman, S. E., Kawachi, I., Fitzmaurice, G. M., & Buka, S. (2003). Family disruption in childhood and risk of adult depression. *American Journal of Psychiatry, 160*, 939–946.

Gleckman, A. D. (1992). *A psychological profile of the learning disabled college student: A cluster analytic assessment as depicted by the MMPI-2*. Unpublished doctoral dissertation, Ball State University, Muncie, IN.

Glutting, J. J., Watkins, M. W., Konold, T. R., & McDermott, P. A. (2006). Distinctions without a difference: The utility of observed versus latent factors from the WISC-IV in estimating reading and math achievement on the WIAT-II. *Journal of Special Education, 40*, 103–114.

Goff, D., Pratt, C., & Ong, B. (2005). The relations between children's reading comprehension, working memory, language skills, and components of reading decoding in a normal sample. *Reading and Writing, 18*, 583–616.

Goldberg, A., Russell, M., & Cook, A. (2003). The effect of computers on student writing: A meta-analysis of studies from 1992 to 2002. *Journal of Technology, Learning, and Assessment, 2*, 1–51.

Goldberg, R. J., Higgins, E. L., Raskind, M. H., & Herman, K. L. (2003). Predictors of success in individuals with learning disabilities: A qualitative analysis of a 20-year longitudinal study. *Learning Disabilities Research and Practice, 18*(4), 222–236.

Gonzales v. National Board of Medical Examiners, 225 F. 3d 620 (6th Cir. 2000).

Gordon, M., Barkley, R. A., & Lovett, B. (2006). Tests and observational measures. In R. A. Barkley, *Attention-deficit hyperactivity disorder: A handbook for diagnosis and treatment* (3rd ed., pp. 369–388). New York: Guilford Press.

Gordon, M., & Keiser, S. B. (1998). *Accommodations in higher education under the Americans with Disabilities Act.* New York: Guilford Press.

Grady, D. L., Chi, H. C., Ding, Y. C., Smith, M., Wang, E., Schuck, S., et al. (2003). High prevalence of rare dopamine receptor D4 alleles in children diagnosed with attention-deficit hyperactivity disorder. *Molecular Psychiatry, 8*, 536–545.

Graesser, A. C. (Ed.). (1993). Inference generation during text comprehension [Special issue]. *Discourse Processes, 16*(1–2).

Graesser, A. C. (2007). An introduction to strategic reading comprehension. In D. S. McNamar (Ed.), *Reading comprehension strategies: Theories, interventions, and technology* (pp. 2–21). Mahwah, NJ: Erlbaum.

Graham, S. (1986). The reliability, validity, and utility of three handwriting measurement procedures. *Journal of Educational Research, 79*, 373–380.

Graham, S. (2006). Strategy instruction and teaching of writing: A meta-analysis. In C. A. MacArthur, S. Graham, & J. Fitzgerald (Eds.), *Handbook of writing research* (pp. 187–207). New York: Guilford Press.

Graham, S., & Harris, K. (1999). Assessment and intervention in overcoming writing difficulties: An illustration from the self-regulated strategy development model. *Language, Speech and Hearing Services in Schools, 30*, 255–264.

Graham, S., Harris, K., & Fink, B. (2000). Is handwriting causally related to learning to write?: Treatment of handwriting problems in beginning writers. *Journal of Educational Psychology, 92*, 620–633.

Graham, S., & Harris, K. R. (2005). *Writing better: Effective strategies for teaching students with learning difficulties.* Baltimore: Brookes.

Graham, S., & Weintraub, N. (1996). A review of handwriting research: Progress and prospects from 1980–1994. *Educational Psychology Review, 8*, 7–86.

Green, D. (2006). Historically underserved students: What we know, what we still need to know. In D. D. Bragg & E. A. Barnett (Eds.), *Academic pathways to and from the community college* (pp. 21–28). San Francisco: Jossey-Bass.

Green, P. (2003). *Word Memory Test.* Edmonton, Alberta, Canada: Green's Publishing.

Green, P., Allen, L., & Astner, K. (1996). *The Word Memory Test: A user's guide to the oral and computer-administered forms, US version 1.1.* Durham, NC: CogniSyst.

Gregg, N. (1985). College learning disabled, normal, and basic writers: A comparison of frequency and accuracy of cohesive ties. *Journal of Psychoeducational Assessment, 3*, 223–231.

Gregg, N. (1994). Eligibility for learning disabilities rehabilitation services:

Operationalizing the definition. *Journal of Vocational Rehabilitation, 4,* 86–95.

Gregg, N. (1996). Research directions, leading toward inclusion, diversity, and leadership in the global economy. In S. C. Cramer & W. Ellis (Eds.), *Learning disabilities: Lifelong issues* (pp. 121–134). Baltimore: Brookes.

Gregg, N. (2007). Underserved and underprepared: Postsecondary learning disabilities. *Learning Disabilities Research and Practice, 22*(4), 219–228.

Gregg, N. (2008). *Evidence-based accommodation research specific to the adolescent and adult population with learning disabilities.* Washington, DC: National Institute for Literacy.

Gregg, N., Bandalos, D., Coleman, C., Davis, M., Robinson, K., & Blake, K. (2008). The validity of a battery of phonemic and orthographic awareness tasks for adults with and without dyslexia and attention deficit/hyperactivity disorder. *Remedial and Special Education, 29,* 175–190.

Gregg, N., & Coleman, C. (2005, June). *Written discourse complexity: A multidimensional analysis.* Paper presented at the meeting of the Society for the Scientific Study of Reading, Toronto.

Gregg, N., Coleman, C., Davis, M., & Chalk, J. (2007). Timed essay writing: Implications for high-stakes tests. *Journal of Learning Disabilities, 40,* 306–318.

Gregg, N., Coleman, C., Davis, M., Lindstrom, W., & Hartwig, J. (2006). Critical issues for the diagnosis of learning disabilities in the adult population. *Psychology in the Schools, 43*(8), 889–899.

Gregg, N., Coleman, C., & Knight, D. (2003). Use of the Woodcock–Johnson III in the diagnosis of learning disabilities. In F. A. Schrank & D. P. Flanagan (Eds.), *WJ III clinical use and interpretation* (pp. 125–174). San Diego, CA: Academic Press.

Gregg, N., Coleman, C., & Lindstrom, J. (2008). Written expression disorders and the adult population with learning disorders. In L. E. Wolf, H. E. Scribner, & J. Wasserstein (Eds.), *Adult learning disorders: Contemporary issues* (pp. 301–332). London: Psychology Press.

Gregg, N., Coleman, C., Lindstrom, J., & Lee, C. (2007). Who are most, average, or high-functioning adults? *Learning Disabilities Research and Practice, 22,* 264–274.

Gregg, N., Coleman, C., Stennett, B., & Davis, M. (2002). Discourse complexity of college writers with and without disabilities: A multidimensional analysis. *Journal of Learning Disabilities, 35*(1), 23–38.

Gregg, N., Coleman, C., Stennett, R., Davis, M., Nielsen, K., Knight, D., et al. (2002). Sublexical and lexical processing of young adults with learning disabilities and attention deficit/hyperactivity disorder. In E. Witruk, A. D. Friederici, & T. Lachmann (Eds.), *Basic functions of language, reading, and reading disability* (pp. 329–358). Dordrecht, The Netherlands: Kluwer Academic.

Gregg, N., & Hartwig, J. (2005). Written expression assessment: An integrated approach. In S. W. Lee (Ed.), *Encyclopedia of school psychology* (pp. 590–600). Thousand Oaks, CA: Sage.

Gregg, N., Heggoy, S., Stapleton, M., Jackson, R., & Morris, R. (1996). Eligibility for college learning disabilities services: A system-wide approach. *Learning Disabilities: A Multidisciplinary Journal, 7*, 29–36.

Gregg, N., Hoy, C., Flaherty, D. A., Norris, P., Coleman, C., Davis, M., et al. (2005). Documenting decoding and spelling accommodations for postsecondary students demonstrating dyslexia: It's more than processing speed. *Learning Disabilities: A Contemporary Journal, 3*, 1–17.

Gregg, N., Hoy, C., King, M., Moreland, C., & Jagota, M. (1992a). The MMPI-2 profile of adults with learning disabilities in university and rehabilitation settings. *Journal of Learning Disabilities, 25*, 386–395.

Gregg, N., Hoy, C., King, M., Moreland, M., Jagota, M., & Nemati, M. (1992b). Performance of adults with learning disabilities at a rehabilitation and a university setting on the MMPI-2, Harris–Lingoes and Social Introversion (SI) Scales. *Rehabilitation Education, 6*, 1–9.

Gregg, N., Hoy, C., McAlexander, P., & Hayes, C. (1991). Written sentence production error patterns of college writers with learning disabilities. *Reading and Writing: An Interdisciplinary Journal, 3*, 169–185.

Gregg, N., & Jackson, R. (1989). Dialogue patterns of the nonverbal learning disabilities population: Mirrors of self-regulation deficits. *Learning Disabilities: A Multidisciplinary Journal, 1*, 63–71.

Gregg, N., Johnson, Y., & McKinley, C. (1996). Learning disabilities policy and legal issues: A consumer and practitioner user-friendly guide. In N. Gregg, C. Hoy, & A. Gay (Eds.), *Adults with learning disabilities: Theoretical and practical perspectives* (pp. 329–367). New York: Guilford Press.

Gregg, N., & Lindstrom, J. (2008). Accommodation of instructional testing situations. In R. J. Morris & N. Mather (Eds.), *Evidence-based interventions for students with behavioral challenges* (pp. 302–320). New York: Routledge.

Gregg, N., & McAlexander, P. (1989). The relation between sense of audience and specific learning disabilities: An exploration. *Annals of Dyslexia, 39*, 206–226.

Gregg, N., Morgan, D., Hartwig, J., & Coleman, C. (2008). Accommodations: Research to practice. In L. E. Wolf, H. E. Scribner, & J. Wasserstein (Eds.), *Adult learning disorders: Contemporary issues* (pp. 389–414). London: Psychology Press.

Gregg, N., Morgan, D., Lindstrom, J., & Coleman, C. (2008). Accommodations: Research to practice. In L. E. Wolf, H. E. Schrieber, & J. Wasserstein (Eds.), *Adult learning disorders: Contemporary issues* (pp. 389–414). New York: Psychology Press.

Gregg, N., & Nelson, J. (2008). *A meta-analysis of the extended time accommodation literature specific to the adolescent and adult populations with LD.* Manuscript submitted for publication.

Gregg, N., & Scott, S. (2000). Definition and documentation: Theory, measurement and the court. *Journal of Learning Disabilities, 33(1)*, 5–13.

Gregg, N., Scott, S., McPeek, D., & Ferri, B. A. (1999). Definitions and eligibility criteria applied to the adolescent and adult populations with learning disabilities across agencies. *Learning Disabilities Quarterly, 22(3)*, 213–223.

Gregg, N., Sigalas, S., Hoy, C., Weisenbaker, J., & McKinley, C. (1996). Sense of audience and the adult writer: A study across competence levels. *Reading and Writing: An Interdisciplinary Journal, 8,* 121–137.

Gregory, M. K. (1977). Sex bias in school referrals. *Journal of School Psychology, 15*(1), 5–8.

Gross-Tsur, V., Manor, O., & Shalev, R. S. (1996). Developmental dyscalculia: Prevalence and demographic features. *Developmental Medicine and Child Neurology, 38,* 25–33.

Guckenberger v. Boston University, 974 F. Supp. 106 (D. Mass. 1997), 8 F. Supp. 2d 82 (D. Mass. 1998).

Guion, R. M. (1995). Commentary on values and standards in performance assessments. *Educational Measurement: Issues and Practice, 14,* 25–57.

Gunter, H. L., Ghaziuddin, M., & Ellis, H. D. (2002). Asperger syndrome: Test of right hemisphere functioning and interhemispheric communication. *Journal of Autism and Developmental Disorders, 32*(4), 263–281.

Gustafsson, J.-E. (2001, November 28). *Schooling and intelligence: Effects of track of study on level and profile of cognitive abilities.* Paper presented at the 3rd International Spearman Seminar, Extending Intelligence Enhancements on New Constructs, Melbourne, Australia. (Abstract retrieved December 7, 2001, from *www.psych.asyd.edu.au/spearman*)

Guthrie, J. T., Weber, S., & Kimmerly, N. (1993). Searching documents: Cognitive processes and deficits in understanding graphs, tables, and illustrations. *Contemporary Educational Psychology, 18,* 186–221.

Hagborg, W. J. (1999). Scholastic competence subgroups among high school students with learning disabilities. *Learning Disability Quarterly, 22*(1), 3–10.

Hager, D., & Vaughn, S. (1995). Parent, teacher, peer, and self-reports of the social competence of students with learning disabilities. *Journal of Learning Disabilities, 28*(4), 205–215.

Hagtret, B. E. (2003). Listening comprehension and reading comprehension in poor decoders: Evidence for the importance of syntactic and semantic skills as well as for phonological skills. *Reading and Writing, 35,* 505–539.

Haladyna, T. M. (2002). Research to improve large-scale testing. In G. Tindal & T. M. Hadadyna (Eds.), *Large-scale assessment programs for all students: Validity, technical adequacy, and implementation* (pp. 341–370). Mahwah, NJ: Erlbaum.

Hale, J. B., Fiorello, C. A., Kavanagh, J. A., Hoeppner, J. B., & Gaitherer, R. A. (2001). WISC-III predictors of academic achievement for children with learning disabilities: Are global and factor scores comparable? *School Psychology Quarterly, 16*(1), 31–35.

Hale, J. B., Naglieri, J. A., Kaufman, A. S., & Kavale, K. A. (2004). Specific learning disability classification in the new Individuals with Disabilities Education Act: The danger of good ideas. *The School Psychologist, 58,* 6–13.

Hallahan, D. P., Lloyd, J. W., Kauffman, J. M., Weiss, M. P., & Martinez, E. A. (2005). *Learning disabilities: Foundations, characteristics, and effective teaching* (3rd ed.). Boston: Pearson/Allyn & Bacon.

Hallenbeck, M. J. (1996). The cognitive strategy in writing: Welcome relief for adolescents with learning disabilities. *Learning Disabilities Research and Practice, 11,* 107–119.

Halliday, M. A. K. (1973). *Explorations in the functions of language.* London: Edward Arnold.

Halliday, M. A. K., & Hasan, R. (1976). *Cohesion in English.* London: Longman.

Hambrick, D., & Engle, R. (2002). Effects of domain knowledge, working memory capacity, and age on cognitive performance: An investigation of the knowledge-is-power hypothesis. *Cognitive Psychology, 44,* 339–387.

Hampton, N. Z., & Mason, E. (2003). Learning disabilities, gender, sources of efficacy, self-efficacy beliefs, and academic achievement in high school students. *Journal of School Psychology, 41,* 101–112.

Handley-More, D., Deitz, J., Billingsley, F. F., & Coggins, T. E. (2003). Facilitating written work using computer word processing and word prediction. *American Journal of Occupational Therapy, 57,* 139–151.

Hartman, D. E. (2002). The unexamined lie is a lie worth fibbing: Neuropsychological malingering and Word Memory Test. *Archives of Clinical Neuropsychology, 17*(7), 709–714.

Harvey, J., & Housman, N. (2004). *Crisis or possibility: Conversations about the American high school.* Washington, DC: National High School Alliance.

Hatcher, J., Snowling, M. J., & Griffiths, Y. M. (2002). Cognitive assessment of dyslexic students in higher education. *British Journal of Educational Psychology, 72,* 119–133.

Hawke, J. L., Wadsworth, S. J., Olson, R. K., & DeFries, J. C. (2006). Etiology of reading difficulties as a function of gender and severity. *Reading and Writing, 20,* 13–25.

Hayes, J. R. (2006). New directions in writing theory. In C. A. MacArthur, S. Graham, & J. Fitzgerald (Eds.), *Handbook of writing research* (pp. 28–40). New York: Guilford Press.

Heath, N. L. (1995). Distortion and deficit: Self-perceived versus actual academic competence in depressed and nondepressed children with and without learning disabilities. *Learning Disabilities Research and Practice, 10,* 2–10.

Heath, S. B. (1983). *Ways with words: Language, life and work in communities and classrooms.* Cambridge, UK: Cambridge University Press.

Heaton, R. K., & Marcotte, T. D. (2000). Clinical and neuropsychological tests and assessment techniques. In F. Boller & J. Grafman (Series Eds.), & G. Rizzolatti (Vol. Ed.), *Handbook of neuropsychology* (2nd ed., Vol. 4, pp. 58–72). Amsterdam: Elsevier.

Heaton, R. K., Taylor, M. J., & Manly, J. (2003). Demographic effects of demographically corrected norms with the WAIS-III and WMS-III. In D. S. Tulsky, G. J. Chelune, R. J. Ivnik, A. Prifitera, D. H. Saklofske, R. K. Heaton, et al. (Eds.), *Clinical interpretation of the WAIS-III and WMS-III* (pp. 183–198). San Diego, CA: Academic Press.

Helwig, R., & Tindal, G. (2003). An experimental analysis of accommodation decisions on large-scale mathematics tests. *Exceptional Children, 69,* 211–225.

Henry, L. A. (2007). *Exploring new literacies, pedagogy, and online reading compre-

hension among middle school students and teachers: Issues of social equity or social exclusion? Unpublished doctoral dissertation, University of Connecticut.

Herr, E. L., & Niles, S. (1997). Perspectives on career assessment of work-bound youth. *Journal of Career Assessment, 5*, 137–150.

Hetzroni, O. E., & Shrieber, B. (2004). Word processing as an assistive technology tool for enhancing academic outcomes of students with writing disabilities in the general classroom. *Journal of Learning Disabilities, 37*(2), 143–154.

Higgins, E. L., & Raskind, M. H. (1995). Compensatory effectiveness of speech recognition on the written composition performance of postsecondary students with learning disabilities. *Learning Disability Quarterly, 18*, 159–174.

Hirsch, E. (2003, Spring). Reading comprehension requires knowledge of words and the world: Scientific insights into the fourth-grade slump and the nation's stagnant comprehension scores. *American Educator*, pp. 10–29.

Hock, M., & Mellard, D. (2005). Reading comprehension strategies for adult literacy outcomes. *Journal of Adolescent and Adult Literacy, 49*(3), 192–200.

Holdnack, J. A., & Weiss, L. G. (2006). IDEA 2004: Anticipated implications for clinical practice: Integrating assessment and intervention. *Psychology in the Schools, 43*, 871–882.

Hollenbeck, K., Tindal, G., Harniss, M., & Almond, P. (1999). Reliability and decision consistency: An analysis of writing mode at two times on a statewide test. *Educational Assessment, 6*(1), 23–40.

Holmes, V. M., & Castles, A. E. (2001). Unexpectedly poor spelling in university students. *Scientific Studies of Reading, 5*(4), 319–350.

Holmes, V. M., & Malone, N. (2004). Adult spelling strategies. *Reading and Writing, 17*(6), 537–566.

Hom, J. (2003). Forensic neuropsychology: Are we there yet? *Archives of Clinical Neuropsychology, 18*, 827–845.

Horn, J. L. (1994). Theory of fluid and crystallized intelligence. In R. J. Sternberg (Ed.), *Encyclopedia of intelligence* (pp. 443–451). New York: Macmillan.

Horn, J. L., & Blankson, N. (2005). Foundations for better understanding of cognitive abilities. In D. P. Flanagan & P. L. Harrison (Eds.), *Contemporary intellectual assessment: Theories, tests, and issues* (2nd ed., pp. 41–68.). New York: Guilford Press.

Horn, J. L., & Noll, J. G. (1997). Human cognitive capabilities: Gf-Gc theory. In D. P. Flanagan, J. L. Genshaft, & P. A. Harrison (Eds.), *Contemporary intellectual assessment: Theories, tests, and issues* (pp. 53–91). New York: Guilford Press.

Horney, M. A., & Anderson-Inman, L. (1994). The Electro Text Project: Hypertext reading patterns of middle school students. *Journal of Educational Multimedia and Hypermedia, 3*, 71–91.

Horney, M. A., & Anderson-Inman, L. (1999). Supported text in electronic reading environments. *Reading and Writing Quarterly, 15*, 127–168.

Howard, K. A., & Tryon, G. S. (2002). Depressive symptoms in and type of classroom placement for adolescents with LD. *Journal of Learning Disabilities, 35*(2), 185–193.

Howlin, P. (2003). Outcome in high-functioning adults with autism with and without early language delays: Implications for the differentiation between autism and Asperger syndrome. *Journal of Autism and Developmental Disorders, 33*, 3–13.

Hoy, C., & Gregg, N. (1994). *Assessment: The special educator's role.* Pacific Grove, CA: Brooks/Cole.

Hoy, C., Gregg, N., Wisenbaker, J., Bonham, S., King, M., & Moreland, C. (1996). Clinical model versus discrepancy model in determining eligibility for learning disabilities services at a rehabilitation setting. In N. Gregg, C. Hoy, & A. Gay (Eds.), *Adults with learning disabilities: Theoretical and practical perspectives* (pp. 55–67). New York: Guilford Press.

Hoza, B., Gerdes, A. C., Hinshaw, S. P., Arnold, L. E., Pelham, W. E., Molina, B. S., et al. (2004). Self-perceptions of competence in children with ADHD and comparison children. *Journal of Consulting and Clinical Psychology, 72*, 382–391.

Hoza, B., Pelham, W. E., Dobbs, J., Owens, J. S.,& Pillow, D. R. (2002). Do boys with attention-deficit/hyperactivity disorders have positive illusory self concepts? *Journal of Abnormal Psychology, 111*, 268–278.

Hoza, B., Pelham, W. E., Waschbusch, D. A., Kipp, H., & Owens, J. S. (2001). Academic task persistence of normally achieving ADHD and control boys: Performance, self-evaluations and attributions. *Journal of Consulting and Clinical Psychology, 69*, 281–283.

Hoza, B., Waschbusch, D. A., Pelham, W. E., Molina, B. S. G., & Milich, R. (2000). Attention-deficit/hyperactive disordered and control boys' responses to social success and failure. *Child Development, 71*, 432–446.

Huber, W. (1989). Text comprehension and production in aphasia: Analysis in terms of micro and macro processing. In Y. Joanette & H. Brownell (Eds.), *Discourse ability and brain damage: Theoretical and empirical perspectives* (pp. 154–179). New York: Springer-Verlag.

Hunt, E. (2002). Let's hear it for crystallized intelligence. *Learning and Individual Differences, 12*(1), 123–129.

Hynd, G. W., Semrud-Clikeman, M., Lorys, A. R., Novey, E. S., Eliopulos, D., & Lyytinen, H. (1991). Corpus callosum morphology in attention deficit hyperactivity disorder: Morphometric analysis of MRI. *Journal of Learning Disabilities, 24*, 141–146.

Individuals with Disabilities Act (IDEA). (2004). Washington, DC: Office of Special Education and Rehabilitation Services. Available at *www.ed.gov/offices/OSERS/policy/IDEA/the_law.html*

Individuals with Disabilities Education Improvement Act of 2004 (IDEA 2004), Public Law No. 108-446, 20 U.S.C. 1462 (2004).

Inhelder, B., & Piaget, J. (1958). *The growth of logical thinking from childhood to adolescence.* New York: Basic Books.

Ivanov, V. V. (1977). The role of semiotics in the cybernetic study of man and collective. In D. P. Lucid (Ed.), *Soviet semiotics: An anthology* (pp. 85–120). Baltimore: Johns Hopkins University Press.

Iverson, G., & Binder, L. M. (2000). Detecting exaggeration and malingering in neuropsychological assessment. *Journal of Head Trauma Rehabilitation, 15*(2), 829–858.

Ives, B. (2007). Graphic organizers applied to secondary algebra instruction for students with learning disabilities. *Learning Disabilities Research and Practice, 22,* 110–118.

Jarrold, C., & Towse, J. N. (2006). Individual differences in working memory. *Neuroscience, 139,* 39–50.

Jastak, S., & Wilkinson, G. (1993). *Wide Range Achievement Test–3 (WRAT3).* Wilmington, DE: Wide Range.

Jensen, A. R. (1998). *The g factor: The science of mental ability.* Westport, CT: Praeger.

Jessor, R., Van Den Bos, J., Vanderryn, J., Costa, F. M., & Turbin, M. S. (1995). Protective factors in adolescent problem behavior: Moderator effects and developmental change. *Developmental Psychopathology, 31,* 923–933.

Job Accommodation Network. (2007). Job accommodations. Retrieved February 2008, from *www.jan.wvu.edu*

John-Steiner, V. (1997). *Notebooks of the mind: Explorations of thinking* (rev. ed.). New York: Oxford University Press.

Johnson, D. J., & Blalock, J. (Eds.). (1987). *Young adults with learning disabilities.* Orlando, FL: Grune & Stratton.

Johnson, D. J., & Myklebust, H. R. (1967). *Learning disabilities: Educational principles and practices.* New York: Grune & Stratton.

Johnson, E. (2000). The effects of accommodations on performance assessments. *Remedial and Special Education, 21,* 261–267.

Johnstone, C. J., Altman, J., Thurlow, M. L., & Thompson, S. J. (2006). *A summary of research on the effects of test accommodations: 2002 through 2004* (Technical Report No. 45). Minneapolis: University of Minnesota, National Center on Educational Outcomes. Retrieved November 11, 2007, from *education.umn.edu/NCEO/OnlinePubs/Tech45/*

Jordan, N. C., Hanich, L. B., & Kaplan, D. (2003). Performance across different areas of mathematical cognition in children with learning disabilities. *Journal of Educational Psychology, 93,* 615–626.

Just, M. A., & Carpenter, P. A. (1987). *The psychology of reading and language comprehension.* Boston: Allyn & Bacon.

Just, M. A., & Carpenter, P. A. (1992). A capacity theory of comprehension: Individual differences in working memory. *Psychological Review, 99,* 122–149.

Kamphaus, R. W. (1993). *Clinical assessment of children's intelligence.* Boston: Allyn & Bacon.

Kamphaus, R. W. (2005). *Clinical assessment of child and adolescent intelligence* (2nd ed.) New York: Springer.

Kanaya, T., Ceci, S. J., & Scullin, M. H. (2003). The rise and fall of IQ in special ed: Historical trends and their implications. *Journal of School Psychology, 41,* 453–465.

Kane, M. J., Conway, R. A., Hambrick, D., & Engle, R. W. (2007). Variation in working memory capacity as variation in executive attention and control. In A. R. A. Conway, C. Jarrold, M. J. Kane, A. Miyake, & J. W. Towse (Eds.), *Variation in working memory* (pp. 21–48). New York: Oxford University Press.

Kane, M. J., & Engle, R. W. (2002). The role of prefrontal cortex in working-memory capacity, executive attention, and general fluid intelligence: An individual-differences perspective. *Psychonomic Bulletin and Review, 9*, 637–671.

Kanwisher, N., McDermott, J., & Chun, M. M. (1997). The fusiform face area: A module in human extrastriate cortex specialized for face perception. *Journal of Neuroscience, 17*, 4302–4311.

Katz, S., Blackburn, A. B., & Lautenschlager, G. J. (1991). Answering reading comprehension items without passages on the SAT when items are quasi-randomized. *Educational and Psychological Measurement, 52*, 747–754.

Kaufman, A. S. (1979). *Intelligent testing with the WISC-R*. New York: Wiley-Interscience.

Kaufman, A. S., & Kaufman, N. (1993). *Kaufman Adolescent and Adult Intelligence Test*. Circle Pines, MN: American Guidance Service.

Kaufman, A. S., & Kaufman, N. (1997). The Kaufman Adolescent and Adult Intelligence Test. In D. P. Flanagan, J. L. Genshaft, & P. L. Harrison (Eds.), *Contemporary intellectual assessment: Theories, tests, and issues* (pp. 209–229). New York: Guilford Press.

Kaufman, A. S., & Lichtenberger, E. O. (2006). *Assessing adolescent and adult intelligence* (3rd ed.). Hoboken, NJ: Wiley.

Kaufman, P., & Alt, M. (2004, October). *Dropout rates in the United States: 2001*. Washington, DC: U.S. Department of Education, National Center for Education Statistics.

Kavale, K. A., & Forness, S. R. (2003). Learning disabilities as a discipline. In H. L. Swanson, K. R. Harris, & S. Graham (Eds.), *Handbook of learning disabilities* (pp. 76–93). New York: Guilford Press.

Kavale, K. A., Fuchs, D., & Scruggs, T. E. (1994). Setting the record straight on learning disability and low achievement: Implications for policy-making. *Learning Disabilities Research and Practice, 9*, 70–77.

Kavale, K. A., Kaufman, A. S., Naglieri, J. A., & Hale, J. (2005). Changing procedures for identifying learning disabilities: The danger of poorly supported ideas. *The School Psychologist, 59*, 16–25.

Keenan, J. M., & Betjemann, R. S. (2006). Comprehending the Gray Oral Reading Test without reading it: Why comprehension tests should not include passage-independent items. *Scientific Studies of Reading, 10*, 363–380.

Keogh, B. K., & Weisner, T. (1993). An ecocultural perspective on risk and protective factors in children's development: Implications for learning disabilities. *Learning Disabilities Research and Practice, 8*, 3–10.

Kim, J., Taft, M., & Davis, C. (2004). Orthographic–phonological links in the lexicon: When lexical and sublexical information conflict. *Reading and Writing: An International Journal, 17*, 187–218.

Kintsch, W. (1998). *Comprehension: A paradigm for cognition*. Cambridge, UK: Cambridge University Press.

Klassen, R. M. (2007). Using predictions to learn about the self-efficacy of early adolescents with and without learning disabilities. *Contemporary Educational Psychology, 32*, 173–187.

Klin, A., McPartland, J., & Volkmar, F. R. (2005). Asperger syndrome. In F. R. Volkmar, R. Paul, A. Klin, & D. Cohen (Eds.), *Handbook of autism and pervasive developmental disorders: Vol. 1. Diagnosis, development, neurobiology, and behavior* (pp. 88–125). Hoboken, NJ: Wiley.

Klin, A., Sparrow, S. S., Volkmar, F. R., Cicchetti, D. V., & Rourke, B. P. (1995). Asperger syndrome. In B. P. Rourke (Ed.), *Syndrome of nonverbal learning disabilities: Neurodevelopmental manifestations* (pp. 93–118). New York: Guilford Press.

Kloomok, S., & Cosden, M. (1994). Self-concept in children with learning disabilities: The relationship between global self-concept, academic "discounting," nonacademic self-concept, and perceived social support. *Learning Disability Quarterly, 17,* 140–153.

Knight, D. (2000). *A cognitive and linguistic model of individual differences in the reading comprehension of college students with and without learning disabilities.* Unpublished doctoral dissertation, University of Georgia.

Kochhar-Bryant, C. A. (2007). The summary of performance as transition "passport" to employment and independent living. *Assessment for Effective Intervention, 32,* 160–170.

Koenig, J. A., & Bachman, L. F. (Eds.). (2004). *Keeping score for all: The effects of inclusion and accommodation policies on large-scale educational assessments.* Washington, DC: National Academies Press.

Konecky, J., & Wolinsky, S. (2000). Through the maze: Legal issues and disability rights. *Learning Disabilities: A Multidisciplinary Journal, 10,* 73–83.

Koone, D. A. (2007). Attention deficit hyperactivity disorder assessment practices by practicing school psychologists: A national survey. *Journal of Psychoeducational Assessment, 25*(4), 319–333.

Koponen, T., Mononen, R., Rasanen, P., & Ahonen, T. (2006). Basic numeracy in children with specific language impairment: Heterogeneity and connections to language. *Journal of Speech, Language, and Hearing Research, 49,* 58–73.

Kopriva, R. (2002). *Taxonomy for testing English language learners.* Funded proposal to the U.S. Department of Education, Grants for Enhanced Assessment Instruments Program.

Kosc, L. (1974). Developmental dyscalculia. *Journal of Learning Disabilities, 7,* 164–177.

Kriss, I., & Evans, B. J. W. (2005). The relationship between dyslexia and Meares–Irlen syndrome. *Journal of Research in Reading, 28*(3), 350–364.

Kwong See, S. J., & Ryan, E. B. (1995). Cognitive mediation of adult age differences in language performance. *Psychology and Aging, 10,* 458–468.

Laanan, F. S. (2006). Editor's notes. In F. S. Laanan (Ed.), *Understanding students in transition: Trends and issues* (pp. 1–5). San Francisco: Jossey-Bass.

Lackaye, T., Margalit, Z., & Zinman, T. (2006). Comparisons of self-efficacy, mood, effort, and hope between students with learning disabilities and their non-LD-matched peers. *Learning Disabilities Research and Practice, 21*(2), 111–121.

Lamb, P. (2006). Transition to employment: Implications for vocational rehabilitation counselors and the summary of performance. *Career Development for Exceptional Individuals, 29*(20), 66–79.

Lambert, N. M. (1988). Adolescent outcomes for hyperactive children. *American Psychologist, 43,* 786–799.

Lambert, N. M., Hartsough, C. S., Sassone, S., & Sandoval, J. (1987). Persistence of hyperactive symptoms from childhood to adolescence and associated outcomes. *American Journal of Orthopsychiatry, 57,* 22–32.

Landerl, K., Bevan, A., & Butterworth, B. (2004). Developmental dyscalculia and basic numerical capacities: A study of 8–9 year old students. *Cognition, 93,* 99–125.

Lee, K., Ng, E. L., Ng, S. F., & Peh, S. (2006). *Individual differences in algebraic problem solving: The roles of executive functions.* Paper presented at the Fourth International Conference on Memory, Sydney, Australia.

Lefly, D., & Pennington, B. F. (2000). Reliability and validity of the Adult Reading History Questionnaire. *Journal of Learning Disabilities, 33*(3), 286–296.

Lehmkuhle, S. (1993). Neurological basis of visual processing in reading. In D. Willows, R. Kruk, & E. Coros (Eds.), *Visual processes in reading and reading disabilities* (pp. 77–94). Hillsdale, NJ: Erlbaum.

Leikin, M., & Hagit, E. Z. (2006). Morphological processing adult dyslexia. *Journal of Psycholinguistic Research, 35,* 1573–6555.

Lenz, K. B., & Deshler, D. D. (2005). Adolescents with learning disabilities: Revisiting the educators' enigma. In B. V. L. Wong (Ed.), *Learning about learning disabilities* (3rd ed., pp. 535–564). San Diego, CA: Academic Press.

Leonard, C. M., Eckert, M. A., Lombardino, L. J., Oakland, T., Kranzler, J., Mohr, C. M., et al. (2001). Anatomical risk factors for phonological dyslexia. *Cerebral Cortex, 11,* 148–157.

Leong, C. K. (1999). Phonological and morphological processing in adult students with learning/reading disabilities. *Journal of Learning Disabilities, 32,* 224–238.

Leu, D. (2006). *Developing new illiteracies: Using the Internet in content area instruction.* Retrieved January 25, 2006, from *web.syr.edu/~djleu/content.html*

Leu, D. J., & Castek, J. (2006). *What skills and strategies are characteristic of accomplished adolescent users of the Internet?* Paper presented at the meeting of the American Educational Research Association, San Francisco.

Leu, D. J., Coiro, J., Castek, J., Hartman, D. K., Henry, L. A., & Reinking, D. (2008). Research on instruction and assessment in the new literacies of online reading comprehension. In C. C. Block & S. R. Parris (Eds.), *Comprehension instruction: Research-based best practices* (2nd ed., pp. 321–346). New York: Guilford Press.

Leu, D. J., & Reinking, D. (2005). *Developing Internet comprehension strategies among adolescent students at risk to become dropouts.* Storrs: New Literacies Research Team, University of Connecticut. Retrieved September 15, 2007, from *www.newliteracies.uconn.edu/ies.html*

Leu, D. J., Reinking, D., Carter, A., Castek, J., Coiron, J., Henry, L. A., et al. (2007, April 9). *Defining online reading comprehension: Using think aloud verbal protocols to refine a preliminary model of Internet reading comprehension processes.* Paper presented at the meeting of the American Educational Research Association, Chicago.

Leu, D. J., Zawilininski, L., Castek, J., Banerjee, M., Housand, B., Liu, Y., et al. (in press). What is new about the new literacies of online reading comprehension? In A. Berger, L. Rush, & J. Eakle (Eds.), *Secondary school reading and writing: What research reveals for classroom practices.* Chicago: National Council of Teachers of English/National Conference on Research in Language and Literacy.

Lewandowski, L., & Arcangelo, K. (1994). The social adjustment and self-concept of adults with learning disabilities. *Journal of Learning Disabilities, 27*(9), 598–605.

Lewinsohn, P. M., Klein, D. N., & Seeley, J. R. (1995). Bipolar disorders in a community sample of older adolescents: Prevalence, phenomenology, comorbidity, and course. *Journal of the American Academy of Child and Adolescent Psychiatry, 34*, 454–463.

Lewis, P. A., & Miall, R. C. (2005). A right hemispheric prefrontal system for cognitive time measurement. *Behavioural Processes, 71*, 226–234.

Lewis, P. A., & Miall, R. C. (2006). Memory for time: A continuous clock. *Trends in Cognitive Sciences, 10*, 406–410.

Li, H., & Hamel, C. (2003). Writing issues in college students with learning disabilities: A synthesis of the literature from 1990 to 2000. *Learning Disability Quarterly, 26*, 29–46.

Liepmann, H. (1900). Das Krankheitsbild der Apraxie [The clinical profile of apraxia]. *Monatsschrift für Psychiatrie und Neurologie, 8*, 15–44, 102–132, 182–192.

Light, J., Pennington, B., Gilger, J., & DeFries, J. (1995). Reading disability and hyperactivity disorders: Evidence for a common genetic etiology. *Developmental Neuropsychiatry, 11*, 323–335.

Lincoln, A., Courchesne, E., Allen, M., Hanson, E. M., & Ene, M. (1998). Neurobiology of Asperger syndrome: Seven case studies and quantitative magnetic resonance imaging findings. In E. Schopler, G. Mesibov, & L. J. Kunce (Eds.), *Asperger syndrome or high functioning autism?* (pp. 145–166). New York: Plenum Press.

Lindstrom, J. H. (2006). *The role of extended time on the SAT reasoning test for students with disabilities.* Unpublished doctoral dissertation, University of Georgia.

Lindstrom, J., & Gregg, N. (2007). The role of extended time on the SAT Reasoning Test for students with learning disabilities and/or attention-deficit/hyperactivity disorder. *Learning Disabilities Research and Practice, 22*, 85–95.

Linn, R. L. (2002). Validation of the uses and interpretation of results of state assessments and accountability systems. In G. Tindal & T. M. Haladyna (Eds.), *Large-scale assessment programs for all students: Validity, technical adequacy, and implementation* (pp. 27–48). Mahwah, NJ: Erlbaum.

Lissitz, R. W., & Samuelsen, J. (2007). Dialogue on validity: A suggested change in terminology and emphasis regarding validity and education. *Educational Researcher, 39*, 437–448.

Livingstone, M. S., Rosen, G. D., Drislane, F. W., & Galaburda, A. M. (1991). Physiological and anatomical evidence for a magnocellular defect in developmental dyslexia. *Proceedings of the National Academy of Sciences USA, 88*, 7943–7947.

Lorch, E. P., Berthiaume, K. S., Milich, R., & van den Broek, P. (2007). Story comprehension impairments in children with attention-deficit/hyperactivity disorder. In K. Cain & J. Oakhill (Eds.), *Children's comprehension problems in oral and written language: A cognitive perspective* (pp. 128–156). New York: Guilford Press.

Love v. Law School Admission Council, Inc., 2007 WL 737788 (E.D. Pa. Mar. 9, 2007).

Lovett, B. J., & Lewandowski, L. J. (2006). Gifted students with learning disabilities: Who are they? *Journal of Learning Disabilities, 39,* 15–27.

Loyd, B. H. (1991). Mathematics test performance: The effects of item type and calculator use. *Applied Measurement in Education, 4,* 11–22.

Luke, A., & Elkins, J. (2000). Re/mediating adolescent literacies. *Journal of Adolescent and Adult Literacy, 43,* 396–398.

Luria, A. R. (1980). *Higher cortical functions in man* (2nd ed., B. Haigh, Trans.). New York: Basic Books.

Lustig, C., Matell, M. S., & Meck, W. H. (2005). Not "just" a coincidence: Frontal–striatal interactions in working memory and interval timing. *Memory, 13,* 441–448.

Maag, J. W., & Reid, R. (2006). Depression among students with learning disabilities: Assessing the risk. *Journal of Learning Disabilities, 39,* 3–10.

MacArthur, C. A. (2006). The effects of new technologies on writing and writing processes. In C. A. MacArthur, S. Graham, & J. Fitzgerald (Eds.), *Handbook of writing research* (pp. 248–262). New York: Guilford Press.

MacArthur, C. A., & Cavalier, A. (2004). Dictation and speech recognition technology as accommodations in large-scale assessments for students with learning disabilities. *Exceptional Children, 71,* 43–58.

MacArthur, C. A., Ferretti, R. P., Okolo, C. M., & Cavalier, A. R. (2001). Technology applications for students with literacy problems: A critical review. *Elementary School Journal, 101,* 273–301.

MacArthur, C. A., & Graham, S. (1987). Learning disabled students' composing under three methods of text production: Handwriting, word processing, and dictation. *Journal of Special Education, 21,* 22–42.

MacArthur, C. A., & Haynes, J. B. (1995). Student Assistant for Learning from Text (SALT): A hypermedia reading aid. *Journal of Learning Disabilities, 28,* 50–59.

Macintosh, K. E., & Dissanayake, C. (2004). Annotation: The similarities and differences between autistic disorder and Asperger's disorder: A review of the empirical evidence. *Journal of Child Psychology and Psychiatry, 45*(3), 421–434.

Madaus, J. W., & Shaw, S. (2007). Transition assessment. *Assessment for Effective Intervention, 32,* 130–132.

Magliano, J. P., Trabasso, T., & Graesser, A. C. (1999). Strategic processing during comprehension. *Journal of Educational Psychology, 91,* 615–629.

Mandinach, E. B., Bridgeman, B., Cahalan-Laitusis, C., & Trapani, C. (2005). *The impact of extended time on SAT test performance* (College Board Research Report No. 2005-8). New York: College Board.

Maniadaki, K., Sonuga-Barke, E., & Kakouros, E. (2006). Adults' self-efficacy beliefs and referral attitudes for boys and girls with AD/HD. *European Child and Adolescent Psychiatry, 15*(3), 132–140.

Mannuzza, S., Gittelman-Klein, R., Bessler, A., Malloy, P., & LaPadula, M. (1993). Adult outcome of hyperactive boys: Educational achievement, occupational rank, and psychiatric status. *Archives of General Psychiatry, 50,* 565–576.

Marin, L. T., Kubzansky, L. D., LeWinn, K. Z., Lipsitt, L. P., Satz, P., & Buka, S. L. (2007). Childhood cognitive performance and risk of generalized anxiety disorder. *International Journal of Epidemiology, 1,* 1–7.

Markus, H., & Wurf, E. (1987). The dynamic self-concept: A social psychological perspective. *Annual Review of Psychology, 38,* 299–337.

Markwardt, F. C. (1989). *Manual for the Peabody Individual Achievement Test— Revised/Normative Update (PIAT-R/NU).* Circle Pines, MN: American Guidance Service.

Masten, A. S. (2001). Ordinary magic: Resilience processes in development. *American Psychologist, 56*(3), 227–238.

Masten, A. S., Hubbard, J. J., Gest, S. D., Tellegen, A., Garmezy, N., & Ramirez, M. (1999). Competence in the context of adversity: Pathways to resilience and maladaptations from childhood to late adolescence. *Development and Psychopathology, 11,* 143–169.

Mastropieri, M. A., & Scruggs, T. E. (1992). Science for students with learning disabilities. *Review of Educational Research, 62,* 377–411.

Mather, N., & Gregg, N. (2006). Specific learning disabilities: Clarifying, not eliminating, a construct. *Professional Psychology: Research and Practice, 37,* 99–106.

Mather, N., Gregg, N., & Simon, J. (2005). The curse of high stakes tests and high abilities: Reactions to *Wong v. Regents of the University of California. Learning Disabilities: A Multidisciplinary Journal, 13,* 139–144.

Mather, N., & Kaufman, N. (Eds.). (2006a). Integration of cognitive assessment and response to intervention [Special issue, Part One]. *Psychology in the Schools, 43*(7).

Mather, N., & Kaufman, N. (Eds.). (2006b). Integration of cognitive assessment and response to intervention [Special issue, Part Two]. *Psychology in the Schools, 43*(8).

Mather, N., & Woodcock, R. (2001). *Woodcock–Johnson III Tests of Achievement: Handwriting Analysis scale: Examiner's manual.* Itasca, IL: Riverside.

Matteucci, N., O'Mahony, M., Robinson, C., & Zwick, T. (2005). Productivity, workplace performance and ICT: Industry and firm-level evidence for Europe and the U.S. *Scottish Journal of Political Economy, 52,* 359–386.

Mazzocco, M. M. M., Murphy, M. M., & McCloskey, M. (2007). The contribution of syndrome research to understanding mathematical learning disability: The case of fragile X and Turner syndromes. In D. B. Berch & M. M. M. Mazzocco (Eds.), *Why is math so hard for some children?: The nature and origins of mathematical learning difficulties and disabilities* (pp. 173–194). Baltimore: Brookes.

McCloskey, M. (2007). Quantitative literacy and developmental dyscalculias. In D. B. Berch & M. M. M. Mazzocco (Eds.), *Why is math so hard for some children?: The nature and origins of mathematical learning difficulties and disabilities* (pp. 415–430). Baltimore: Brookes.

McCutchen, D. (2006). Cognitive factors in the development of children's writing. In C. A. MacArthur, S. Graham, & J. Fitzgerald (Eds.), *Handbook of writing research* (pp. 115–130). New York: Guilford Press.

McGee, R., & Share, D. L. (1988). Attention deficit disorder–hyperactivity and academic failure: Which comes first and what should be treated? *Journal of the American Academy of Child and Adolescent Psychiatry, 27*, 318–327.

McGrew, K., & Woodcock, R. W. (2001). *Woodcock–Johnson III technical manual.* Itasca, IL: Riverside.

McGrew, K. S. (1997). Analysis of the major intelligence batteries according to a proposed comprehensive Gf-Gc framework. In D. P. Flanagan, J. L. Genshaft, & P. L. Harrison (Eds.), *Contemporary intellectual assessment: Theories, tests, and issues* (pp. 151–180). New York: Guilford Press.

McGrew, K. S. (2005). The Cattell–Horn–Carroll theory of cognitive abilities: Past, present, and future. In D. P. Flanagan & P. L. Harrison (Eds.), *Contemporary intellectual assessment: Theories, tests, and issues* (2nd ed., pp. 136–182). New York: Guilford Press.

McGrew, K. S., & Flanagan, D. P. (1998). *The intelligence test desk reference: Gf-Gc cross-battery assessment.* Boston: Allyn & Bacon.

McGrew, K. S., Woodcock, R. W., & Ford, L. (2002). The Woodcock–Johnson Battery—Third Edition (WJ III). In A. S. Kaufman & E. O. Lichtenberger (Eds.), *Assessing adolescent and adult intelligence* (2nd ed.). Boston: Allyn & Bacon.

McIntyre, L. L. (1988). Teacher gender: A predictor of special education referral? *Journal of Learning Disabilities, 21*, 382–383.

McLaughlin, M. J., Embler, S., & Nagle, K. (2004). *Students with disabilities and accountability: The promise and the realities should there be alternatives* (Prepared for Center on Education Policy). Retrieved August 1, 2006, from *www.ncrel.org/sdrs/areas/issues/methods/technlgy/te8refer*

McNamara, D. S., Ozuru, Y., Best, R., & O'Reilly, T. (2007). The 4-pronged comprehension strategy framework. In D. S. McNamara (Ed.), *Reading comprehension strategies: Theories, interventions, and technology* (pp. 465–496). Mahwah, NJ: Erlbaum.

McNamara, J. K., Willoughby, T., Chalmers, H., & Youth Lifestyle Choices–Community University Research Alliance. (2005). Psychosocial status of adolescents with learning disabilities with and without comorbid attention deficit hyperactivity disorders. *Learning Disabilities Research and Practice, 20*(4), 234–244.

McPhail, J. C., & Stone, C. A. (1995). The self-concept of adolescents with learning disabilities: A review of the literature and a call for theoretical elaboration. In T. E. Scruggs & M. A. Mastropieri (Eds.), *Advances in learning and behavioral disabilities* (Vol. 9, pp. 193–226). Greenwich, CT: JAI Press.

Meade, A. W., & Lautenschlager, G. J. (2004). A Monte Carlo study of confirmatory factor analytic tests of measurement equivalence/invariance. *Structural Equation Modeling, 11*(1), 60–72.

Mellard, D., Patterson, M. B., & Prewett, S. (2007). Reading practices among adult education participants. *Reading Research Quarterly, 42*, 188–213.

Meltzer, L. J., Katzir, T., Miller, L., Reddy, R., & Roditi, B. (2004). Academic self-perceptions, effort, and strategy use in students with learning disabilities: Changes over time. *Learning Disabilities Research and Practice, 19*(2), 99–108.

Meltzer, L. J., Roditi, B., Houser, R. F., & Perlman, M. (1998). Perceptions of academic strategies and competence in students with learning disabilities. *Journal of Learning Disabilities, 31,* 437–451.

Messick, S. (1995). Validity of psychological assessment: Validation of inferences from persons' responses and performances as scientific inquiry into score meaning. *American Psychologist, 50,* 741–749.

Michaels, S. (1987). "Sharing time": Children's narrative styles and differential access to literacy. *Language in Society, 10,* 423–442.

Microsoft. (2002). *Accessible technology in today's business.* Redmond, WA: Author.

Milberger, S., Biederman, J., Faraone, S. V., Murphy, J., & Tsuang, M. T. (1995). Attention deficit hyperactivity disorder and comorbid disorders: Issues of overlapping symptoms. *American Journal of Psychiatry, 152,* 1873–1800.

Miller, S. P. (1996). Perspectives on mathematics instruction. In D. D. Deshler, E. S. Ellis, & K. Lenz (Eds.), *Teaching adolescents with learning disabilities: Strategies and methods* (2nd ed., pp. 313–367). Denver, CO: Love.

Moll, L. (Ed.). (1990). *Vygotsky and education: Instructional applications of sociohistorical psychology.* Cambridge, UK: Cambridge University Press.

Monastra, V. J., Lubar, J. F., & Linden, M. (2001). The development of a quantitative electroencephalographic scanning process for attention deficit-hyperactivity disorders: Reliability and validity studies. *Neuropsychology, 15*(1), 136–144.

Morgan, D. L., & Huff, K. (2002). *Reliability and dimensionality of the SAT for examinees tested under standard timing conditions and examinees tested with extended time* (Unpublished research report). Princeton, NJ: Educational Testing Service.

Morocco, C. C., Aguilar, C. M., Clay, K., Brigham, N., & Zigmond, N. (2006). Good high schools for students with disabilities: Introduction to the special issue. *Learning Disabilities Research and Practice, 21*(3), 135–145.

Mortensen, T. (2001, October). *High school graduation rate by family income quartile for dependent 18–24 year olds* [Graph]. Oskaloosa, IA: Postsecondary Education Opportunity. Retrieved from *www.postsecondary.org*

Munger, G. F., & Loyd, B. H. (1991). Effect of speededness on test performance of handicapped and nonhandicapped examinees. *Journal of Educational Research, 85,* 53–57.

Murphy, K. R. (2006). Psychological counseling of adults with ADHD. In R. A. Barkley, *Attention-deficit hyperactivity disorder: A handbook for diagnosis and treatment* (3rd ed., pp. 692–703). New York: Guilford Press.

Murphy, K. R., & Barkley, R. A. (1996). Prevalence of DSM-IV symptoms of ADHD in adult licensed drivers: Implications for clinical diagnosis. *Journal of Attention Disorders, 1,* 147–161.

Murphy, K. R., Barkley, R. A., & Bush, T. (2002). Young adults with ADHD: Subtype differences in comorbidity, educational, and clinical history. *Journal of Nervous and Mental Disease, 190,* 147–157.

Murphy, K. R., & Gordon, M. (2006). Assessment of adults with ADHD. In R. A. Barkley, *Attention-deficit hyperactivity disorder: A handbook for diagnosis and treatment* (3rd ed., pp. 425–453). New York: Guilford Press.

Murphy, M. M., Mazzocco, M. M. M., Hanich, L. B., & Early, M. C. (2007). Cognitive characteristics of children with mathematics learning disability (MLD) vary as a function of the cutoff criterion used to define MLD. *Journal of Learning Disabilities, 40,* 458–478.

Murray, C., & Naranjo, J. (2008). Poor, black, learning disabled, and graduating: An investigation of factors and processes associated with school completion among high-risk urban youth. *Remedial and Special Education, 29*(3), 145–160.

Murray, D. (1978). Internal revision: A process of discovery. In C. Cooper & L. Odell (Eds.), *Research on composing: Points of departure* (pp. 85–103). Urbana, IL: National Council of Teachers of English.

Myklebust, H. R. (1965). *Development and disorders of written language: Studies of normal and exceptional children.* New York: Grune & Stratton.

Myklebust, H. R. (1975). Nonverbal learning disabilities. In H. R. Myklebust (Ed.), *Progress in learning disabilities* (Vol. 3, pp. 85–121). New York: Grune & Stratton.

Nagarajan, S., Mahncke, H., Salz, T., Tallal, P., Roberts, T., & Merzenich, M. (1999). Cortical auditory signal processing in poor readers. *Proceedings of the National Academy of Sciences USA, 96,* 6483–6488.

Nagy, W., Berninger, V., Abbott, R., Vaughan, K., & Vermeulen, K. (2003). Relationship of morphology and other language skills to literacy skills in at-risk second graders and at-risk fourth grade writers. *Journal of Educational Psychology, 95,* 730–742.

Nagy, W. E., Anderson, R., Schommer, M., Scott, J., & Stallman, A. C. (1989). Morphological families and word recognition. *Reading Research Quarterly, 24,* 262–282.

Naiden, N. (1976). Ratio of boys to girls among disabled readers. *The Reading Teacher, 92,* 432–442.

Nation, K., Adams, J. W., Bowyer-Crane, A., & Snowling, M. J. (1999). Working memory deficits in poor comprehenders reflect underlying language impairments. *Journal of Experimental Child Psychology, 73,* 139–158.

Nation, K., & Snowling, M. J. (1998). Semantic processing and the development of word-recognition skills: Evidence from children with reading comprehension difficulties. *Journal of Memory and Language, 37,* 85–101.

National Association for College Admission Counseling. (2006). *State of college admission.* Retrieved April 2007, from *www.nacacnet.org*

National Center for Education Statistics (NCES). (2007). *The condition of education 2007 in brief.* Retrieved May 2007, from *www.nces.ed.gov/programs/coe*

National Commission on Writing for America's Families, Schools, and Colleges. (2003). *The neglected "R": The need for a writing revolution.* New York: College Board.

National Commission on Writing for America's Families, Schools, and Colleges. (2004). *Writing: A ticket to work . . . or a ticket out: A survey of business leaders.* New York: College Board.

National Commission on Writing for America's Families, Schools, and Colleges. (2005). *Writing: A powerful message from state government.* New York: College Board.

National Council on Disability. (2003, May). *Addressing the needs of youth with disabilities in the juvenile justice system: The current status of evidence-based research.* Retrieved February 1, 2005, from *www.ncd.gov/newsroom/publications/2003/juvenile.htm*

National High School Alliance. (2005). *A call to action: Transforming high school for all youth.* Washington, DC: Institute for Educational Leadership. Available at *www.iel.org.*

National Joint Committee on Learning Disabilities (NCJLD). (1997). *Operationalizing the NJCLD definition of learning disabilities for ongoing assessment.* Retrieved July 17, 2006, from *www.ldonline.org/nicld/operationalizing.html*

National Joint Committee on Learning Disabilities (NJCLD). (2007). *The documentation disconnect for students with learning disabilities: Improving access to postsecondary disability services.* Retrieved July 2007 from *www.ldonline.org*

National Reading Panel. (2000). *Teaching children to read: An evidence-based assessment of the scientific research literature on reading and its implications for reading instruction.* Washington, DC: National Institute of Child Health and Human Development, National Institutes of Health.

National Science Foundation. (2006). *Women, minorities, and persons with disabilities in science and engineering.* Available at *www.nsf.gov/statistical/wmpd/disablity/htm#underenroll*

National Transition Assessment Summit. (2005). *Nationally ratified summary of performance template.* Retrieved June 5, 2007, from *www.unr.edu/educ/ceds*

Neisser, U., Boodoo, G., Bouchard, T. J., Boykin, A. W., Brody, N., Ceci, S. J., et al. (1996). Intelligence: Knowns and unknowns. *American Psychologist, 51,* 77–101.

Nelson, J. M., Canivez, G. L., Lindstrom, W., & Hatt, C. V. (2007). Higher-order exploratory factor analysis of the Reynolds Intellectual Assessment Scales with a referred sample. *Journal of School Psychology, 45,* 439–456.

Nelson, J., Denis, D., Canivez, G. L., & Hatt, C. V. (2007). *Hierarchical confirmatory factor analysis of the Reynolds Intellectual Assessment Scales using a learning disabled sample.* Unpublished manuscript, University of Georgia.

New Literacies Research Team. (2007). New literacies, new challenges, and new opportunities. In M. B. Sampson, S. Szabo, F. Falk-Ross, M. M. Foote, & P. E. Linder (Eds.), *Multiple literacies in the 21st century: The twenty-eighth yearbook of the College Reading Association* (pp. 31–50). Logan, UT: College Reading Association.

New London Group. (2000). A pedagogy of multiliteracies: Designing social futures. In B. Cope & M. Kalantzis (Eds.), *Multiliteracies: Literacy learning and the design of social futures* (pp. 9–38). London: Routledge.

Nicolson, R. I., Fawcett, A. J., Berry, E. L., Jenkins, I. H., Dean, P., & Brooks, D. J. (1999). Association of abnormal cerebellar activation with motor learning difficulties in dyslexic adults. *Lancet, 353,* 1662–1667.

Nigg, J. T., Goldsmith, H. H., & Sacheck, J. (2004). Temperament and attention deficit hyperactivity disorders: The development of a multiple pathway model. *Journal of Clinical Child and Adolescent Psychology, 33,* 42–53.

No Child Left Behind (NCLB) Act of 2001, Public Law No. 107-110, 115 Stat. 1425 (2002).

Noeth, R., & Wimberly, G. (2002). *Creating seamless educational transitions for urban African American and Hispanic students* (ACT Policy Report). Iowa City, Iowa: ACT.

Norman, S., Kiemper, S., & Kynette, D. (1992). Adults' reading comprehension: Effects of syntactic complexity and working memory. *Journal of Gerontology, 47,* 258–265.

Ofiesh, N., Mather, N., & Russell, A. (2005). Using speeded cognitive, reading, and academic measures to determine the need for extended test time among university students with learning disabilities. *Journal of Psychoeducational Assessment, 23,* 35–52.

Olson, C., & Land, R. (2007). A cognitive strategies approach to reading and writing instruction for English language learners in secondary school. *Research in the Teaching of English, 41*(30), 269–303.

Olson, R. K. (2007). Introduction to the special issue on genes, environment, and reading. *Reading and Writing, 20,* 1–11.

Olson, R. K., Forsberg, H., & Wise, B. (1994). Genes, environment, and the development of orthographic skills. In V. W. Berninger (Ed.), *The varieties of orthographic knowledge: Vol. 1. Theoretical and developmental issues* (pp. 27–71). Dordrecht, The Netherlands: Kluwer Academic.

Osmon, D. C., Plambeck, E., Klein, L., & Mano, Q. (2006). The Word Reading Test of effort in adult learning disability: A simulation study. *The Clinical Neuropsychologist, 20,* 315–324.

Osmon, D., Smerz, J. M., Braun, M. M., & Plambeck, E. (2006). Processing abilities associated with math skills in adult learning disability. *Journal of Clinical and Experimental Neuropsychiatry, 28,* 1–12.

Padget, S. Y. (1998). Lessons from research on dyslexia: Implications for a classification system for learning disabilities. *Learning Disability Quarterly, 21,* 167–178.

Pagani, L., Tremblay, R., Vitaro, F., Boulerice, B., & McDuff, P. (2001). Effects of grade retention on academic performance and behavioral development. *Development and Psychopathology, 13,* 297–315.

Pajares, F., & Valiante, G. (2006). Self-efficacy beliefs and motivation in writing development. In C. A. MacArthur, S. Graham, & J. Fitzgerald (Eds.), *Handbook of writing research* (pp. 158–170). New York: Guilford Press.

Paris, S. G. (2005). Reinterpreting the development of reading skills. *Reading Research Quarterly, 40,* 184–202.

Paris, S. G., & Stahl, S. S. (Eds.). (2005). *Children's reading comprehension and assessment.* Mahwah, NJ: Erlbaum.

Parker, R. I., Tindal, G., & Hasbrouck, J. (1989). Initial validation of two classroom-based measures of reading comprehension. *Diagnostique, 14,* 222–240.

Patton, J. R., Cronin, M. E., Bassett, D. S., & Koppel, A. E. (1997). A life skills approach to mathematics instruction: Preparing students with learning disabilities for the real-life math demands of adulthood. *Journal of Learning Disabilities, 30,* 178–187.

Pearson, P. D., & Hamm, D. N. (2005). The assessment of reading comprehension: A review of practices—past, present, and future. In S. G. Paris & S. S. Stahl (Eds.), *Children's reading comprehension and assessment* (pp. 13–69). Mahwah, NJ: Erlbaum.

Pennington, B. F., & Olson, R. K. (2005). Genetics of dyslexia. In M. Snowling & C. Hulme (Eds.), *The science of reading: A handbook* (pp. 453–472). Oxford, UK: Blackwell.

Perels, F., Gurtler, T., & Schmits, B. (2005). Training of self-regulation and problem solving. *Learning and Instruction, 15*(2), 123–139.

Perfetti, C. A. (1985). *Reading ability.* New York: Oxford University Press.

Perfetti, C. A. (2007). Reading ability: Lexical quality to comprehension. *Scientific Studies of Reading, 11,* 357–383.

Perfetti, C. A., Marron, M. A., & Foltz, P. W. (1996). Sources of comprehension failure: Theoretical perspectives and case studies. In C. Coroldi & J. Oakhill (Eds.), *Reading comprehension difficulties: Processes and intervention* (pp. 137–165). Mahwah, NJ: Erlbaum.

Peterson, B. S., Pine, D. S., Cohen, P., & Brook, J. S. (2001). Prospective, longitudinal study of tic, obsessive–compulsive, and attention deficit/hyperactivity disorders in an epidemiological sample. *Journal of the American Academy of Child and Adolescent Psychiatry, 40,* 685–695.

Pfiffner, L. J., Barkley, R. A., & DuPaul, J. G. (2006). Treatment of ADHD in school settings. In R. A. Barkley, *Attention-deficit hyperactivity disorder: A handbook for diagnosis and treatment* (3rd ed., pp. 547–589). New York: Guilford Press.

Pfiffner, L. J., McBurnett, K., Lahey, B. B., Loeber, R., Green, S., Frick, P. J., et al. (1999). Association of parental psychopathology to the comorbid disorders of boys with attention-deficit hyperactivity disorder. *Journal of Consulting and Clinical Psychology, 67,* 881–893.

Phelps, L. A., & Hanley-Maxwell, C. (1997). School-to-work transitions for youth with disabilities: A review of outcomes and practices. *Review of Educational Research, 67,* 197–226.

Piaget, J. (1972). Intellectual evolution from adolescence to adulthood. *Human Development, 15,* 1–12.

Pintrich, P. R. (2000). The role of goal orientation in self-regulated learning. In M. Boekaerts, P. Pintrich, & M. Zeidner (Eds.), *Handbook of self-regulation* (pp. 452–502). San Diego, CA: Academic Press.

Pitoniak, M., & Royer, J. (2001). Testing accommodations for examinees with disabilities: A review of psychometric, legal, and social policy issues. *Review of Educational Research, 71*(1), 53–104.

Postle, B. R. (2006). Working memory as an emergent property of the mind and brain. *Neuroscience, 139,* 23–38.

Price et al. v. National Board of Medical Examiners, 1997 WL 323998 (S.D. W. Va. June 6, 1997).

Prior, P. (2006). A sociocultural theory of writing. In C. A. MacArthur, S. Graham, & J. Fitzgerald (Eds.), *Handbook of writing research* (pp. 54–66). New York: Guilford Press.

Proctor, B. E., Floyd, R. G., & Shaver, R. B. (2005). Cattell–Horn–Carroll broad cognitive ability profiles of low math achievers. *Psychology in the Schools, 42,* 1–11.

Prout, H. T., Marcal, S. D., & Marcal, D. C. (1992). A meta-analysis of self-reported personality characteristics of children and adolescents with learning disabilities. *Journal of Psychoeducational Assessment, 10*(1), 59–64.

Pugh, K., Mencl, W., Shaywitz, B., Shaywitz, S., Fulbright, R., Constable, R., et al. (2000). The angular gyrus in developmental dyslexia: Task-specific differences in functional connectivity within posterior cortex. *Psychological Science, 11,* 51–56.

Ramaa, S., & Gowramma, I. P. (2002). A systematic procedure for identifying and classifying children with dyscalculia among primary school children in India. *Dyslexia, 8,* 67–88.

Ramus, E. (2001). Dyslexia: Talk of two theories. *Nature, 412,* 393–395.

Ramus, F., Rosen, S., Dakin, S. C., Day, B. L., Castellote, J. M., White, S., et al. (2003). Theories of developmental dyslexia: Insights from a multiple case study of dyslexic adults. *Brain, 126,* 841–865.

RAND Reading Study Group. (2003). *Reading for understanding: Toward an R & D program in reading comprehension.* Santa Monica, CA: RAND.

Rasch, G. (1980). *Probabilistic models for some intelligence and attainment tests.* Chicago: University of Chicago Press.

Rasmussen, K., Almik, R., & Levander, S. (2001). Attention-deficit hyperactivity disorder, reading disabilities, and personality disorders in a prison population. *Journal of the American Academy of Psychiatry and the Law, 29,* 186–193.

Ray, N. J., Fowler, S., & Stein, J. F. (2005). Yellow filters can improve magnocellular function: Motion sensitivity convergence, accommodation and reading. *Annals of the New York Academy of Sciences, 1039,* 283–293.

Rayner, K. (1978). Eye movements in reading and information processing. *Psychological Bulletin, 85,* 618–660.

Recht, D. R., & Leslie, V. (1988). Effects of prior knowledge on good and poor readers memory of text. *Journal of Educational Psychology, 33,* 477–514.

Reese, J. E., & Cummings, G. (1996). Evaluating speech-based composition methods: Planning, dictation, and the listening word processor. In C. M. Levy & S. Ransdell (Eds.), *The science of writing: Theories, methods, individual differences, and applications* (pp. 361–380). Mahwah, NJ: Erlbaum.

Rehabilitation Act of 1973, Public Law No. 93-112, 87 Stat. 355 (1973).

Rehabilitation Act Amendments of 1992, Public Law No. 102-569, 106 Stat. 4430 (1992).

Rehabilitation Act Amendments of 1998: Incorporated into Workforce Investment Act of 1998, Public Law No. 105-220, 112 Stat. 936 (1998).

Reiff, H. B., & Gerber, P. J. (1995). Social/emotional and daily living issues for adults with learning disabilities. In P. J. Gerber & H. B. Reiff (Eds.), *Learning disabilities in adulthood: Persisting problems and evolving issues* (pp. 72–81). Austin, TX: Pro-ED.

Reinking, D. (1998). Synthesizing technological transformation in a post-typographic world. In D. Reinking, M. McKenna, L. Labbo, & R. Kiefer (Eds.), *Handbook of literacy and technology: Transformation in a post-typographic world* (pp. xi–xx). Mahwah, NJ: Erlbaum.

Repovs, G., & Baddeley, A. (2006). The multi-component model of working memory: Explorations in experimental cognitive psychology. *Neuroscience, 139,* 5–21.

Reynolds, A. W. (1999). *High risk college students with emotional disorders as well as learning disabilities.* Unpublished doctoral dissertation, University of Georgia.

Reynolds, C. R., & Kamphaus, R. W. (2003). *Reynolds Intellectual Assessment Scales (RIAS).* Lutz, FL: Psychological Assessment Resources.

Reynolds, C. R., & Kamphaus, R. W. (2004). *Behavior Assessment System for Children—Second Edition (BASC-2).* Circle Pines, MN: American Guidance Service.

Reynolds, T. H., & Bonk, C. J. (1996). Facilitating college writers' revisions within a generative–evaluative computerized prompting framework. *Computers and Composition, 13,* 93–108.

Riccio, C. A., Reynolds, C. R., & Lowe, P. A. (2001). *Clinical applications of continuous performance tests: Measuring attention and impulsive responding in children and adults.* New York: Wiley.

Richters, J. E., & Martinez, P. E. (1993). Violent communities, family choices, and children's chances: An algorithm for improving the odds. *Development and Psychopathology, 5,* 609–627.

Roach, N. W., & Hogben, J. H. (2004). Attentional modulation of visual processing in adult dyslexia: A spatial cuing deficit. *Psychological Science, 15,* 650–654.

Roberts, R., & Mather, N. (1997). Orthographic dyslexia: The neglected subtype. *Learning Disabilities Research and Practice, 12*(4), 236–250.

Robinson, G. L., & Conway, R. N. F. (2000). Irlen lenses and adults: A small-scale stud of reading speed, accuracy comprehension and self-image. *Australian Journal of Learning Disabilities, 5,* 4–12.

Robison, L. M., Skaer, T. L., Sclar, D. A., & Galin, R. S. (2002). Is attention deficit hyperactivity disorder increasing among girls in the U.S.? *CNS Drugs, 16,* 129–137.

Rogan, L. L., & Hartman, L. D. (1990). Adult outcome of learning disabled students ten years after initial follow-up. *Learning Disabilities Focus, 5,* 91–102.

Rogers, R. (2008). *Clinical assessment of malingering and deception* (3rd ed.). New York: Guilford Press.

Roid, G. H. (2003). *Stanford–Binet Intelligence Scales, Fifth Edition.* Itasca, IL: Riverside.

Roid, G. H., & Pomplun, M. (2005). Interpreting the Stanford–Binet Intelligence Scales, Fifth Edition. In D. P. Flanagan & P. L. Harrison (Eds.), *Contemporary intellectual assessment: Theories, tests, and issues* (2nd ed., pp. 325–343). New York: Guilford Press.

Rojewski, J. W., & Kim, H. (2003). Career choice patterns and behavior of work-bound youth during early adolescence. *Journal of Career Development, 30,* 89–108.

Rosaen, C. (2003). Preparing teachers for divers classrooms: Creating public and private spaces to explore culture through poetry writing. *Teachers College Record, 105,* 1437–1485.

Rosenblum, S., Weiss, P. L., & Parush, S. (2004). Handwriting evaluation for developmental dysgraphia: Process versus product. *Reading and Writing: An Interdisciplinary Journal, 17,* 433–458.

Ross-Gordon, J. M. (1996). Sociocultural issues affecting the identification and service delivery models for adults with learning disabilities. In N. Gregg, C. Hoy, & A. Gay (Eds.), *Adults with learning disabilities: Theoretical and practical perspectives* (pp. 85–126). New York: Guilford Press.

Rothman, H., & Cosden, M. (1995). The relationship between self-perception of a learning disability and achievement, self-concept, and social support. *Learning Disability Quarterly, 18,* 203–221.

Rothstein, L. R. (2002). Judicial intent and legal precedents. In L. Brincker-hoff, J. McGuire, & S. Shaw (Eds.), *Postsecondary education and transition for students with learning disabilities* (pp. 71–106). Austin, TX: Pro-Ed.

Rourke, B. (1989). *Nonverbal learning disabilities: The syndrome and the model.* New York: Guilford Press.

Rourke, B. (Ed.). (1995). *Syndrome of nonverbal learning disabilities: Neurodevelopmental manifestations.* New York: Guilford Press.

Rourke, B. P., & Conway, J. A. (1997). Disabilities of arithmetic and mathematical reasoning: Perspectives from neurology and neuropsychology. *Journal of Learning Disabilities, 30,* 34–46.

Rowley, K., Carsons, P., & Miller, T. (1998). A cognitive technology to teach composition skills: Four studies with the R-WISE writing tutor. *Journal of Educational Computing Research, 18,* 259–296.

Rowley, K., & Meyer, N. (2003). The effect of a computer tutor for writers on student writing achievement. *Journal of Educational Computing Research, 29,* 169–187.

Roy-Byrne, P., Scheele, L., Brinkley, J., Ward, N., Wiatrak, C., Russo, J., et al. (1997). Adult attention-deficit hyperactivity disorder: Assessment guidelines based on clinical presentation to a specialty clinic. *Comprehensive Psychiatry, 38,* 133–140.

Rubin, D. (1984). Social cognition and written communication. *Written Communication, 1*(2), 211–245.

Rubin, D., & Looney, J. (1990). Facilitation of audience awareness: Revision processes of basic writers. In G. Kirsch, & D. Roen (Eds.), *A sense of audience in written communication* (pp. 280–292). Newbury Park, CA: Sage.

Rubin, L. M., McCoach, B., McGuire, J. M., & Reis, S. M. (2003). The differential impact of academic self-regulatory methods on academic achievement among university students with and without learning disabilities. *Journal of Learning Disabilities, 36,* 270–286.

Rucklidge, J. J., & Tannock, R. (2002). Neuropsychological profiles of adolescents with ADHD: Effects of reading difficulties and gender. *Journal of Child Psychology and Psychiatry, 43,* 988–1003.

Rumelhart, D. E. (1994). Toward an interactive model of reading. In R. B. Ruddell, M. R. Ruddell, & H. Singer (Eds.), *Theoretical models and processes of reading* (4th ed., pp. 864–894). Newark, DE: International Reading Association.

Rumsey, M. H., Donohue, C., Nace, K., Maisong, M., & Andreason, P. (1997). Phonological and orthographic components of word recognition: A PET-rCBF scan study. *Brain, 120,* 739–759.

Russell, B., & Cook, C. (2002). *Meta-analysis: Writing with computers 1992–2002.* Chestnut Hill, MA: Boston College, Technology and Assessment Study Collaborative. Retrieved September 1, 2004, from *www.intasc.org*

Salahu-Din, D., Persky, H., & Miller, J. (2008). *The nation's report card: Writing 2007* (NCES Publication No. 2008-468). Washington, D.C.: U.S. Department of Education, National Center for Education Statistics. Retrieved April 16, 2008, from *nces.ed.gov/nationsreportcard/pubs/main2007/2008468. asp*

Samuels, S. J. (1982). Understanding the reading process. *School Psychology Review, 11,* 230–238.

Scheuneman, J. D., Camara, W. J., Cascallar, C. W., & Lawrence, I. (2002). Calculator access, use, and type in relation to performance on the SAT I: Reasoning test in mathematics. *Applied Measurement in Education, 15,* 95–112.

Schiff, R., & Raveh, M. (2006). Deficient morphological processing in adults with developmental dyslexia: Another barrier to efficient word recognition. *Dyslexia, 13,* 110–129.

Schmidt, M. H., & Moll, G. H. (1995). The course of hyperkinetic disorders and symptoms: A ten-year prospective longitudinal field study. In J. Sergeant (Ed.), *Eunethydis: European approaches to hyperkinetic disorder* (pp. 191–207). Amsterdam: University of Amsterdam.

Schrank, F., Miller, J., Caterino, L. C., & Desrochers, J. (2006). American Academy of School Psychology survey on the independent educational evaluation for a specific learning disability: Results and discussion. *Psychology in the Schools, 43,* 771–780.

Schrank, F. A., Telgasi, H., Wolf, L. L., Miller, J., Caterino, L. C., & Reynolds, C. R. (2005). American Academy of School Psychologists reply to the response-to-intervention perspective. *The School Psychologist, 58*(1), 30–33.

Schraw, G., & Dennison, R. (1994). Assessing metacognitive awareness. *Contemporary Educational Psychology, 19,* 460–475.

Schumaker, J. B., & Deshler, D. D. (1992). Validation of learning strategy interventions for students with learning disabilities. Results of a programmatic research effort. In B. Y. L. Wong (Ed.), *Contemporary intervention research in learning disabilities: An international perspective* (pp. 22–46). New York: Springer-Verlag.

Schumaker, J., & Deshler, D. (2006). Teaching adolescents to be strategic learners. In D. Deshler & J. Schumaker (Eds.), *Teaching adolescents with disabilities: Accessing the general education curriculum* (pp. 128–156). Thousand Oaks, CA: Corwin Press.

Schunk, D. H., & Zimmerman, B. J. (1998). *Self-regulated learning: From teaching to self-reflective practice.* New York: Guilford Press.

Schwarzer, R., & Born, A. (1997). Optimistic self-beliefs: Assessment of general perceived self-efficacy in thirteen cultures. *World Psychology, 3,* 177–190.

Schweitzer, J. B., & Sulzer-Azaroff, B. (1995). Self-control in boys with attention-deficit hyperactivity disorder: Effects of added stimulation and time. *Journal of Child Psychology and Psychiatry, 36,* 671–686.

Scott, S. (2002). The dynamic process of providing accommodations. In L. C. Brinckerhoff, J. M. McGuire, & S. Shaw (Eds.), *Postsecondary education and transition for students with learning disabilities* (pp. 295–332). Austin, TX: Pro-ED.

Scruggs, T. E., & Mastropieri, M. A. (2002). On babies and bathwater: Addressing the problems of identification of learning disabilities. *Learning Disability Quarterly, 25,* 155–168.

Semrud-Clikeman, M., Biederman, J., Sprich-Buckminster, S., Lehman, B. K., Faraone, S. V., & Norman, D. (1992). Comorbidity between ADHD and learning disability: A review and report in a clinically referred sample. *Journal of the American Academy of Child and Adolescent Psychiatry, 31,* 439–448.

Semrud-Clikeman, M., Guy, K., Griffin, J. D., & Hynd, G. W. (2000). Rapid naming deficits in children and adolescents with reading disabilities and attention deficit hyperactivity disorder. *Brain and Language, 74,* 70–83.

Serafini, S., Steury, K., Richards, T., Corina, D., Abbott, R., & Berninger, V. (2001). Comparison of FMRI and FMR spectroscopic imaging during language processing in children. *Magnetic Resonance in Medicine, 45,* 217–225.

Shalev, R. S., Manor, O., & Gross-Tsur, V. (2005). Developmental dyscalculia: A prospective six-year follow-up. *Developmental Medicine and Child Neurology, 47,* 121–125.

Shanahan, T. (2006). Relations among oral language, reading, and writing development. In C. A. MacArthur, S. Graham, & J. Fitzgerald (Eds.), *Handbook of writing research* (pp. 171–186). New York: Guilford Press.

Shanahan, T., Kamil, M. L., & Tobin, A. W. (1984). The relationship of concurrent and construct validities to cloze. *National Reading Conference Yearbook, 33,* 252–256.

Shaywitz, S. E. (2003). *Overcoming dyslexia: A new and complete science-based program for reading problems at any level.* New York: Knopf.

Shaywitz, S. E., Shaywitz, B. A., Fletcher, J. M., & Escobar, M. D. (1990). Prevalence of reading disabilities in boys and girls: Results of the Connecticut Longitudinal Study. *Journal of the American Medical Association, 264*(8), 998–1002.

Shaywitz, S. E., Shaywitz, B. A., Fulbright, R. K., Skudlarski, P., Mencl, W. E., Constable, R. T., et al. (2003). Neural systems for compensation and persistence: Young adult outcome of childhood reading disability. *Biological Psychiatry, 54,* 25–33.

Shea, V., & Mesibov, G. (2005). Adolescents and adults with autism. In F. R. Volkmar, P. Rhea, A. Klin, & D. Cohen (Eds.), *Handbook of autism and pervasive developmental disorders: Diagnosis, development, neurobiology, and behavior* (Vol. 1, pp. 288–311). New York: Wiley.

Shepard, L., Taylor, G., & Betebenner, D. (1998). *Inclusion of limited-English-proficient students in Rhode Island's Grade 4 mathematics performance assessment.* Los Angeles: University of California, Center for the Study of Evaluation/National Center for Research on Evaluation, Standards, and Student Testing.

Shiner, R., Tellegen, A., & Masten, A. S. (2003). Childhood personality foreshadows adult personality and life outcomes two decades later. *Journal of Personality, 71*(6), 1145–1170.

Shinn, M. R., Good, R. H., Knutson, N., Tilly, W. D., & Collins, V. L. (1992). Curriculum-based measurement of oral reading fluency: A confirmatory analysis of its relation to reading. *School Psychology Review, 21,* 459–479.

Shinn, M. R., Tindal, G. A., & Spira, D. A. (1987). Special education referral as an index of teacher tolerance: Are teachers imperfect tests? *Exceptional Children, 54,* 32–40.

Siegel, L. S. (1990). IQ and learning disabilities: R.I.P. In H. L. Swanson & B. Keogh (Eds.), *Learning disabilities: Theoretical and research issues* (pp. 111–128). Hillsdale, NJ: Erlbaum.

Singleton, C., & Henderson, L. (2007). Computerized screening for visual stress in reading. *Journal of Research in Reading, 30*(3), 316–331.

Sireci, S. G. (2004). *Validity issues in accommodating NAEP reading tests.* Paper presented at the NAGB Conference on Increasing the Participation of SD and LEP Students in NAEP. Retrieved July 25, 2006, from *www.nagb.org/pubs/conferences/sireci.co*

Sireci, S. G., Li, S., & Scarpati, S. (2003). *The effects of test accommodation on test performance: A review of the literature* (Center for Educational Assessment Research Report No. 485). Amherst: School of Education, University of Massachusetts, Amherst.

Sireci, S. G., & Parker, P. (2005). Validity on trial: Psychometric and legal conceptualizations of validity. *Educational Measurement: Issues and Practice, 25,* 27–34.

Sireci, S. G., & Pitoniak, M. (2006). *Assessment accommodations: What have we learned from research?* Paper presented at the 2006 Educational Testing Service Symposium on Accommodating Students with Disabilities on State Assessments, Princeton, NJ.

Sireci, S. G., Scarpati, S. E., & Li, S. (2005). Test accommodations for students with disabilities: An analysis of the interaction hypothesis. *Review of Educational Research, 75,* 457–490.

Sireci, S. G., Zanetti, M., & Berger, J. (2003). Recent and anticipated changes in postsecondary admissions: A survey of New England colleges and universities. *Review of Higher Education, 26,* 323–342.

Siskind, T. (2004). *Achieving accurate results for diverse learners: Accommodations and access-enhanced formats for English language learners and students with disabilities.* Funded proposal to the U.S. Department of Education, Grants for Enhanced Assessment Instruments Program.

Sitlington, P. L., & Frank, A. R. (1990). Are adolescents with learning disabilities successfully crossing the bridge into adult life? *Learning Disability Quarterly, 13,* 17–111.

Skottun, B. C. (2000). The magnocellular deficit theory of dyslexia: The evidence from contrast sensitivity. *Visual Research, 40*, 111–127.

Skottun, B. C. (2007). Yellow filters, magnocellular responses, and reading. *International Journal of Neuroscience, 117*, 287–293.

Skottun, B. C., & Skoyles, J. (2007). Yellow filters, magnocellular responses, and reading. *International Journal of Neuroscience, 117*, 287–293.

Sliffe, B. D., Weiss, J., & Bell, T. (1985). Separability of metacognition and cognition: Problem solving in learning disabled and regular students. *Journal of Learning Disabilities, 77*, 437–445.

Smith, L., & Wilkins, A. (2007). How many colours are necessary to increase the reading speed of children with visual stress?: A comparison of two systems. *Journal of Research in Reading, 30*, 332–343.

Smythe, I., Everatt, J., & Salter, R. (2004). *International book of dyslexia: A cross-language comparison and practice guide.* Hoboken, NJ: Wiley.

Snow, C., & Strucker, J. (2000). Lessons from preventing reading difficulties in young children for adult learning and literacy. In J. Coming, B. Garner, & C. Smith (Eds.), *Annual review of adult learning and literacy: A project of the National Center for the Study of Adult Learning and Literacy* (Vol. 1, pp. 25–73). San Francisco: Jossey-Bass.

Solan, H. A., Ficarra, A., Brannan, J. R., & Rucker, F. (1998). Eye movement efficiency in normal and reading disabled elementary school children: Effect of varying luminance and wavelength. *Journal of the American Optomology Association, 69*, 455–464.

Sparks, R. (1995). Examining the linguistic coding differences hypothesis to explain individual differences in foreign language learning. *Annals of Dyslexia, 45*, 187–214.

Spear-Swerling, L., & Sternberg, R. J. (1996). *Off track: When poor readers become "learning disabled."* Boulder, CO: Westview Press.

Spekman, N. J., Goldberg, R. J., & Herman, K. L. (1992). Learning disabled children grow up: A search for factors related to success in the young adult years. *Learning Disabilities Research and Practice, 7*, 161–170.

Spencer, T. J. (Ed.). (2004). Adult attention-deficit/hyperactivity disorder [Special issue]. *Psychiatric Clinics of North America, 27*(2).

Spencer, T. J. (2006). Antidepressant and specific norepinephrine reuptake inhibitor treatments. In R. A. Barkley, *Attention-deficit hyperactivity disorder: A handbook for diagnosis and treatment* (3rd ed., pp. 648–657). New York: Guilford Press.

Spencer, T. J., Wilens, T., Biederman, J., Wozniak, J., & Harding-Crawford, M. (2000). Attention-deficit/hyperactivity disorder with mood disorders. In T. E. Brown (Ed.), *Attention-deficit disorders and comorbidities in children, adolescents, and adults* (pp. 79–124). Washington, DC: American Psychiatric Press.

Stanovich, K. E. (1980). Toward an interactive–compensatory model of individual differences in the development of ready fluency. *Reading Research Quarterly, 16*, 32–35.

Stanovich, K. E. (1999). *Who is rational?: Studies of individual differences in reasoning.* Mahwah, NJ: Erlbaum.

Stanovich, K. E. (2000). *Progress in understanding reading: Scientific foundations and new frontiers.* New York: Guilford Press.

Stanovich, K. E., & Cunningham, A. E. (1993). Where does knowledge come from?: Specific associations between print exposure and information acquisition. *Journal of Educational Psychology, 85,* 211–229.

Stanovich, K. E., & West, R. F. (1989). Exposure to print and orthographic processing. *Reading Research Quarterly, 24,* 402–484.

Stanovich, K. E., & West, R. F. (2000). Individual differences in reasoning: Implications for the rationality debate? *Behavioral and Brain Sciences, 23,* 645–726.

Stanovich, K. E., West, R. F., & Cunningham, A. E. (1991). Beyond phonological processes: Print exposure and orthographic processing. In S. A. Brady & D. P. Shankweiler (Eds.), *Phonological processes in literacy: A tribute to Isabelle Y. Liberman* (pp. 219–235). Hillsdale, NJ: Erlbaum.

Stavy, R., Goel, V., Critchley, H., & Dolan, R. (2006). Intuitive interference in quantitative reasoning. *Brain Research, 1073–1074,* 383–388.

Steele, C. (1999). Thin ice: "Stereotype threat" and black college students. Retrieved January 4, 2004, from *www.theatlantic.com/issues/99aug/9908stereotype.htm*

Steele, C. M., & Aronson, J. (1995). Stereotype threat and the intellectual test performance of African Americans. *Journal of Personality and Social Psychology, 69,* 797–985.

Steen, L. A. (Ed.). (1997). *Why numbers count: Quantitative literacy for tomorrow's America.* New York: College Entrance Examination Board.

Stein, J., & Walsch, V. (1997). To see but not to read: The magnocellular theory of dyslexia. *Trends in Neuroscience, 20,* 147–152.

Stenhjem, P. (2005, February). *Youth with disabilities in the juvenile justice system: Prevention and intervention strategies.* Minneapolis, MN: National Center on Secondary Education and Transition. Retrieved April 5, 2007, from *www.ncset.org/publications/viewdesc.asp?id=1929*

Stevenson, J., Pennington, B. F., Gilger, J. W., DeFries, J. C., & Gillis, J. J. (1993). Hyperactivity and spelling disability: Testing for shared genetic aetiology. *Journal of Child Psychology and Psychiatry, 14,* 1137–1152.

Stodden, R., Jones, M., & Chang, K. (2002). *Services, supports and accommodations for individuals with disabilities: An analysis across secondary education, postsecondary education, and employment* (White Paper). Manoa: University of Hawaii at Manoa, National Center on Secondary Education and Transition. Retrieved March 24, 2003, from *ncset.hawaii.edu*

Stone, C. A. (1997). Correspondences among parent, teacher, and student perceptions of adolescents' learning disabilities. *Journal of Learning Disabilities, 30,* 660–669.

Stone, C. A., & May, A. L. (2002). The accuracy of academic self-evaluations in adolescents with learning disabilities. *Journal of Learning Disabilities, 35*(4), 370–383.

Stone, D. B., Fisher, S. K., & Elito, J. (1999). Adults' prior exposure to print as a predictor of the legibility of text on paper and laptop computers. *Reading and Writing: An Interdisciplinary Journal, 11,* 1–28.

Stoodley, C. J., Talcott, J. B., Carter, E. L., Witton, C., & Stein, J. F. (2000). Selective deficits of vibrotactile sensitivity in dyslexic readers. *Neuroscience Letters, 295,* 16–16.

Stothard, S. E., & Hulme, C. (1996). A comparison of reading comprehension and decoding difficulties in children. In C. Cornoldi & J. Oakhill (Eds.), *Reading comprehension difficulties: Processes and intervention* (pp. 93–112). Mahwah, NJ: Erlbaum.

Sturm, J. M., & Rankin-Erickson, J. L. (2002). Effects of hand-drawn and computer-generated concept mapping on the expository writing of students with learning disabilities. *Learning Disabilities Research and Practice, 17,* 124–139.

Swanson, H. L. (1993). An information processing analysis of learning disabled children's problem solving. *American Education Research Journal, 30,* 861–893.

Swanson, H. L., & Alexander, J. E. (1997). Cognitive processes as predictors of word recognition and reading comprehension in learning disabled and skilled readers: Revisiting the specificity hypothesis. *Journal of Educational Psychology, 89,* 128–158.

Swanson, H. L., & Ashbaker, H. (2000). Working memory, short-term memory, speech rate, word recognition, and reading comprehension in learning disabled readers: Does the executive system have a role? *Intelligence, 28,* 1–30.

Swanson, H. L., Howard, C. B., & Saez, L. (2007). Reading comprehension and working memory in children with learning disabilities in reading. In K. Cain & J. Oakhill (Eds.), *Children's comprehension problems in oral and written language: A cognitive perspective* (pp. 157–190). New York: Guilford Press.

Swanson, H. L., & Jerman, O. (2006). Math disabilities: A selective meta-analysis of the literature. *Review of Educational Research, 76,* 249–274.

Swanson, H. L., & Sachse-Lee, C. (2001). Mathematical problem solving and working memory in children with learning disabilities: Both executive and phonological processes are important. *Journal of Experimental Child Psychology, 79,* 294–321.

Swanson, H. L., & Siegel, L. (2001). Learning disabilities as a working memory deficit. *Issues in Education, 7,* 1–48.

Sweet, A. P., & Snow, C. E. (Eds.). (2003). *Rethinking reading comprehension.* New York: Guilford Press.

Szatmari, P. (1998). Differential diagnosis of Asperger disorder. In E. Schopler, G. B. Mesibov, & L. J. Kunce (Eds.), *Asperger syndrome or high-functioning autism?* (pp. 61–76). New York: Plenum Press.

Szatmari, P. (2000). Perspectives on the classification of Asperger syndrome. In A. Klin, F. R. Volkmar, & S. S. Sparrow (Eds.), *Asperger syndrome* (pp. 403–417). New York: Guilford Press.

Szpara, M. Y., & Wylie, E. C. (2007). Writing differences in teacher performance assessments: An investigation of African American language and edited American English. *Applied Linguistics, 28,* 1–23.

Tannock, R. (2000). Attention-deficit/hyperactivity disorder with anxiety disorders. In T. E. Brown (Ed.), *Attention-deficit disorders and comorbidities in children, adolescents, and adults* (pp. 125–170). Washington, DC: American Psychiatric Press.

Technology-Related Assistance for Individuals with Disabilities Act (Tech Act) of 1988, Public Law No. 100-407, 102 Stat. 1044 (1988).

Technology-Related Assistance for Individuals with Disabilities Act (Tech Act) of 1994, Public Law No. 103-128, 29 U.S.C. 2201 (1994).

Thomas, A., & Chess, S. (1977). *Temperament and development.* New York: Brunner/Mazel.

Thompson, B. (2006). *Foundations of behavioral statistics: An insight-based approach.* New York: Guilford Press.

Thompson, S. J., Blount, A., & Thurlow, M. L. (2002). *A summary of research on the effects of test accommodations: 1999 through 2001* (Technical Report No. 34). Minneapolis: University of Minnesota, National Center on Educational Outcomes, Retrieved January 4, 2004, from *www.education.umn.edu/ NCEO/OnlinePubs/Technical34.htm*

Thompson, S. J., Johnstone, C. J., Thurlow, M. L., & Altaian, J. R. (2005). *2005 State special education outcomes: Steps forward in a decade of change.* Minneapolis: University of Minnesota, National Center on Educational Outcomes. Retrieved August 1, 2006, from *education.umn.edu/NCEO/ OnlinePubs/2005StateReport.htm*

Thompson, S. J., Thurlow, M. L., Quenemoen, R. F., & Lehr, C. A. (2002). *Access to computer-based testing for students with disabilities* (Synthesis Report No. 45). Minneapolis: University of Minnesota, National Center on Educational Outcomes. Retrieved January 18, 2007, from *education.umn.edu/ NCEO/OnlinePubs/synthesis45.html*

Thorley, G. (1984). Review of follow-up and follow-back studies of childhood hyperactivity. *Psychological Bulletin, 96,* 116–132.

Thurlow, M. (2006). *Accommodations in state policies: What a wonderful world of diversity: Issues and implications.* Paper presented at the 2006 Educational Testing Service Symposium on Accommodating Students with Disabilities on State Assessments, Princeton, NJ.

Timmer, S. (2007, February). *Assistive technology for text summarization.* Paper presented at the 44th annual meeting of the International Learning Disabilities Association of America, Pittsburgh, PA.

Tindal, G., & Fuchs, L. (1999). *A summary of research on test changes: An empirical basis for defining accommodations.* Lexington: University of Kentucky, Mid-South Regional Resource Center.

Tindal, G., & Ketterlin-Geller, L. R. (2004). *Research on mathematics test accommodations relevant to NAEP testing.* Paper presented at the NAGB Conference on Increasing the Participation of SD and LEP Students in NAEP. Retrieved July 25, 2006, from *www.nagb.org/pubs/conferences/tindal*

Tombaugh, T. N. (1996). *Test of Memory Malingering.* Toronto: Multi-Health Systems.

Torgesen, J. K., Wagner, R. K., & Rashotte, C. A. (1999). *Test of Word Reading Efficiency.* Austin, TX: Pro-ED.

Torrance, M., & Galbraith, D. (2006). The processing demands of writing. In C. A. MacArthur, S. Graham, & J. Fitzgerald (Eds.), *Handbook of writing research* (pp. 67–82). New York: Guilford Press.

Tucker, M. (2004). *High school and beyond: The system is the problem—and the solution.* Washington, DC: National Center on Education and the Economy.

Tufte, E. (1990). *Envisioning information.* Cheshire, CT: Graphics Press.

Turner et al. v. American Association of Medical Colleges. (2006).

Turner, M. L., & Engle, R. W. (1989). Is working memory capacity task dependent? *Journal of Memory and Language, 28,* 127–134.

Twigg, C. (2006, May). *Increasing success for underserved students: Redesigning introductory courses.* Saratoga Springs, NY: National Center for Academic Transformation. Retrieved April 1, 2007, from *www.thencat.org/Monographs/IncSuccess.htm*

U.S. Bureau of the Census. (2004). *Population estimates.* Retrieved June 30, 2005, from *www.census.gov/popest/AAAAstates/tables/NST-EST2004-01.pdf*

U.S. Department of Labor, Bureau of Labor Statistics. (2002). *Tomorrow's jobs* (Bulletin No. 2540-1). Washington, DC: Author.

U.S. Employment and Training Administration. (1991). *The learning disabled in employment and training programs* (Research and Evaluation Series No. 91-E). Washington, DC: U.S. Department of Labor.

U.S. General Accounting Office. (2003, July). *Special education federal actions can assist states in improving postsecondary outcomes for youth* (GAO Report No. 03-773). Retrieved May 5, 2003, from *www.gao.gov/new.items/do3773.pdf*

van Ark, B., Inklaar, R., & McGuckin, R. H. (2003). ICT productivity in Europe and the United States: Where do the differences come from? *CESifo Economic Studies, 49,* 295–318.

Vandenberg, R. J., & Lance, C. E. (2000). A review and synthesis of the measurements invariance literature: Suggestions, practices, and recommendations for organizational research. *Organizational Research Methods, 3,* 4–69.

Vanderberg, R., & Swanson, H. L. (2007). Which components of working memory are important in the writing process? *Reading and Writing, 20,* 721–752.

Van der Linden, M. (1999). Cognitive mediators of age-related differences in language comprehension and verbal memory performance. *Aging, Neuropsychology, and Cognition, 6,* 32–36.

Vanderploeg, R. D., Schinka, J. A., Baum, K. M., Tremont, G., & Mittenberg, N. (1998). WISC-III premorbid prediction strategies: Demographic and best performance approaches. *Psychological Assessment, 10*(3), 77–84.

Van Dijk, T. A., & Kintsch, W. (1983). *Strategies of discourse comprehension.* New York: Academic Press.

Van Ingelghem, M., van Wieringen, A., Wouters, J., Vandenbussche, E., Onghena, P., & Ghesquirere, P. (2001). Psychophysical evidence for a general temporal processing deficit in children with dyslexia. *NeuroReport, 12,* 3603–3607.

Vaughn, S., & Elbaum, B. E. (1999). The self-concept and friendships of students with learning disabilities: A developmental perspective. In R. Gallimore, L. Bernheimer, D. L. MacMillan, D. L. Speece, & S. Vaughn (Eds.), *Developmental perspectives on children with high incidence disabilities* (pp. 81–110). Mahwah, NJ: Erlbaum.

Vellutino, F. R. (2003). Individual differences as sources of variability in reading comprehension in elementary school children. In A. P. Sweet & C. E. Snow (Eds.), *Rethinking reading comprehension* (pp. 51–81). New York: Guilford Press.

Vellutino, F. R., Scanlon, D. M., & Chen, R. S. (1994). The increasingly inextricable relationship between orthographic and phonological coding in learning to read: Some reservations about current methods of operationalizing orthographic coding. In V. W. Berninger (Ed.), *The varieties of orthographic knowledge: Vol. 1. Theoretical and developmental issues* (pp. 47–112). Dordrecht, The Netherlands: Kluwer Academic.

Vellutino, F. R. Tunmer, N. E., Jaccard, J. J., & Chen, R. (2007). Components of reading ability: Multivariate evidence for a convergent skills model of reading development. *Scientific Studies of Reading, 11*, 3–21.

Vest, C. M. (2006, May–June). Open content and the emerging global meta-university. *EDUCAUSE Review, 41*(3). Retrieved August 11, 2006, from *www.educause.eduapps/er/erm06/erm0630.asp*

Vogel, S. A. (1990). Gender differences in intelligence, language, visual–motor abilities, and academic achievement in students with learning disabilities: A review of the literature. *Journal of Learning Disabilities, 23*, 44–52.

Vogel, S. A., & Adelman, P. B. (1992). The success of college students with learning disabilities: Factors related to educational attainment. *Journal of Learning Disabilities, 25*(7), 430–441.

Vogel, S. A., Hruby, P. J., & Adelman, P. B. (1993). Educational and psychological factors in successful and unsuccessful college students with learning disabilities. *Learning Disabilities Research and Practice, 8*(1), 35–43.

Volkmar, F. R., & Klin, A. (2000). Diagnostic issues in Asperger syndrome. In A. Klin, F. R. Volkmar, & S. S. Sparrow (Eds.), *Asperger syndrome* (pp. 25–71). New York: Guilford Press.

Vygotsky, L. S. (1962). *Thought and language.* Cambridge, MA: Massachusetts Institute of Technology Press.

Wagner, M., Cameot, R., & Newman, L. (2003). *Youth with disabilities: A changing population: A report of findings from the National Longitudinal Transition Study (NLTS) and the National Longitudinal Transition Study–2 (NLTS2).* Menlo Park, CA: SRI International. Retrieved November 10, 2006, from *www.nltsw.org/pdfs/full_report_changepop.pdf*

Wagner, M., Newman, L., & Cameto, R. (2004). *Changes over time in the secondary school experiences of students with disabilities. A report of findings from the national Longitudinal Transition Study (NLTS) and the National Longitudinal Transition Study–2 (NLTS2).* Menlo Park, CA: SRI International. Retrieved November 15, 2006, from *www.nlts2.org/pdfs/changestime_compreport.pdf*

Wagner, M., Newman, L., Cameto, R., Garza, N., & Levine, P. (2005). *After high school: A report from the National Longitudinal Transition Study–2 (NLTS-2).* Menlo Park, CA: SRI International. Retrieved February 7, 2007, from *www.nlts2.org*

Wagner, R. K., Torgesen, J. K., & Rashotte, C. A. (1999). *Comprehensive Test of Phonological Processing.* Austin, TX: Pro-ED.

Walsh, D. A., & Hershey, D. A. (1993). Mental models and the maintenance of complex problem solving skills in old age. In J. Cerella, J. Rybash, W. Hoyer, & M. Commons (Eds.), *Adult information processing: Limits on loss* (pp. 553–584). San Diego, CA: Academic Press.

Ward, M., & Berry, H. (2005, Summer). Students with disabilities and postsecondary education: A tale of two data sets. *Heath Quarterly Newsletter.*

Washington, DC: The George Washington University HEATH Resource Center. Retrieved December 3, 2005, from *www.heath.gwu.edu/newsletter/ issue%2014/issue%2014.htm*

Watkins, M. W., Glutting, J. J., & Youngstrom, E. A. (2005). Issues in subtest profile analysis. In D. P. Flanagan & P. L. Harrison (Eds.), *Contemporary intellectual assessment: Theories, tests, and issues* (2nd ed., pp. 251–268). New York: Guilford Press.

Wechsler, D. (1997a). *Wechsler Adult Intelligence Scale—Third Edition (WAIS-III)*. San Antonio, TX: Psychological Corporation.

Wechsler, D. (1997b). *Wechsler Memory Scale—Third Edition (WMS-III)*. San Antonio, TX: Psychological Corporation.

Wechsler, D. (2001). *Wechsler Individual Achievement Test—Second Edition (WIAT-II)*. San Antonio, TX: Psychological Corporation.

Wechsler, D. (2008). *Wechsler Adult Intelligence Scale—Fourth Edition (WAIS-IV)*. San Antonio, TX: Pearson Education.

Weiss, G., & Hechtman, L. (1993). *Hyperactive children grown up* (2nd ed.). New York: Guilford Press.

Wentzel, K. R. (1999). Social-motivational processes and interpersonal relationships: Implications for understanding students' academic success. *Journal of Educational Psychology, 91,* 76–97.

Werner, E. F. (1993). Risk and resilience in individuals with learning disabilities: Lessons learned from the Kauai longitudinal study. *Learning Disabilities Research and Practice, 8,* 28–35.

Wertsch, J. V. (1985). *Vygotsky and the social formation of mind.* Cambridge, MA: Harvard University Press.

West, R. F., Stanovich, K. E., & Mitchell, H. R. (1993). Reading in the real world and its correlates. *Reading Research Quarterly, 28,* 35–50.

Westby, C. (2002). Beyond decoding: Critical and dynamic literacy for students with dyslexia, language learning disabilities (LLD), or attention deficit–hyperactivity (ADHD). In K. G. Butler & E. R. Silliman (Eds.), *Speaking, reading, and writing in children with language learning disabilities: New paradigms in research and practice* (pp. 73–107). Mahwah, NJ: Erlbaum.

Wetherby, A., & Prizant, B. (2001). *Communicative and Symbolic Behavior Scales Developmental Profile.* Baltimore: Brookes.

White, E. M. (2001). The opening of the modern era of writing assessment: A narrative. *College English, 63,* 306–320.

Wiederholt, J. L., & Bryant, B. R. (2001). *Gray Oral Reading Tests—Fourth Edition (GORT-4).* San Antonio, TX: Pearson.

Wigfield, A., Eccles, J. S., & Pintrich, P. R. (1996). Development between the ages of 11 and 25. In D. C. Berliner & R. C. Calfee (Eds.), *Handbook of educational psychology* (pp. 148–185). New York: Macmillan.

Wigfield, A., Eccles, J. S., Schiefele, U., Roeser, R., & Davis-Kean, P. (2006). Development of achievement motivation. In W. Damon & R. M. Lerner (Series Eds.), & N. Eisenberg (Vol. Ed.), *Handbook of child psychology* (6th ed., Vol. 3, pp. 933–1002). Hoboken, NJ: Wiley.

Wigfield, A., & Wentzel, K. R. (2007). Introduction to motivation at school: Interventions that work. *Educational Psychologist, 42*(4), 191–196.

Wightman, L. (1993). *Test takers with disabilities: A summary of data from special administrations of the LSAT* (LSAC Research Report No. 93-03). Newton, PA: Law School Admissions Council.

Wilens, T. E. (2004). Attention-deficit/hyperactivity disorder and the substance use disorders: The nature of the relationship, subtypes at risk, and treatment issues. *Psychiatric Clinics of North America, 27*(2), 283–302.

Wilkinson, G. S., with Robertson, G. J. (2004). *Wide Range Achievement Test–4 (WRAT4)*. Lutz, FL: Psychological Assessment Resources.

Wilkoff, W. L., & Abed, L. W. (1994). *Practicing universal design: An Interpretation of the ADA*. New York: Van Nostrand Reinhold.

Willcutt, E. G., Betjemann, R. S., Wadsworth, S. J., Samuelsson, S., Corley, R., DeFries, J. C., et al. (2007). Preschool twin study of the relation between attention-deficit/hyperactivity disorder and prereading skills. *Reading and Writing, 20*, 103–125.

Willcutt, E. G., & Gaffney-Brown, R. (2002). Etiology of dyslexia, ADHD, and related difficulties: Using genetic methods to understand comorbidity. *Perspectives of the International Dyslexia Association, 30*, 12–15.

Willcutt, E. G., Pennington, B. F., Smith, S. D., Cardon, L. R., Gayan, J., Knoopik, V. S., et al. (2002). Quantitative trait locus for reading disability on chromosone 6p is pleiotropic for ADHD. *American Journal of Medical Genetics, Part B: Neuropsychiatric Genetics, 114*(3), 260–268.

Williams, M. C., LeCluyse, K., & Rock-Faucheux, A. (1992). Effective interventions for reading disability. *Journal of the American Optometric Association, 63*, 411–417.

Willingham, W. W., Ragosta, M., Bennett, R. E., Braun, H., Rock, D. A., & Powers, D. E. (1988). *Testing handicapped people*. Needham Heights, MA: Allyn & Bacon.

Wilson, K. M., & Swanson, H. L. (2001). Are mathematics disabilities due to a domain-general or a domain-specific working memory deficits? *Journal of Learning Disabilities, 34*, 237–248.

Wing, L. (2000). Past and future of research on Asperger syndrome. In A. Klin, F. R. Volkmar, & S. S. Sparrow (Eds.), *Asperger syndrome* (pp. 418–432). New York: Guilford Press.

Winnie, P. H. (2001). Self-regulated learning viewed from models of information processing. In B. J. Zimmerman & D. H. Schunk (Ed.), *Self-regulated learning and academic achievement: Theoretical perspectives* (pp. 153–190). Mahwah, NJ: Erlbaum.

Winnie, P. H., & Hadwin, A. F. (1998, August). *Using CoNoteS2 to study and support self-regulated learning*. San Francisco: International Association of Applied Psychology.

Wolf, G., & Lee, C. (2007). Promising practices for providing alternative media to postsecondary students with print disabilities. *Learning Disabilities Research and Practice, 22*, 256–264.

Wolinsky, S., & Whelan, A. (1999). Federal law and the accommodation of students with LD: The lawyers' look at the BU decision. *Journal of Learning Disabilities, 32*(4), 286–291.

Wong v. Regents of the University of California, WL 1837752 (9th Cir. 2004).

Wong, B. Y. L. (2003). General and specific issues for researchers' consideration in applying the risk and resilience framework to the social domain of learning disabilities. *Learning Disabilities Research and Practice, 18*(2), 68–76.

Woodcock, R. W., McGrew, K. S., & Mather, N. (2001a). *Woodcock–Johnson III Tests of Achievement.* Itasca, IL: Riverside.

Woodcock, R. W., McGrew, K. S., & Mather, N. (2001b). *Woodcock–Johnson III Tests of Cognitive Abilities.* Itasca, IL: Riverside.

Workforce Investment Act of 1998, Public Law 105-220, 112 Stat. 936, 29 U.S.C. § 2801.

Wright, B. D., & Lineacre, J. M. (1999). *WINSTEPS: Rasch analysis for all two-facet models.* Chicago: MESA Press.

Wright, P. W., & Wright, P. D. (2007). *Special education law* (2nd ed.). Hartfield, VA: Harbor House Law Press.

Yeargin-Allsopp, M., Rice, C., Karapurkar, T., Doernberg, N., Boyle, C., & Murphy, C. (2003). Prevalence of autism in a U.S. metropolitan area. *Journal of the American Medical Association, 289*(1), 49–55.

Young, G., & Browning, J. (2005). Learning disabilities/dyslexia and employment—A mythical view. In G. Reid & A. Fawcett (Eds.), *Dyslexia in context: Research, policy and practice* (pp. 25–59). London: Whurr.

Young, G., Kim, J., & Gerber, P. (1999). Gender bias and learning disabilities: School age and long-term consequences for females. *Learning Disabilities: A Multidisciplinary Journal, 9*(3), 107–114.

Zametkin, A. J., Nordahl, T. E., Gross, M., King, A. C., Semple, W. E., Reumsey, J., et al. (1990). Cerebral glucose metabolism in adults with hyperactivity of childhood onset. *New England Journal of Medicine, 323,* 1361–1366.

Zellermayer, M., Salomon, G., Globerson, T., & Givon, H. (1991). Enhancing writing-related metacognitions through a computerized writing partner. *American Educational Research Journal, 28,* 373–391.

Zimmerman, B. J., & Schunk, D. H. (2001). *Self-regulated learning and academic achievement* (2nd ed.). Mahwah, NJ: Erlbaum.

Zurcher, R., & Bryant, D. P. (2001). The validity and comparability of entrance examination scores after accommodations are made for students with LD. *Journal of Learning Disabilities, 43,* 462–471.

Zuriff, G. E. (2000). Extra examination time for students with learning disabilities: An examination of the maximum potential thesis. *Applied Measurement in Education, 13,* 99–117.

Index

Cognitive ability measures, 70–75, 75–80
  profiles of, 72*f*, 73*f*, 83
Cognitive efficiency, in reading decoding,
  139–140
Cognitive impairment, malingering and,
  117–119
Cognitive pluralism, 194
Cognitive processes
  in different symbol systems, 194
  in math learning disability, 199, 200*t*
  in mathematical tasks, 207–209
  in reading comprehension, 149–154
  sense of audience and, 190*t*
  in spelling, 177*t*
  in syntax performance, 182*t*
  in written text, 186–187, 186*t*
  See also Brain regions
Cognitive processing, 55–87
  Cattell–Horn–Carroll theory of, 62, 63*f*
  developmental influences, 66–67
  efficiency of, 85–86
  implications for assessment and
    accommodation, 87
  measurement of
    decision making and, 67–70
    tools used for, 75–80
    validity and efficacy and, 70–75
  process-oriented view of, 61–67
  sense of time and, 86
  speed of, 84–85
  verbal ability and, 86
  WMC models of, 62, 64–66, 65*f*
Cognitive Strategy Instruction in Writing,
  188–189
Cognitive tests, in assessment of ADHD,
  117
Coherence
  cognitive and linguistic processes
    influencing, 186*t*
  written text and, 187
Cohesion
  cognitive and linguistic processes
    influencing, 186*t*
  written text and, 187
College Board
  documentation guidelines and eligibility
    criteria of, 45
  test accommodations and, 246–247
Color filters, for accommodating LD
  students, 146–147
Communication skills
  monologic versus dialogic, 108–109
  in nonverbal learning disorder, 107–108
Compensatory readers, 59
Composition, 185–189
  assessment of, 188
  See also Writing; Writing competence

Composition deficits, accommodations for,
  173*t*, 188–189
Comprehension. *See* Reading
  comprehension
Comprehensive Test of Phonological
  Processing, 138
Computer-based testing, accommodations
  in, 239–240
Concentration impairment,
  accommodations for, 120
Conduct disorder, comorbidity with LD
  and ADHD, 105
Confidence intervals, 70
Conners' Continuous Performance
  Test II, in assessment of ADHD,
  117
Counting, 198, 199*t*
Cultural diversity, writing competency and,
  166–167
Cutoff methods, 25–26

Depressive disorders, comorbidity with LD
  and ADHD, 103–104
Developmental issues in cognitive
  processing, 66–67
Dialogic speech, 108–109
Different symbol systems, 193–223
  implications for assessment and
    accommodation, 222–223
  See also Mathematics; Science
    underachievement; Second
    language learning
Differential Ability Scales–II, 79
Differential item functioning, 247
Differential-boost hypothesis, defined,
  225*t*
Digital Divide Measurement Scale for
  Students, 157
Digital learning, 142, 156–157
  workplace and, 125–128
Direct observations, in assessment of LD
  and ADHD, 112–113
Disability, ADA definition of, 39
Discrepancy methods, 24–25, 35
Documentation
  in postsecondary setting, 37–50
  in secondary setting, 31–37
Documentation checklist
  for ADHD, 44*f*
  for learning disabilities, 43*f*
Documentation guidelines, 39–40
  for higher education, 41–45
  of testing agencies, 45–47
  for vocational rehabilitation, 40–41
Dropouts with LD/ADHD
  rate of, 2–3
  services for, 12–13